Veterinary Medical Terminology Guide and Workbook

Angela Taibo

WILEY Blackwell

This edition first published 2014 © 2014 by John Wiley & Sons, Inc

Editorial Offices

1606 Golden Aspen Drive, Suites 103 and 104, Ames, Iowa 50010, USA

The Atrium, Southern Gate, Chichester, West Sussex, PO19 8SQ, UK

9600 Garsington Road, Oxford, OX4 2DQ, UK

For details of our global editorial offices, for customer services and for information about how to apply for permission to reuse the copyright material in this book please see our website at www.wiley.com/wiley-blackwell.

Library of Congress Cataloging-in-Publication Data

Taibo, Angela, author.

Veterinary medical terminology guide and workbook / Angela Taibo.

p. ; cm.

Includes bibliographical references and index.

ISBN 978-1-118-52748-1 (pbk.)

I. Title. [DNLM: 1. Veterinary Medicine–Problems and Exercises.   2. Veterinary Medicine–Terminology–English.   SF 610]

SF610

636.089001′4–dc23

2013039718

A catalogue record for this book is available from the British Library.

Wiley also publishes its books in a variety of electronic formats. Some content that appears in print may not be available in electronic books.

Cover images: Dog image – courtesy of Greg Martinez; rabbit image – iStock #22953871 © NiDerLander; cat image – courtesy of Amy Johnson

Cover design by Matt Kuhns

Set in 10/12pt Sabon by SPi Publisher Services, Pondicherry, India

Printed and bound in Singapore by Markono Print Media Pte Ltd

1   2014

Dedication

To Mom: You are my constant inspiration, my idol, and my best friend.

To Alisha: You continue to show me that if you put your mind to something, there's nothing you can't do.

To Daddy: La persona más inteligente que conozco, y la que me ha enseñado valentía y perseverancia.

Y'all are my rock.

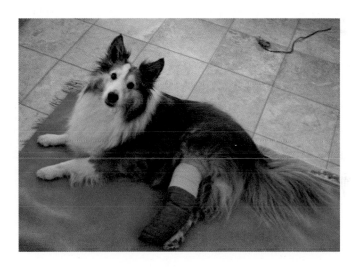

Contents

Contents

Preface

After teaching medical terminology and various other subjects for many years, I've noticed the lack of retention of medical terminology as students progressed into their upper-level courses. In turn, I've come to appreciate the need for workbook-based materials. My quest began to find a decent medical terminology textbook that would aid the students in retention through repetition as well as act as a useful reference. The books I found for the beginner veterinary technician student and veterinary student were written at a higher level than the beginner student could comprehend or the books would go into greater detail than what was required. Perhaps it was a bit of frustration on my part and the part of my students that finally led me to this project.

Medical terminology is essential to basic understanding in the veterinary and medical fields. As students, it can be difficult to avoid the mindset that you simply just need to pass the course. However you will use these terms every day in practice as you speak with clients and co-workers, and as you write in patient files.

A basic understanding of anatomy and physiology is required to better comprehend the medical terms. Students can be easily overwhelmed with the learning of a new language coupled with the anatomy and physiology required. It is my hope that this book helps to better organize the material and ultimately simplify your learning experience. Each chapter includes exercises and case studies that will help you apply what you have learned in each chapter. It's my recommendation that you make multiple copies of these exercises so that you can treat them as quizzes, and I hope the Website material will complement your learning experience through this book.

Writing this book was an amazing experience for me. I sent mass emails to graduates, former co-workers, and total strangers that I knew were working in the field. I was pleasantly surprised by the response I received. Veterinarians and veterinary technicians alike were excited and anxious to help donate images and information for the textbook. I consistently received the same response: "I wish we had something like this when I was a student." Several contributors remembered the lack of organization and examples in their own textbooks when they were in school. The response has simply been amazing. The veterinary community is an amazing family to be a part of. We all strive for the same goal: to create quality medicine.

I would like to thank my image contributors including Dr. Greg Martinez, Dr. Alison Traylor, Beth Romano, Amy Johnson, Nora Vanatta, Irene Chou, Deanna Roberts, and Dr. Patrick Hemming. I couldn't have completed the more specialized chapters without the aid of my co-teachers, former teachers, and former co-workers Tammy Schneider, Dr. Debra Van Houten, Gina Stonier, Janet King, Michaela Witcher, Scott Newman, Cyndi Rideout, Amy Perez, Jan Lyons-Barnett, Jessie Loberg, Dr. Sam Mersfelder, Dr. Earl Wenngren, Dr. Debra Singleton, Dr. Donna Anglin, and Beverly Gollehon. Finally, I'd like to thank VCA Wingate Animal Hospital. There is no substitute for working in the field and you gave me my start. You hired me as a volunteer at the age of 11 and patiently molded me for 16 years.

This book was written based on the feedback that I've received over the years from students and instructors. I welcome your feedback and recommendations in the future so that I may use them to improve subsequent editions. The veterinary field is an exciting field because the information is constantly changing. Newer and more improved methods are always being introduced. My goal is that this book will help you to stay current with the changes and challenges that meet you in the future.

About the Companion Website

This book is accompanied by a companion website:

www.wiley.com/go/taibo/terminology

The website includes:

- A crossword puzzle
- Flashcards
- Audio clips to show how to pronounce terms
- Case studies
- Review questions
- The figures from each chapter in PowerPoint

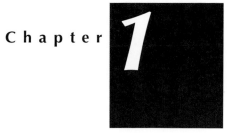

Chapter **1**

Introduction

Understanding the language of medicine is basic to comprehension and competency in the world of veterinary medicine. Medical terms are often heard on various television shows and movies and are seen in novels. What you may not realize is that these medical terms are variations of Greek and Latin terminology.

When we see medical terms we should look at them differently from other words in the English language. Your task in learning medical terminology is to break these big words into smaller components, understand the meaning of those components, and then create an overall definition for the medical term.

Basic knowledge of anatomy and physiology is essential for the understanding of these medical terms. Therefore, this textbook will use various diagrams and photographs to help you to learn this new language. This book will not go into further detail other than the basics. You must learn medical terminology before focusing on more complicated curriculum.

Ultimately the use of proper medical terminology is a key to a professional work environment. Proper spelling and pronunciation of medical terms is essential for communication with the professional staff as well as clients.

Anatomy of a Medical Term

There are five components to medical terms. Typically a medical term will use two or three of these components. There is no rule that states how many parts a medical term must use. Your goal is to break down a medical term into its component parts, then define each part separately. These components were derived from Greek or Latin, so when defining these parts we are in essence translating them to the English language. This book does not nearly cover all the medical terms that have ever existed. Instead, it will prepare you for any terms that you may encounter by teaching you how to translate their component parts.

Veterinary Medical Terminology Guide and Workbook, First Edition. Angela Taibo.
© 2014 John Wiley & Sons, Inc. Published 2014 by John Wiley & Sons, Inc.
Companion website: www.wiley.com/go/taibo/terminology

The Root

The root is the foundation of the term. It is the basic essential part of the word that other words are derived from. Think of it as the root of a tree. Like the roots of a tree holding it in place, the root of a medical term holds the main meaning of the word.

You are probably already familiar with some roots of medical terms that you've probably heard from friends, family, and television shows. The following are examples of roots:

Root	Meaning	Example of Use	
Cardi	= Heart	Cardiology	Study of the heart
Hemat	= Blood	Hematology	Study of blood
Dermat	= Skin	Dermatology	Study of skin
Gastr	= Stomach	Gastrology	Study of the stomach
Enter	= Small intestine	Enterology	Study of the small intestine

The Combining Vowel

The combining vowel is a vowel that is used to link the root to its suffix. In most cases it is the letter "o." The combining vowel has no meaning and therefore will not alter the meaning of the term. The following is an example of how the combining vowel is used:

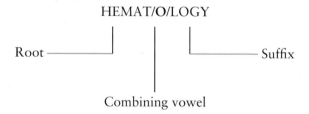

Notice that in order to attach the root "Hemat" to the suffix "-logy," we must use a combining vowel. In this case it is the letter "o."

The Combining Form

The combining form is the root plus its combining vowel. The meaning of the root is not altered by adding the combining vowel. Let's use roots from previous examples:

Combining Form	Meaning
Cardi/o	= Heart
Hemat/o	= Blood
Dermat/o	= Skin
Gastr/o	= Stomach
Enter/o	= Small intestine

The Prefix

The prefix precedes the root (comes before the root) and modifies its meaning. Not all terms will have a prefix.

Prefix	Meaning	Example of Use	
Sub-	Below	Subgastric	Pertaining to below the stomach
Epi-	Above	Epigastric	Pertaining to above the stomach
Trans-	Across	Transgastric	Pertaining to across the stomach

The Suffix

The suffix follows the root and modifies its meaning. Not all medical terms will have a suffix.

Suffix	Meaning	Example of Use	
-ic	Pertaining to	Gastric	Pertaining to the stomach
-logy	Study of	Hematology	Study of blood
-itis	Inflammation	Enteritis	Inflammation of the small intestine

Five Rules to Medical Terminology

There are five basic rules to medical terminology. If you can remember these rules then understanding the terms and their meanings will be much easier.

1. **If a suffix begins with a vowel, drop the combining vowel.** The following are two different examples to illustrate this rule. In the first example we'll come up with the medical term that means "pertaining to the stomach." If you refer to the previous examples under their word parts you'll see that the suffix for "pertaining to" is "-ic," and the combining form for stomach is "gastr/o."

    Gastr/o = Stomach
    -ic = Pertaining to

    Now we need to combine these parts. Because the suffix "-ic" begins with a vowel, then we must drop the combining vowel in the combining form gastr/o. Therefore we drop the letter "o."

    GASTR/~~O~~ + -IC = GASTRIC

    In the second example we look at the definition "study of the stomach."

    Gastr/o = Stomach
    -logy = Study of

Because the suffix does not begin with a vowel, we can keep the combining vowel.

GASTR/O + -LOGY = GASTROLOGY

2. **Read the parts to define the term from back, then to the beginning, and follow through.** You have probably noticed by now that when we define a medical term, we begin at the suffix, then look at the beginning of the term, and follow through. The following is an example of this rule:

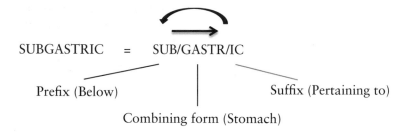

SUBGASTRIC   =   SUB/GASTR/IC

Prefix (Below)   Suffix (Pertaining to)

Combining form (Stomach)

Define the suffix, followed by the prefix, and then follow through.

SUBGASTRIC = PERTAINING TO BELOW THE STOMACH

Not all medical terms will use this rule; however, the rule will apply 90% of the time.

3. **Keep the combining vowel between roots.** Some medical terms have more than one root. When attaching roots together we leave the combining vowel between them.

GASTR/O/ENTER/O/LOGY

In this example we have combined the combining forms "gastr/o" for stomach and enter/o for small intestine. Because we have two roots in the term, "gastr" and "enter," we must leave the combining vowel between them. In this case it's the letter "o."

Using our previous rule of how to break down a medical term we get the following:

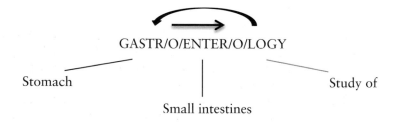

GASTR/O/ENTER/O/LOGY

Stomach   Study of

Small intestines

Definition: Study of the stomach and small intestines.

4. **List the roots in anatomical order.** By now you've already used this rule without even realizing it. If we look at the previous term, gastroenterology, the roots are listed in anatomical order. The stomach comes before the small intestines in the order of the organs of the gastrointestinal (GI) tract. It wouldn't make sense to have the term enterogastrology because the intestines are not before the stomach. If you're asking how I know this, don't worry, this textbook will teach you basic anatomy so you will also know how to place certain roots in anatomical order.

5. **Not all terms break down exactly.** This rule—knowing when to define a medical term literally or use a "special" definition—can be the most frustrating for students. Unfortunately, this knowledge only comes with practice and memorization. You will notice that common sense will become useful with some of these terms. To illustrate this rule, we will look at the term orthopedic.

ORTH/O/PED/IC

You or a friend may have been seen by an orthopedic surgeon or orthopedic specialist. Usually people associate this term with bones and joints. However, if you break the term down literally, that doesn't make sense.

Word Part	Meaning
Orth/o	Straight
Ped/o	Child
-ic	Pertaining to

If using the basic rules of medical terminology to define this term, then the definition would be "pertaining to a straight child." It is for this reason that we must create special definitions for certain terms.

Study Tips

Understanding medical terminology comes down to memorization. You must find the study technique that works best for you. Memorizing the component parts and their definitions is essential to understanding and defining medical terms. Techniques that may help with memorization include:

- Writing the combining forms, suffixes, and prefixes on one side of a page and then their definitions on the other side. Repetition is the key. Also try to write out definitions first and then come up with the combining forms, prefixes, and suffixes. Learn the terms both ways.
- Make up flashcards with the component parts on one side and their meaning on the other side. By the end of this textbook, your pile of note cards will probably be more than six feet tall.
- Write and speak the terms over and over again.

- Learn the pronunciation of the terms. You can use the textbook Website, which offers a list of the terms in this book and enables you to listen to how they are pronounced, or refer to the pronunciation sections in Appendix A. Sound out the terms.
- Conduct group studies, which work well for subjects like medical terminology. Bring a dry-erase board to the study group and write the terms or definitions on the board, one at a time. The members of the group can say their answers and how they remembered them. Hearing classmates use these terms helps you to remember them. Memorization is both a visual and audio technique.
- Relate the terms to a specific body part or body function. Whether you use this technique while thinking of your pet's body or even your own, it can be quite useful.
- Ask for help. Students don't do this enough. I realize that this subject can be overwhelming and some of you may be afraid to ask for help. The sooner you ask someone for help, the easier your learning experience will be. If you fail to ask then you will feel as if you're drowning halfway through the book.
- Use the review exercises at the end of each chapter.
- Make up your own terms using the component parts you've already learned.
- Create your own review exercises and mock quizzes. This can be a very useful tool when working in study groups.
- Make multiple copies of the workbook pages and then each day, try to fill them in.

Building the Terms

Combining Forms

For combining forms with multiple meanings, the context in which the term is used determines which definition to choose.

Prefixes

Prefixes alter the meaning of the term. For prefixes with multiple meanings, the combining form the prefix is attached to determines which meaning to use.

Suffixes

Suffixes also alter the meaning of the term. For suffixes with multiple meanings, the combining form the suffix is attached to determines which meaning to use.

Table 1.1 Chapter 1 Combining Forms.

Combining Forms	Definition	Combining Forms	Definition
Arthr/o	Joint	Hemat/o	Blood
Bi/o	Life	Hepat/o	Liver
Carcin/o	Cancer	Hist/o	Tissue
Cardi/o	Heart	Iatr/o	Treatment
Cephal/o	Head	Leuk/o	White
Cis/o	To cut	Nephr/o	Kidney
Col/o; Colon/o	Large intestine (colon)	Neur/o	Nerve
Cyst/o	Urinary bladder; cyst	Ophthalm/o	Eye
Cyt/o	Cell	Opt/o	Eye; vision
Derm/o	Skin	Oste/o	Bone
Dermat/o	Skin	Path/o	Disease
Electr/o	Electricity	Radi/o	X-rays
Encephal/o	Brain	Ren/o	Kidney
Enter/o	Small intestine	Rhin/o	Nose
Erythr/o	Red	Sarc/o	Connective tissue
Gastr/o	Stomach	Sect/o	To cut
Glyc/o	Sugar	Thromb/o	Clot; clotting
Gnos/o	Knowledge	Ur/o	Urine; urinary tract
Hem/o	Blood		

TECH TIP 1.1 Do you know when to use Ren/o vs. Nephr/o? Ren/o may only be used with the suffix -al. Nephr/o can be used with a variety of suffixes to describe a condition (usually abnormal) of the kidney.

Table 1.2   Chapter 1 Prefixes.

Prefix	Definition	Prefix	Definition
a-, an-	no; not; without	hypo-	deficient; below; under; less than normal
brachy-	short	in-	in; into; not
dia-	through; complete	intra-	within; into
dolicho-	long	meso-	middle
endo-	in; within	pro-	before; forward
epi-	above; upon; on	re-	back; again; backward
ex-, exo-	out; away from	retro-	behind; back; backward
extra-	outside	sub-	under; below
hyper-	above; excessive	trans-	across; through

Table 1.3   Chapter 1 Sufffixes.

Suffix	Definition	Suffix	Definition
-ac, -al, -ic, -ical	pertaining to	-ion	process
-algia	pain	-ist	specialist
-centesis	surgical puncture to remove fluid or gas	-itis	inflammation
-cyte	cell	-logy	study of
-cytosis	increase in cell number	-oma	tumor; mass; fluid collection
-drome	to run	-oma	tumor; mass; fluid collection
-ectomy	removal; excision; resection	-opsy	view of
-emia	blood condition	-osis	abnormal condition
-emic	pertaining to a blood condition	-pathy	disease condition; emotion
-genic	produced by or in	-scope	instrument for visual examination
-gram	record	-scopy	visual examination
-graph	instrument for recording	-sis	state of; condition
-graphy	process of recording	-tomy	incision; process of cutting

Now it's time to put these word parts together. If you memorize the meaning of the combining forms, prefixes, and suffixes then this will get easier each time. Remember your five basic rules to medical terminology when building and defining these terms.

Parts			Medical Term	Definition
Arthr/o	+ -ectomy		= Arthrectomy	: _____
Arthr/o	+ -itis		= Arthritis	: _____
Arthr/o	+ -centesis		= Arthrocentesis	: _____
Arthr/o	+ -logy		= Arthrology	: _____
Arthr/o	+ -pathy		= Arthropathy	: _____
Arthr/o	+ -scope		= Arthroscope	: _____
Arthr/o	+ -scopy		= Arthroscopy:	_____
Arthr/o	+ -osis		= Arthrosis	: _____
Arthr/o	+ -tomy		= Arthrotomy	: _____

Notice that the combining vowel was dropped with the suffix "-osis," but kept with the suffix "-tomy."

Parts			Medical Term	Definition
Bi/o	+ -logy	+ -ical	= Biological	: _____
Bi/o	+ -logy	+ -ist	= Biologist	: _____
Bi/o	+ -logy		= Biology	: _____
Carcin/o	+ -genic		= Carcinogenic	: _____
Cardi/o	+ -ac		= Cardiac	: _____
Cardi/o	+ -logy		= Cardiology	: _____
Cardi/o	+ -pathy		= Cardiopathy	: _____
intra-	+ Cardi/o	+ -ac	= Intracardiac	: _____
retro-	+ Cardi/o	+ -ac	= Retrocardiac	: _____
Cephal/o	+ -ic		= Cephalic	: _____
ex-	+ Cis/o	+ -ion	= Excision	: _____
in-	+ Cis/o	+ -ion	= Incision	: _____
Col/o	+ -ectomy		= Colectomy	: _____
Colon/o	+ -ectomy		= Colonectomy	: _____
Col/o	+ -itis		= Colitis	: _____
Colon/o	+ -itis		= Colonitis	: _____
Colon/o	+ -ic		= Colonic	: _____
Colon/o	+ -pathy		= Colonopathy	: _____
Colon/o	+ -scopy		= Colonoscopy	: _____
Cyst/o	+ -algia		= Cystalgia	: _____
Cyst/o	+ -ectomy		= Cystectomy	: _____
Cyst/o	+ -itis		= Cystitis	: _____
Cyst/o	+ -centesis		= Cystocentesis	: _____
Cyst/o	+ -gram		= Cystogram	: _____
Cyst/o	+ -tomy		= Cystotomy	: _____

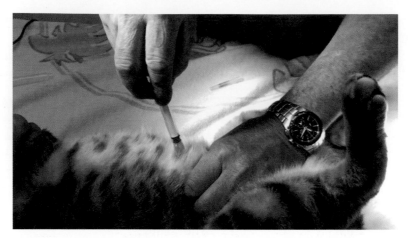

Figure 1.1   Cystocentesis on a cat. Courtesy of Greg Martinez DVM; www.youtube.com/drgregdvm.

Cyt/o	+ -logy		= Cytology	:_____
Cyt/o	+ -logy	+ -ical	= Cytological	:_____
Dermat/o	+ -itis		= Dermatitis	:_____
Dermat/o	+ -logy		= Dermatology	:_____
Derm/o	+ -al		= Dermal	:_____
hypo-	+ Derm/o	+ -ic	= Hypodermic	:_____
intra-	+ Derm/o	+ -al	= Intradermal	:_____
Electr/o	+ Cardi/o	+ -gram	= Electrocardiogram	:_____
Electr/o	+ Cardi/o	+ -graphy	= Electrocardiography	:_____
Electr/o	+ Encephal/o	+ -gram	= Electroencephalogram	:_____
Encephal/o	+ -ic		= Encephalic	:_____
Encephal/o	+ -itis		= Encephalitis	:_____
Encephal/o	+ -gram		= Encephalogram	:_____
Encephal/o	+ -graphy		= Encephalography	:_____
Endo-	+ -scope		= Endoscope	:_____
Endo-	+ -scopy		= Endoscopy	:_____
Enter/o	+ -ic		= Enteric	:_____
Enter/o	+ -itis		= Enteritis	:_____
Enter/o	+ -logy		= Enterology	:_____
Enter/o	+ -pathy		= Enteropathy	:_____
Erythr/o	+ -cyte		= Erythrocyte	:_____
Erythr/o	+ -cytosis		= Erythrocytosis	:_____

*This condition is also
known as polycythemia.*

Gastr/o	+ -ectomy		= Gastrectomy	:_____
Gastr/o	+ -ic		= Gastric	:_____
Gastr/o	+ -itis		= Gastritis	:_____
Gastr/o	+ -tomy		= Gastrotomy	:_____
Gastr/o	+ Enter/o	+ -itis	= Gastroenteritis	:_____
epi-	+ Gastr/o	+ -ic	= Epigastric	:_____

hypo-	+ Gastr/o + -ic	= Hypogastric	:_____
Glyc/o	+ -emic	= Glycemic	:_____
hyper	+ Glyc/o + -emia	= Hyperglycemia	:_____
hypo-	+ Glyc/o + -emia	= Hypoglycemia	:_____
Hemat/o	+ -logy	= Hematology	:_____
Hemat/o	+ -oma	= Hematoma	:_____
Hepat/o	+ -ic	= Hepatic	:_____
Hepat/o	+ -itis	= Hepatitis	:_____
Hepat/o	+ -oma	= Hepatoma	:_____
sub-	+ Hepat/o + -ic	= Subhepatic	:_____
trans-	+ Hepat/o + -ic	= Transhepatic	:_____
Hist/o	+ -logy	= Histology	:_____
Hist/o	+ -logy + -ist	= Histologist	:_____
Hist/o	+ Path/o + -logy + -ist	= Histopathologist	:_____
Iatr/o	+ -genic	= Iatrogenic	:_____
Leuk/o	+ -cyte	= Leukocyte	:_____
Leuk/o	+ -cytosis	= Leukocytosis	:_____
Nephr/o	+ -algia	= Nephralgia	:_____
Nephr/o	+ -ectomy	= Nephrectomy	:_____
Nephr/o	+ -itis	= Nephritis	:_____
Nephr/o	+ -osis	= Nephrosis	:_____
Nephr/o	+ -gram	= Nephrogram	:_____
Nephr/o	+ -oma	= Nephroma	:_____
Nephr/o	+ -logy	= Nephrology	:_____
Neur/o	+ -al	= Neural	:_____
Neur/o	+ -algia	= Neuralgia	:_____
Neur/o	+ -ectomy	= Neurectomy	:_____
Neur/o	+ -itis	= Neuritis	:_____
Neur/o	+ -logy	= Neurology	:_____
Ophthalm/o	+ -ic	= Ophthalmic	:_____
Ophthalm/o	+ -logy + -ist	= Ophthalmologist	:_____
Ophthalm/o	+ -logy	= Ophthalmology	:_____
Ophthalm/o	+ -scope	= Ophthalmoscope	:_____
Opt/o	+ -ic	= Optic	:_____
Opt/o	+ -ical	= Optical	:_____
Oste/o	+ -ectomy	= Ostectomy	:_____
Oste/o	+ -itis	= Osteitis	:_____
Oste/o	+ Arthr/o + -itis	= Osteoarthritis	:_____
Oste/o	+ -genic	= Osteogenic	:_____
Oste/o	+ -logy	= Osteology	:_____
Oste/o	+ -tomy	= Osteotomy	:_____
Path/o	+ -genic	= Pathogenic	:_____
Path/o	+ -logy	= Pathology	:_____
Path/o	+ -logy + -ist	= Pathologist	:_____
Radi/o	+ -graph	= Radiograph	:_____
Radi/o	+ -graphy	= Radiography	:_____

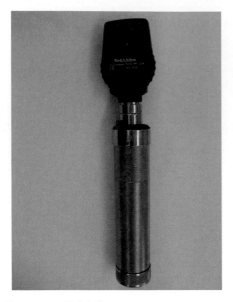

Figure 1.2 Ophthalmoscope.

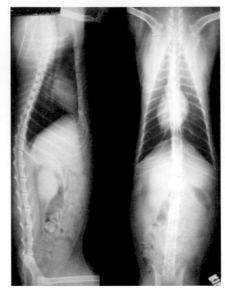

Figure 1.3 Radiograph of a cat.

Radi/o   + -logy   = Radiology   :_____
Ren/o   + -al   = Renal   :_____
re-   + sect/o   + -ion   = Resection   :_____
Rhin/o   + -itis   = Rhinitis   :_____
Thromb/o   + -cyte   = Thrombocyte   :_____
                                              Also known as a platelet.
Thromb/o   + -cytosis   = Thrombocytosis   :_____
Ur/o   + -logy   = Urology   :_____

Special Terms

The following medical terms do not break down correctly. Therefore, we must create new and more specific definitions.

Anemia   Decrease in red blood cells and/or hemoglobin.
Biopsy   Removal of tissue for microscopic examination.
Brachycephalic   Pertaining to a short, wide head (i.e. Persians, Pugs, Boston Terriers).

TECH TIP 1.2 Various breeds have a variety of skull shapes. Brachycephalics are of greatest concern because they are predisposed to various medical conditions. These animals are an anesthetic risk so additional precautions must be taken with surgery.

Dolichocephalic   Pertaining to a narrow, long head (i.e., Greyhounds, Collies).
Mesocephalic   Pertaining to an average width head (i.e., Golden Retrievers).

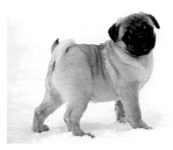

Figure 1.4A A Pug is an example of a brachyce-phalic breed. Courtesy of shutterstock/Utekhina Anna.

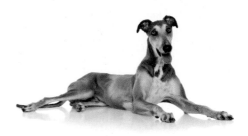

Figure 1.4B Greyhounds are dolichocephalics. Courtesy of shutterstock/Jagodka.

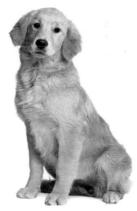

Figure 1.4C Golden Retrievers are mesocephalics. Courtesy of shutterstock/Eric Isselee.

Carcinoma	Malignant tumor arising from epithelial tissue.
Prodrome	Symptoms run together before the onset of a more specific disease.
Syndrome	Symptoms that run together and point to a specific disease.
Sarcoma	Malignant tumor arising from connective tissue.
Leukemia	Increase in the number of cancerous white blood cells.

TECH TIP 1.3 Leukocytosis vs. Leukemia

At first glance the definitions for these terms are very similar. However, there is one word that makes a huge difference: cancerous. Leukocytosis is simply an increase in the number of white blood cells, whereas leukemia is an increase in the number of cancerous white blood cells.

Diagnosis	Estimation of the cause of disease.
Prognosis	Estimation of disease outcome.
Canine	Dog.
Feline	Cat.

Bovine	Cattle.
Ovine	Sheep.
Caprine	Goat.
Aggressive	Eager to fight.
Alert	Energetic, quick, and responsive.
Docile	Relaxed, easy to handle.
Feral	Wild.
Submissive	Willing to submit.

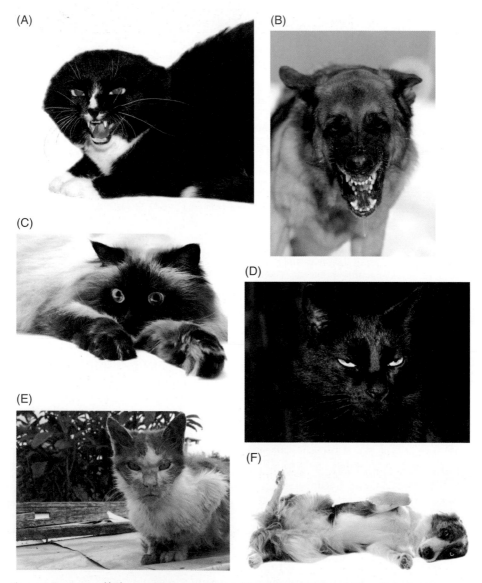

Figure 1.5 Types of behavior. (A) Aggressive cat. Courtesy of shutterstock/Kuzmin Andrey. (B) Aggressive dog. Courtesy of shutterstock/Antonova Victoria. (C) Alert cat. Courtesy of shutterstock/Adisa. (D) Docile cat. Courtesy of shutterstock/Jennifer Nickert. (E) Feral cat. Courtesy of shutterstock/Andre Blais. (F) Submissive dog. Courtesy of shutterstock/cynoclub.

Chapter Abbreviations

At the end of each chapter there is a set of abbreviations that are commonly used in veterinary medicine. These abbreviations can be used to communicate with other professionals on cage cards, files, appointment books, and prescription labels.

Table 1.4   Chapter 1 Abbreviations.

Abbreviation	Definition
BAR	Bright, alert, responsive
CCU	Critical care unit
ICU	Intensive care unit
CWPM	Continue with previous medication
DLH	Domestic long hair (This a mixed-breed cat with long hair)
DMH	Domestic medium hair (This a mixed-breed cat with medium hair)
DSH	Domestic short hair (This a mixed-breed cat with short hair)
DOA	Dead on arrival
DOB	Date of birth
ER	Emergency room
OR	Operating room
GROS	Gross review of systems
K-9	Canine
ISO	Isolation unit
NAF	No abnormalities found
NSF	No significant findings
P/E	Physical examination
PPH	Past pertinent history
R/O	Rule out
SOAP	Subjective, objective, assessment, plan *(See explanation below)*
TPR(W)	Temperature, pulse, respiration, (weight)
WNL	Within normal limits

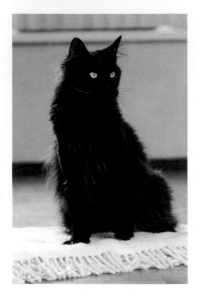

Figure 1.6A   Domestic long hair (DLH). Courtesy of shutterstock/Jeroen van den Broek.

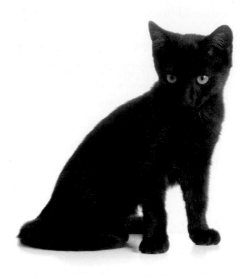

Figure 1.6B   Domestic short hair (DSH). Courtesy of shutterstock/Jiri Hera.

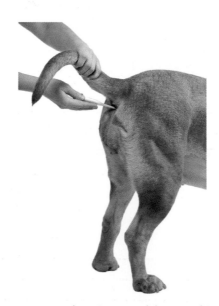

Figure 1.7   Dog having its temperature taken. Courtesy of shutterstock/Vitaly Titov & Maria.

SOAP:

When the veterinary technician goes into the exam room to perform the TPR(W) and to speak with the owner, the tech begins to fill out a patient record. (See Figure 1.8). As you can see, the tech recorded the patient's TPR(W) and began a

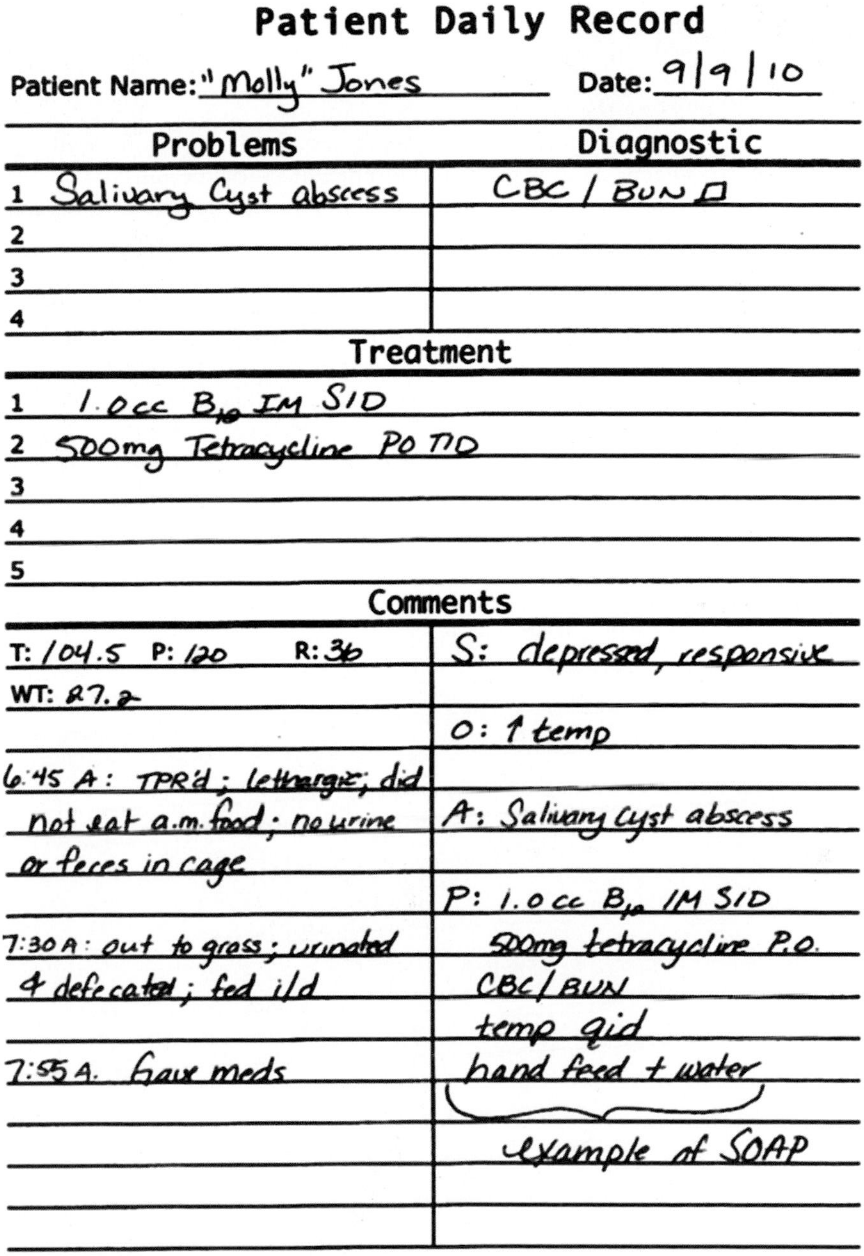

Patient Daily Record

Patient Name: "Molly" Jones _____   Date: 9/9/10

Problems	Diagnostic
1 Salivary Cyst abscess	CBC / BUN ▢
2	
3	
4	

Treatment

1 1.0 cc B₁₂ IM SID
2 500mg Tetracycline PO TID
3
4
5

Comments

T: 104.5 P: 120 R: 36	S: depressed, responsive
WT: 27.2	
	O: ↑ temp
6:45 A: TPR'd; lethargic; did not eat a.m. food; no urine or feces in cage	A: Salivary Cyst abscess
	P: 1.0 cc B₁₂ IM SID
7:30 A: out to gross; urinated & defecated; fed i/d	500mg tetracycline P.O. CBC/BUN temp qid
7:55 A. Gave meds	hand feed + water
	example of SOAP

Figure 1.8   Example of using SOAP in a patient file.

SOAP. There are parts of the SOAP that can be filled out by the technician and other parts to be filled out by the veterinarian. The type of information is as follows:

S (Subjective):   How the animal appears; opinions.
                   For example, is he/she depressed, BAR, not eating well
O (Objective):   Facts. Things that can be reproduced or measured.
                   For example, an increased temperature or white blood cell count.
A (Assessment):   Initial diagnosis. This aspect is for the doctor only.
                   As technicians, you will not diagnose.
P (Plan):   This is the technician's focus. Lab tests, treatments, and radiographs are ordered. Surgery is recommended. As technicians, it is our job to carry out these tests.

Case Study: Define the medical terms and abbreviations in bold print in the case below

Maverick, a 12-year-old **K-9**, comes in to your clinic for a yearly exam. His owners have just moved from Texas to your state. As the veterinary technician, you are the first into the exam room to perform the **TPR(W)** and to speak with the owner about their visit today. Maverick appears **BAR** and his TPR is normal. His **DOB** is May 5, 2000. The owner, Mrs. Nethery, mentions that Maverick was seen by a different veterinarian a few months ago because he was limping. After obtaining a **PPH**, the owner gives you the copies of Maverick's records and **radiographs** from the previous clinic.

According to Maverick's records, he was previously **diagnosed** with **cardiopathy**, **arthritis**, and **hepatitis**. The veterinarian, Dr. Rojas, enters the exam room to perform the **P/E**. He immediately notices that Maverick has **dermatitis** on his abdomen. Dr. Rojas decides to perform a **cytology** on the affected area of skin. The skin scrape shows **NSF**. While speaking to Mrs. Nethery, the doctor feels a mass in the **hypogastric** region. After discussing the options, Mrs. Nethery agrees to let Dr. Rojas obtain a **gastric biopsy** the following day.

The following day, Maverick checks in for surgery and has a pre-surgical **hematology** panel done. His **erythrocytes, leukocytes, and thrombocytes** are **WNL**. **Hepatic** enzymes are slightly elevated, but Dr. Rojas isn't too concerned about it. An **electrocardiogram** is also done because Maverick was previously diagnosed with a cardiopathy. The results were unremarkable. He's taken to the **OR** where an **incision** is made into the abdomen and the mass is **excised**. Dr. Rojas asks you to send the mass to a reference lab for a biopsy. Maverick is sent to the **ICU** for recovery after surgery because of his age. The recovery goes well and Maverick is sent home. You tell Mrs. Nethery that the biopsy results will be back in three to five working days.

After a week has passed, Mrs. Nethery has returned with Maverick for a post-surgical exam. Maverick's incision is healing nicely. Dr. Rojas explains that the mass was a **sarcoma**. His **prognosis** is guarded.

Exercises

1-A: Match the combining forms with their meaning.

1.	_____ Heart	A.	Arthr/o
2.	_____ Small intestine	B.	Cardi/o
3.	_____ Brain	C.	Col/o
4.	_____ Liver	D.	Cyst/o
5.	_____ Electricity	E.	Dermat/o
6.	_____ Urinary bladder	F.	Electr/o
7.	_____ Stomach	G.	Encephal/o
8.	_____ Sugar	H.	Enter/o
9.	_____ Joint	I.	Gastr/o
10.	_____ Blood	J.	Glyc/o
11.	_____ Skin	K.	Hemat/o
12.	_____ Large intestine	L.	Hepat/o

1-B: Write the correct medical term in the blank.

1. _____: Study of tissue
2. _____: Mass or collection of blood
3. _____: Inflammation of the brain
4. _____: Disease condition of the heart
5. _____: Tumor on the liver
6. _____: Inflammation of the liver
7. _____: Incision into bone
8. _____: Increase in platelets
9. _____: Specialist in the study of disease
10. _____: Abnormal condition of the kidney
11. _____: Instrument to visually examine the eye
12. _____: Record of electricity in the heart
13. _____: Pertaining to nerves
14. _____: Red blood cell
15. _____: Pertaining to below the skin
16. _____: Pertaining to below the liver
17. _____: Blood condition of excessive sugar
18. _____: Estimation of the cause of disease
19. _____: Inflammation of skin
20. _____: Pertaining to outside the liver

1-C: Complete the definition for the following terms.

1. Arthralgia: Pain in the _____.
2. Neuritis: _____ of nerves.
3. Arthrocentesis: _____ from a joint.

4. Rhinitis: Inflammation of the _____.
5. Cephalic: Pertaining to the _____.
6. Anemic: Pertaining to a decrease in _____ and/or

_____.
7. Ophthalmology: Study of the _____.
8. Colectomy: Removal of the _____.
9. Incision: Process of _____.
10. Nephrectomy: Removal of the _____.

1-D: Define the following suffixes.

1. _____: -itis   7. _____: -ist
2. _____: -ectomy   8. _____: -graph
3. _____: -tomy   9. _____: -pathy
4. _____: -gram   10. _____: -algia
5. _____: -scopy   11. _____: -centesis
6. _____: -osis   12. _____: -emia

1-E: Circle the correct answer.

1. A dog named Brutus presents to your clinic with an abnormal heart rhythm.
    After further testing it was recommended that Brutus be referred to a:
    a. Pathologist
    b. Histpathologist
    c. Ophthalmologist
    d. Cardiologist

2. Mrs. Potter calls your clinic worried about her cat, Harry. She says that
    Harry has had blood in his urine. She makes an appointment for Harry to
    come in for an exam and to have his urine checked. When Harry comes for
    his appointment, the doctor asks you to obtain urine from Harry. What
    procedure would you perform?
    a. Arthrocentesis
    b. Cystocentesis
    c. Osteocentesis
    d. Gastrocentesis

3. A horse named Desperado was rushed to your clinic unable to put weight
    on one of his legs. Apparently fell during a race. The veterinarian suspects
    a fracture (broken bone). What would confirm this?
    a. Encephalograph
    b. Radiograph
    c. Nephrogram
    d. Cardiogram

4. Mr. Manning has just rushed into your clinic with his dog, Peyton. Peyton hasn't felt like playing with his ball like he usually does. Upon examination, you notice that he has pale gums. A blood test reveals that his erythrocyte count is decreased. Peyton has:
   a. Leukemia
   b. Thrombocytosis
   c. Leukocytosis
   d. Anemia

5. A boxer named Rosie presents to your clinic with a mass on her shoulder. The owner is worried that it might be cancerous. What procedure would be performed to see if the cells in the mass are cancerous?
   a. Electrocardiogram
   b. Biopsy
   c. Cystocentesis
   d. Osteocentesis

1-F: Define the following abbreviations.

1. _____: BAR
2. _____: OR
3. _____: DSH
4. _____: ICU
5. _____: TPR(W)
6. _____: DOB

7. _____: P/E
8. _____: R/O
9. _____: ISO
10. _____: NSF
11. _____: PPH
12. _____: WNL

1-G: Define the following prefixes.

1. _____: intra-
2. _____: extra-
3. _____: trans-
4. _____: epi-
5. _____: sub-
6. _____: hyper-

7. _____: pro-
8. _____: re-
9. _____: endo-
10. _____: retro-
11. _____: a-, an-
12. _____: ex-

1-H: Define the following medical terms.

1. _____: Hyperglycemia
2. _____: Prognosis
3. _____: Incision
4. _____: Cytology
5. _____: Carcinoma
6. _____: Thrombocytosis
7. _____: Gastroenterology

8. _____: Biology
9. _____: Brachycephalic
10. _____: Iatrogenic
11. _____: Optic
12. _____: Osteitis
13. _____: Rhinitis
14. _____: Urology

Answers can be found starting on page 571.

Go to www.wiley.com/go/taibo/terminology to find additional learning materials for this chapter:

- A crossword puzzle
- Flashcards
- Audio clips to show how to pronounce terms
- Case studies
- Review questions
- The figures from the chapter in PowerPoint

Chapter 2

Anatomical Organization

This chapter will focus on the anatomical divisions and structural organization of the body. Because you'll be learning how to use directional and positional terms, basic skeletal anatomy will be introduced. The book will go into more detail on anatomy in later chapters.

Structural Organization

We can divide the body into four basic groups: cells, tissues, organs, and systems. Within each general group are more specialized structures with specific functions.

The Cell

The cell is the basic structure of all things. Cells can be found everywhere in the body, where they exist in specific organs and tissues. While the functions of cells differ based on their anatomical location, their basic anatomy is the same. Label the cell diagram in Figure 2.1 below using the structures in Table 2.1.

Chemical Process of the Cell

There are three basic processes that occur within a cell. They are as follows:

Anabolism   Process of building up complex proteins from simpler substances.
Catabolism   Process of breaking down complex foods into simpler substances.
Metabolism   The total of the chemical processes in a cell:
            anabolism + catabolism.

Veterinary Medical Terminology Guide and Workbook, First Edition. Angela Taibo.
© 2014 John Wiley & Sons, Inc. Published 2014 by John Wiley & Sons, Inc.
Companion website: www.wiley.com/go/taibo/terminology

Structure of a typical animal cell

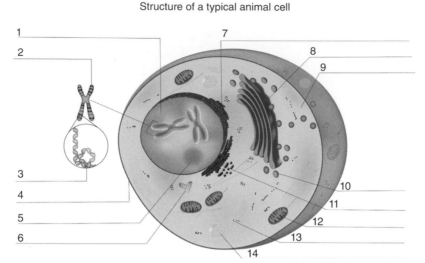

Figure 2.1A   Anatomy of a cell. Courtesy of shutterstock/Alila Sao Mai, blamb, and SSCREATIONS.

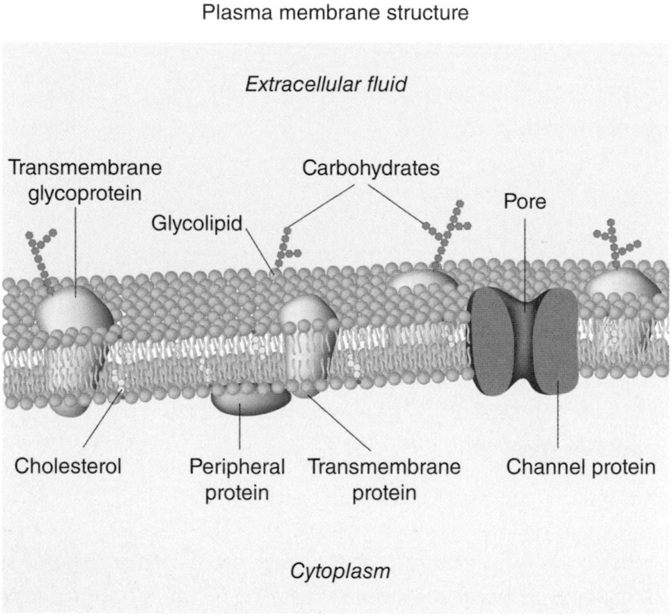

Plasma membrane structure

Extracellular fluid

Transmembrane
glycoprotein   Carbohydrates

                                                        Pore

          Glycolipid

Cholesterol   Peripheral   Transmembrane   Channel protein
                   protein   protein

Cytoplasm

Figure 2.1B   Semipermeable cell membrane. Courtesy of shutterstock/Alila Sao Mai.

Cell Types

There are many different types of cells in the body. Each has a specific function. Although the types share similar internal structures, their morphologies (shapes) differ (Figure 2.2).

Table 2.1 Cellular Anatomy.

Cell membrane (4)	Semipermeable structure that surrounds and protects the cell.
Centrioles (6)	Tubular structures that maintain the cell's shape and move chromosomes during mitosis.
Chromosomes (2)	Rod-like structures containing regions of DNA called genes.
Cytoplasm (9)	Material inside the cell membrane that surrounds the nucleus
DNA (3)	The basic structure of genes that directs cell activity and transmits genetic information; Deoxyribonucleic acid.
Endoplasmic reticulum	Protein factory where proteins are made from simple materials. (11) **Smooth endoplasmic reticulum** synthesizes lipids. (7) **Rough endoplasmic reticulum** synthesizes proteins.
Golgi apparatus (8)	Processing factory where proteins are stored, modified, and transported.
Lysosome (14)	Site of intracellular digestion containing enzymes to disintegrate microorganisms and damaged tissue.
Mitochondria (12)	Energy factory of the cell in which foods are burned for energy.
Nucleoplasm	Material within the nucleus.
Nucleus (1)	The control center of the cell that contains chromosomes.
Nucleolus (5)	Site of RNA synthesis. Plural form is nucleoli.
Protoplasm	Cell membrane, cytoplasm, and nucleus.
Ribosomes (13)	Structures found in endoplasmic reticulum containing RNA, and the site of protein synthesis. Note the ribosomes also found on the **rough endoplasmic reticulum** (7).
Vacuole (10)	Fluid-filled cavity containing food, water, or waste products.

TECH TIP 2.1 Did you know that the number of chromosomes is different from species to species? Some examples are as follows:

Humans:	46		Sheep:	54
Dogs:	78		Goats:	60
Cats:	38		Pigs:	38
Horses:	64		Chickens:	20
Donkeys:	62		Birds:	69
Cattle:	60			

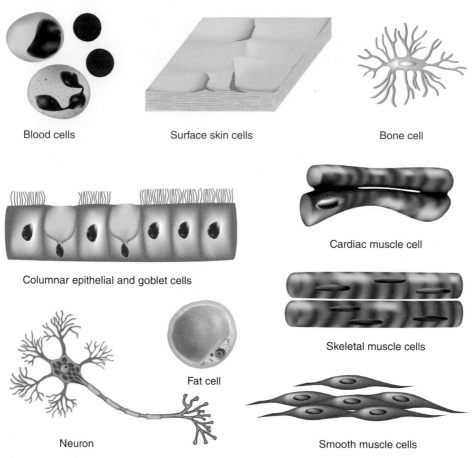

Blood cells

Surface skin cells

Bone cell

Columnar epithelial and goblet cells

Cardiac muscle cell

Skeletal muscle cells

Fat cell

Neuron

Smooth muscle cells

Figure 2.2   Cell and tissue types. Courtesy of shutterstock/Alila Sao Mai.

Tissue

Tissues are groups of similar cells working together for a specific function. The following are examples of tissue types.

Adipose tissue	Collection of fat cells.
Connective tissue	Binds and supports various structures. Examples include fat, bone, blood, cartilage.
Epithelial tissue	Consists of **epithelium**, which lines external and internal body surfaces.
	Consists of **endothelium**, which lines organs and blood vessels.
	Consists of **mesothelium**, which lines cavities such as the peritoneum.
Muscle tissue	**Skeletal muscle**, which is striated, voluntary muscle controlling movement.

Cardiac muscle, which is striated, involuntary muscle controlling the heart.

Visceral muscle, which is smooth, involuntary muscle controlling the internal organs (viscera).

Nerve tissue Cells that conduct electrical impulses all over the body.

Organs

Organs are different tissues working together for a specific function. For example, the organs of the abdomen and chest use nervous tissue, muscle tissue, and epithelial tissue to function. The medical term for internal organs is viscera. Examples of viscera include the heart, lungs, stomach, liver, and spleen.

System

A system is a group of different organs working together for a complex function (Figure 2.3). For example, the respiratory system consists of the nose, throat, voice box, windpipe, and lungs working together to help an animal breathe. Table 2.2 is a list of the different systems of the body. The following chapters will focus on each system individually.

Cavities

The body can be divided into different areas that contain organs working together. Each area is referred to as a cavity. This book will discuss each body cavity in detail in the later chapters. This chapter introduces the body cavities (Figure 2.3).

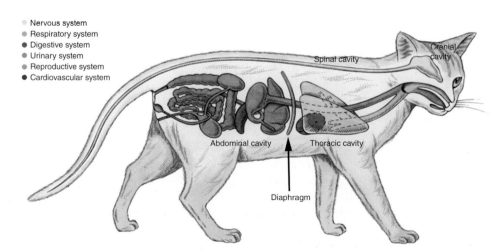

Figure 2.3 Body systems of a cat. Courtesy of Getty Images/John Woodcock.

Table 2.2 Systems.

System	Definition
Cardiovascular	Consists of organs such as the heart, veins, arteries, capillaries, and spleen.
Digestive	Consists of organs such as the mouth, throat, esophagus, stomach, intestines, pancreas, liver, and gallbladder.
Endocrine	Consists organs such as the pancreas, pituitary gland, thyroid gland, ovaries, testes, and adrenal glands.
Integumentary	Consist of organs such as the skin, hair (fur), nails, and glands.
Musculoskeletal	Consists of organs such as the bones, muscle, and joints.
Nervous	Consists of organs such as the brain and spinal cord.
Reproductive	Consists of organs such as the ovaries, vagina, uterus, testes, and penis.
Respiratory	Consists of organs such as the windpipe, lungs, and heart.
Urogenital	Consists of organs such as the kidneys, ureters, urinary bladder, and urethra.

Abdominal   Cavity containing organs such as the stomach, intestines, spleen, and pancreas.
Cranial   Cavity containing the brain.
Spinal   Cavity containing the spinal cord.
Thoracic   Cavity containing organs such as the heart, lungs, esophagus, and trachea.

Additional Terminology for Structural Organization

Anatomy   The form and structure of the body.
Benign   Not malignant, non-invasive; not spreading.
Cartilage   Flexible connective tissue attached to bones at a joint.
Diaphragm   Thin, muscular partition separating the thoracic and abdominal cavities.
Endocrine   Glands that secrete hormones directly into the bloodstream
glands   (Figure 2.4).
Exocrine   Glands that secrete chemicals through tubes everywhere in the
glands   body (Figure 2.4).
Larynx   Voice box (Figure 2.5).

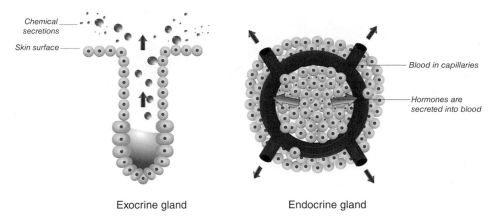

Exocrine gland   Endocrine gland

Figure 2.4 Endocrine and exocrine glands. Courtesy of shutterstock/GRei.

Lavage	Irrigation or washing out of an organ or cavity.
Malignant	Tending to become progressively worse.
Membrane	Thin layer of tissue that covers a surface, lines a cavity, or divides a space or an organ.
Peritoneum	Membrane surrounding the organs in the abdomen.
Pharynx	Throat
Physiology	Study of the body's function.
Trachea	Windpipe (Figure 2.5).
Umbilicus	The navel (Figure 2.6).

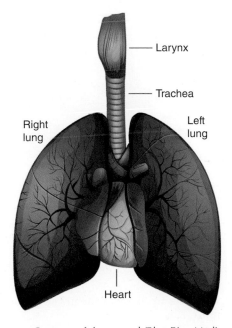

Figure 2.5 Respiratory system. Courtesy of shutterstock/Blue Ring Media.

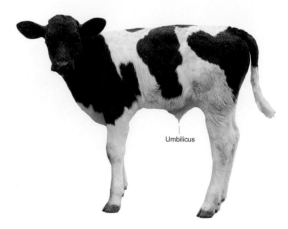

Figure 2.6   Umbilicus on a calf. Courtesy of shutterstock/Damian Palus.

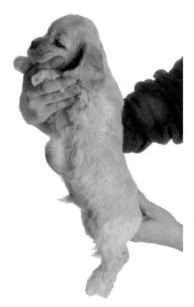

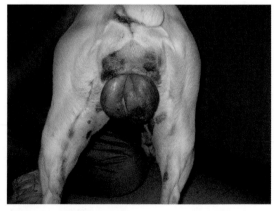

Figure 2.7A   Umbilical hernia in a
Cocker Spaniel puppy. Courtesy of
shutterstock/Willee Cole.

Figure 2.7B   Vaginal prolapse in an American Pit Bull
Terrier. Courtesy of AK Traylor, DVM; Microscopy
Learning Systems.

Ureter	Tube that carries urine from the kidneys to the urinary bladder.
Urethra	Tube that carries urine from the urinary bladder to the outside of the body.
Viscera	Internal organs.

Pathology of Structures

Evisceration	Displacement of internal organs outside the cavity that should contain them.
Hernia	Abnormal protrusion of an organ or tissue through the structure that should contain it (Figure 2.7A).
Prolapse	Abnormal protrusion of an organ or tissue through a natural opening (Figure 2.7B).

Introduction to the Skeletal Anatomy

Below is a diagram of the cat skeleton. Knowing the location of these bones is essential in understanding how to use directional terminology. This chapter merely introduces the location of these bones (Figure 2.8). Chapter 3 will go into more detail on skeletal anatomy.

Directional Terms

We use directional terms when describing the location of various structures in the body and when comparing the relationship of one structure to another in the body (Table 2.3). These terms, for the most part, are widely used in veterinary medicine. To better understand their application, try picturing yourself on all fours. You'd be surprised how much this helps.

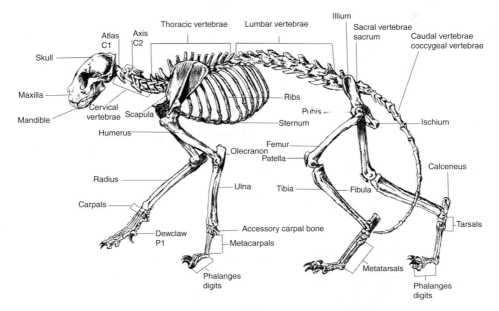

Figure 2.8   Cat skeleton. Courtesy of shutterstock/The Paper Street Design Co.

Table 2.3　Directional Terms.

Directional Term	Definition	Example
Dorsal	Pertaining to the back; closer to the back; away from the ground	The spine is dorsal to the sternum. The spine is dorsal to the heart.
Ventral	Pertaining to the belly; closer to the belly; toward the ground	The heart is ventral to the spine. The sternum is ventral to the heart.
Cranial	Pertaining to the head; closer to the head	The neck is cranial to the tail. The heart is cranial to the stomach.
Caudal	Pertaining to the tail; closer to the tail	The hindlimb is caudal to the forelimb. The lumbar vertebrae are caudal to the cervical vertebrae.
Medial	Pertaining to middle; closer to the median plane; closer to the midline	The dewclaw is medial to the other digits. The heart is medial to the ribs.
Lateral	Pertaining to the side; further from the median plane; further from the midline	The ribs are lateral to the heart. Your pinky toe is lateral to your big toe.
Proximal	Pertaining to the beginning; nearer the point of attachment	The femur is proximal to the tibia. The ulna is proximal to the carpals.
Distal	Pertaining to far from the beginning; farther from the point of attachment	The patella is distal to the femur. The phalanges are distal to the humerus.
Superficial	Nearer the surface of the body	A paper cut is superficial. The biceps are superficial to the humerus.
Deep	Farther from the surface of the body	A stab wound is deep. The humerus is deep to the biceps muscle.
Plantar	Pertaining to the caudal surface of the rear paw (pes) and tarsus	The dog has a laceration on the plantar aspect of its left paw.
Palmar	Pertaining to the caudal surface of the front paw (manus) and carpus	The dog has a laceration on the palmar aspect of its left paw.
Rostral	Pertaining to the nose; closer to the nose	The hard palate is rostral to the soft palate.
Anterior	Pertaining to the front side of the body	The toe of the hoof is anterior to the heal.
Posterior	Pertaining to the back side of the body	The heal of the hoof is posterior to the toe.

Recumbency

Recumbent is defined as lying down. Certain procedures require an animal to be positioned in a particular recumbency. The following are examples of recumbency:

Dorsal recumbency   Animal is lying on its back. This is also known as supine recumbency (Figure 2.9).

Ventral recumbency   Animal is lying on its belly. This is also known as sternal recumbency or prone recumbency.

Lateral recumbency   Animal is lying on its side. An animal lying on its right side is said to be in right lateral recumbency.

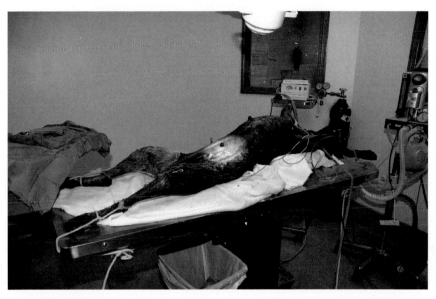

Figure 2.9   Animal prepped for surgery in dorsal recumbency. Courtesy of shutterstock/Julie Keen.

Table 2.4   Planes of the Body.

Plane	Definition
Dorsal plane	Divides the body into a belly side (ventral) and a back side (dorsal).
Median plane	Divides the body into equal right and left halves. This is also known as a **midsagittal plane**.
Sagittal plane	Divides the body into unequal right and left halves.
Transverse plane	Divides the body into cranial and caudal halves.

Planes of the Body

Planes are imaginary flat surfaces that divide the body into different sections (Figure 2.10).

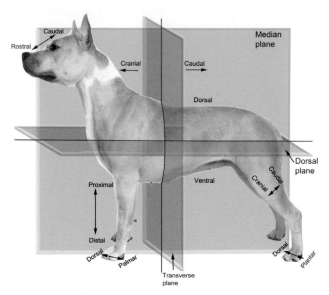

Figure 2.10   Medical planes and directional terms on a pit bull. Courtesy of shutterstock/serg741.

The Spinal Column

As you've probably noticed in the cat skeleton diagram, there are different kinds of bones in the back called vertebrae. In between these backbones are cartilage pads called intervertebral discs (Figure 2.11).

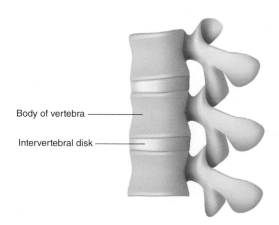

Figure 2.11   Intervertebral disc. Courtesy of shutterstock/Alila Sao Mai.

Intervertebral disk   Cartilage pad between vertebrae used for cushion and support.

Spinal cord   Nervous tissue within the spinal cavity.

Spinal column   Bones surrounding the spinal cavity.

Vertebra   Back bone.

Vertebrae   Back bones.

Below is a list of the different vertebrae and where they fall along the spinal column (Table 2.5).

Table 2.5   Vertebrae.

Vertebrae	Location
Cervical (C)	Neck area
Thoracic (T)	Chest area
Lumbar (L)	Lower back area (waist)
Sacral (S)	Sacrum
Caudal; coccygeal (Ca, Cy)	Tail area

TECH TIP 2.2 The different kinds of vertebrae differ in numbers in each species. Instead of merely writing out the numbers of each type in a table, we write them into **vertebral formulas**. They are as follows:

Dog and cat	$C_7T_{13}L_7S_{3fused}Ca\ (Cy)_{3-24}$
Horse	$C_7T_{18}L_6S_{5fused}Ca\ (Cy)_{15-21}.$ Some Arabians have five lumbar
Cattle	$C_7T_{13}L_6S_5Ca\ (Cy)_{18-20}$
Pigs	$C_7T_{14-15}L_{6-7}S_4Ca\ (Cy)_{20-23}$
Sheep and goats	$C_7T_{13}L_{6-7}S_4Ca\ (Cy)_{16-18}$
Chickens	$C_{14}T_7LS_{14fused}Ca\ (Cy)_6$

From the Outside In

Anatomical terms change when describing structures and landmarks on the outside of the body (Figure 2.12).

Cheek   Fleshy portion on either side of the face, forming the sides of the mouth and continuing rostrally to the lips.

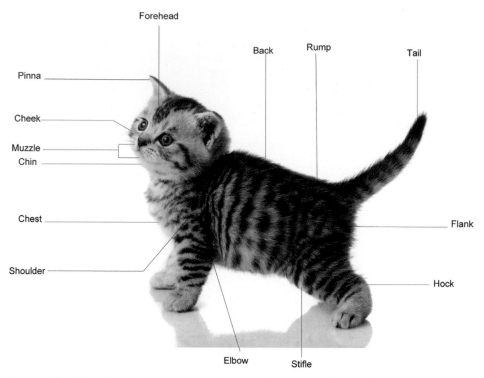

Figure 2.12   External landmarks on a kitten. Courtesy of shutterstock/Ewa Studi.

Chest	Part of the body between the neck and abdomen; also called the thorax.
Chin	Anterior prominence of the mandible.
Elbow	Joint where the humerus, radius, and ulna meet; medically known as the humeroradioulnar joint.
Flank	Lateral aspect of the body between the ilium and ribs.
Forehead	Region between the eyes and ears.
Hock	Common name for the tarsus joint.
Muzzle	Skin, muscles, and fascia of the upper and lower lip and including the nasal bones.
Pinna	Flap of the ear; also known as the auricle.
Rump	Region around the pelvis, hindquarters, and buttocks; also known as the croup or gluteal region.
Shoulder	Joint where the scapula and humerus meet; medically known as the scapulohumeral joint.
Stifle	Joint where the femur and tibia meet; medically known as the femorotibial joint.
Tail	Caudal appendage of the vertebral column made up of caudal vertebrae.

Table 2.6 Chapter 2 Combining Forms.

Combining Forms	Definition	Combining Forms	Definition
Abdomin/o	Abdomen	**Medi/o**	Middle
Aden/o	Gland	**My/o**	Muscle
Adip/o	Fat	**Neur/o**	Nerve
Anis/o	Unequal(in size)	**Nucle/o**	Nucleus
Anter/o	Front	**Path/o**	Disease
Bol/o	To cast (throw)	**Pelv/o**	Pelvis (hip)
Caud/o	Tail	**Peritone/o**	Peritoneum
Cervic/o	Neck	**Pharyng/o**	Pharynx; throat
Chondr/o	Cartilage	**Poster/o**	Back; behind
Chrom/o	Color	**Prot/o**	First
Coccyg/o	Tailbone	**Proxim/o**	Nearest
Crani/o	Skull	**Rhin/o**	Nose
Crin/o	To secrete	**Sacr/o**	Sacrum
Cyt/o	Cell	**Sarc/o**	Connective tissue
Dist/o	Far; distant	**Spin/o**	Spine; backbone
Dors/o	Back of body	**Stern/o**	Sternum
Duct/o	To lead or carry	**Thel/o**	Nipple
Hist/o	Tissue	**Thorac/o**	Chest
Inguin/o	Groin	**Trache/o**	Trachea; windpipe
Kary/o	Nucleus	**Umbilic/o**	Umbilicus; navel
Laryng/o	Larynx; voice box	**Vertebr/o**	Vertebrae; back bones
Later/o	Side	**Viscer/o**	Viscera; internal organs
Lumb/o	Lower back		

Table 2.7   Chapter 2 Prefixes.

Prefix	Definition	Prefix	Definition
a-, an-	no; not; without	hypo-	deficient; below; under; less than normal
ana-	up	inter-	between
cata-	down	meta-	change
endo-	in; within	neo-	new
epi-	above; upon; on	uni-	one

Table 2.8   Chapter 2 Suffixes.

Suffix	Definition	Suffix	Definition
-ac, -al-, -ar, -eal, -iac, -ic, -ical, -ior, -ose	pertaining to	-oma	tumor; mass; fluid collection
-algia	pain	-osis	abnormal condition
-centesis	surgical puncture to remove fluid or gas	-plasia	development; formation; growth
-ectomy	removal; excision; resection	-plasm	formation
-ism	process; condition	-plasty	surgical repair
-ist	specialist	-somes	bodies
-itis	inflammation	-tomy	incision; process of cutting
-logy	study of		

Building the Terms

Now it's time to put these word parts together. If you memorize the meaning of the combining forms, prefixes, and suffixes, then this will get easier each time. Remember your five basic rules to medical terminology when building and defining these terms. You'll notice some word parts are repeated from the previous chapter.

Parts			Medical Term	Definition
Abdomin/o + -al			= Abdominal	: _____
Abdomin/o + -centesis			= Abdominocentesis	: _____
ana-	+ Bol/o	+ -ic	= Anabolic	: _____
cata-	+ Bol/o	+ -ic	= Catabolic	: _____
meta-	+ Bol/o	+ -ic	= Metabolic	: _____
Adip/o	+ -ose		= Adipose	: _____
Caud/o	+ -al		= Caudal	: _____
Cervic/o	+ -al		= Cervical	: _____
Chondr/o	+ -al		= Chondral	: _____
Chondr/o	+ -algia		= Chondralgia	: _____
Chondr/o	+ -ectomy		= Chondrectomy	: _____
Chondr/o	+ -oma		= Chondroma	: _____
Chondr/o	+ Sarc/o	+ -oma	= Chondrosarcoma	: _____

TECH TIP 2.3 Rules for Using Sarcoma

When a combining form is attached to the term sarcoma, then it is inserted into the definition for sarcoma. As an example, the term osteosarcoma has the combining form "oste/o" attached to the term sarcoma. Therefore, the definition is a malignant tumor of bone arising from connective tissue.

Remember your definition for sarcoma from Chapter 1 and use the following guide: A malignant tumor of _____ arising from connective tissue.

---

hypo-	+ Chondr/o + -iac	= Hypochondriac	: _____
Coccyg/o	+ -eal	= Coccygeal	: _____
Crani/o	+ -al	= Cranial	: _____
Crani/o	+ -tomy	= Craniotomy	: _____
Crani/o	+ Sacr/o + -al	= Craniosacral	: _____

TECH TIP 2.4 Did You Know?

We have all heard of or used the term hypochondriac when describing a person who thinks they are sick frequently. The origin of the term's usage stems from ancient Greece. In ancient times, the most common complaints of sickness were related to the viscera in the hypochondriac region: the stomach, liver, and spleen. In most cases, these people were truly sick. They usually had eaten something they shouldn't have and were treated with medications to induce vomiting. However, with the limited knowledge of medicine in those times, many complaints went untreated and were believed to be lies created by the patients. Because these common complaints of the hypochondriac region were believed to be imaginary, these people became known as hypochondriacs-people suffering from hypochondriasis.

Crani/o	+ -plasty			= Cranioplasty	: _____
Cyt/o	+ -logy			= Cytology	: _____
Cyt/o	+ -logy	+ -ist		= Cytologist	: _____
Cyt/o	+ -logy	+ -ical		= Cytological	: _____
Hist/o	+ -logy			= Histology	: _____
Hist/o	+ -logy	+ -ist		= Histologist	: _____
Hist/o	+ -logy	+ -ical		= Histological	: _____
Hist/o	+ Path/o	+ -logy		= Histopathology	: _____
Hist/o	+ Path/o	+ -logy	+ -ist	= Histopathologist	: _____
Inguin/o	+ -al			= Inguinal	: _____
Anis/o	+ Kary/o	+ -osis		= Anisokaryosis	: _____
Laryng/o	+ -eal			= Laryngeal	: _____
Laryng/o	+ -itis			= Laryngitis	: _____
Lumb/o	+ -ar			= Lumbar	: _____
Lumb/o	+ Sacr/o	+ -al		= Lumbosacral	: _____
neo-	+ -plasia			= Neoplasia	: _____
neo-	+ -plasm			= Neoplasm	: _____
Nucle/o	+ -ar			= Nuclear	: _____
Nucle/o	+ -ic			= Nucleic	: _____
Path/o	+ -logy			= Pathology	: _____
Path/o	+ -logy	+ -ist		= Pathologist	: _____
Pelv/o	+ -ic			= Pelvic	: _____
Peritone/o	+ -al			= Peritoneal	: _____
Peritone/o	+ -itis			= Peritonitis	: _____
Pharyng/o	+ -eal			= Pharyngeal	: _____
Pharyng/o	+ -itis			= Pharyngitis	: _____
Rhin/o	+ -itis			= Rhinitis	: _____
Sacr/o	+ -al			= Sacral	: _____
Sacr/o	+ -algia			= Sacralgia	: _____
Sacr/o	+ Caud/o	+ -al		= Sacrocaudal	: _____
Sacr/o	+ Coccyg/o	+ -eal		= Sacrococcygeal	: _____
Sacr/o	+ Pelv/o	+ -ic		= Sacropelvic	: _____
Spin/o	+ -al			= Spinal	: _____
Trache/o	+ -al			= Tracheal	: _____
Trache/o	+ -tomy			= Tracheotomy	: _____
endo-	+ Trache/o	+ -al		= Endotracheal	: _____
Thorac/o	+ -centesis			= Thoracocentesis	: _____

Also known as thoracentesis.

Thorac/o	+ -ic			= Thoracic	: _____
Thorac/o	+ -tomy			= Thoracotomy	: _____
Vertebr/o	+ -al			= Vertebral	: _____
inter	+ Vertebr/o	+ -al		= Intervertebral	: _____
Viscer/o	+ -al			= Visceral	: _____
Viscer/o	+ -algia			= Visceralgia	: _____
uni-	+ Later/o	+ -al		= Unilateral	: _____

Abbreviations

Table 2.9   Chapter 2 Abbreviations.

Abbreviation	Definition
c̄	With
s̄	Without
CBA	Cat bite abscess (Figure 2.13A)
DHLPP-C	Distemper, hepatitis, leptospirosis, parvovirus, parainfluenza, coronavirus–Canine vaccine set
ET tube	Endotracheal tube (Figure 2.14)
FeLV	Feline leukemia virus
FIP	Feline infectious peritonitis
FIV	Feline immunodeficiency virus
FVRCP	Feline viral rhinotracheitis, calicivirus, panleukopenia–Feline vaccine set
HBC	Hit by car (Figure 2.13B)
IVD	Intervertebral disk (disc)
MM	Mucous membranes
neg or ⊖	Negative
pos or ⊕	Positive
pt.	Patient
PT	Physical therapy
RV	Rabies vaccine
stat	Immediately
V/D	Vomiting/diarrhea

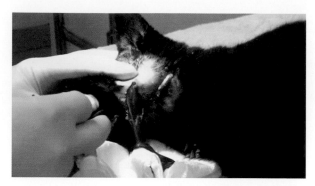

Figure 2.13A   Draining a cat bite abscess on a cat's cheek. Courtesy of Greg Martinez, DVM; www.youtube.com/drgregdvm.

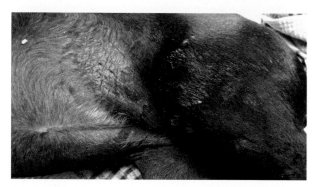

Figure 2.13B   Dog that has been hit by a car. Note the road rash and grease on the hair. Courtesy of Greg Martinez, DVM; www.youtube.com/drgregdvm.

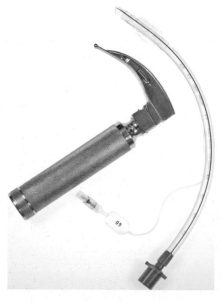

Figure 2.14A   Endotracheal tube and laryngoscope. Courtesy of shutterstock/Chris Pole.

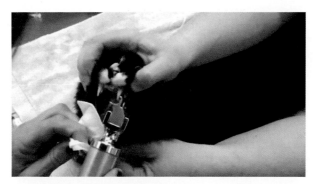

Figure 2.14B Endotracheal tube placement in a cat using a laryngoscope. Courtesy of Greg Martinez, DVM; www.youtube.com/drgregdvm.

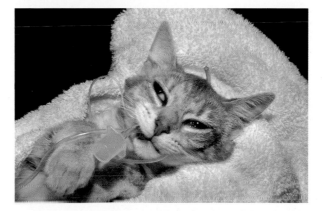

Figure 2.14C Cat waking up after surgery with an endotracheal tube still in place. Courtesy of shutterstock/Julie Keen.

Case Study: Define the medical terms and abbreviations in bold print. You'll notice some terms from the previous chapter

You hear a page over the intercom stating that you are needed in the emergency room, **stat**. The **pt.** is Bungee, a 4-year-old male **DLH** with an **abdominal evisceration**. Apparently Bungee had been fighting with the neighbor's cat and fell from the top of the fence onto the gardening tools below. A quick check of his file shows that he is current on his **FVRCP, FeLV, and RV**. Upon **P/E**, a mass is found on the **lateral** aspect of his right stifle. The mass was warm to the touch. The veterinarian confirms that Bungee also has a **CBA**. His **MM** are pale and he's breathing rapidly. Pre-surgical bloodworm is run, which shows **anemia**.

Bungee is taken into surgery to repair the evisceration. An **endotracheal** tube is placed and Bungee is positioned in **dorsal recumbency** for the procedure. After replacing the abdominal **viscera**, the veterinarian performs an abdominal **lavage** to try to prevent **peritonitis**. Bungee was moved to the recovery room after surgery.

After waking up from the surgery, Bungee begins coughing. The owner should be told that Bungee will have short-term laryngitis because of the ET tube.

Exercises

2-A: Match the combining forms with their meaning.

1.	_____ Throat	A.	Abdomin/o
2.	_____ Disease	B.	Adip/o
3.	_____ Nose	C.	Chondr/o
4.	_____ Abdomen	D.	Crani/o
5.	_____ Groin	E.	Cyt/o
6.	_____ Voice box	F.	Hist/o
7.	_____ Cartilage	G.	Inguin/o
8.	_____ Fat	H.	Laryng/o
9.	_____ Skull	I.	Path/o
10.	_____ Tissue	J.	Pelv/o
11.	_____ Cell	K.	Pharyng/o
12.	_____ Hip	L.	Rhin/o

2-B: Write the correct medical term in the blank.

1. _____: Study of disease
2. _____: New formation
3. _____: Incision into the skull
4. _____: Pertaining to the internal organs
5. _____: Tumor of cartilage
6. _____: Pertaining to the groin
7. _____: Specialist in the study of cells
8. _____: Pertaining to the throat
9. _____: Inflammation of the voice box
10. _____: Pertaining to between the back bones
11. _____: Incision into the windpipe
12. _____: Incision into the chest
13. _____: Surgical repair of the skull
14. _____: Pertaining to the hip
15. _____: Pertaining to the sacrum and tail
16. _____: Pertaining to the lower back
17. _____: Pain in cartilage
18. _____: Irrigation of organ or cavity
19. _____: Not malignant; non-invasive
20. _____: Study of the body's function

2-C: Circle the correct spelling for each word.

1.	Diaphragm	Diaphram	Diafram
2.	Larynx	Layrnx	Larnyx
3.	Diarrea	Diahrrea	Diarrhea
4.	Abcess	Absess	Abscess

5. Cartalige   Cartilage   Cartlaje
6. Maligent   Malignent   Malignant
7. Thorasic   Thoracic   Thoraxic
8. Vertibrea   Vertibra   Vertebrae
9. Cerival   Cervical   Cervicle
10. Vommitting   Vomiting   Vomitting

2-D: Define the following suffixes.

1. _____: -plasty   7. _____: -plasia
2. _____: -ose   8. _____: -ism
3. _____: -logy   9. _____: -osis
4. _____: -algia   10. _____: -ar
5. _____: -centesis   11. _____: -oma
6. _____: -ist   12. _____: -itis

2-E: Match the following directional terms to complete the sentences. Some terms are used more than once.

A. Cranial   F. Lateral
B. Caudal   G. Medial
C. Deep   H. Proximal
D. Distal   I. Superficial
E. Dorsal   J. Ventral

1. The xiphoid process is _____ to the thoracic vertebrae.
2. The tarsus is _____ to the carpus.
3. A cat scratch is _____; a stab wound is _____.
4. The humerus is _____ to the metacarpals.
5. The atlas is _____ to the ilium.
6. The ribs are _____ to the heart.
7. The dewclaw is _____ to the other digits.
8. A dog lying on its side is in _____ recumbency.
9. The intestines are _____ to the heart.
10. The phalanges are _____ to the stifle.
11. The tibia is _____ to the fibula.
12. The thoracic vertebrae are _____ to the sacral vertebrae.
13. The lumbar vertebrae are _____ to the umbilicus.
14. The accessory carpal bone is on the _____ aspect of the carpus.
15. The humerus is _____ to the muscles.

2-F: Define the following abbreviations.

1. _____: CBA   3. _____: V/D
2. _____: FIP   4. _____: stat

5. _____: P.T.
6. _____: ⊖
7. _____: FIV
8. _____: DHLPP-C
9. _____: s̄
10. _____: pos
11. _____: c̄
12. _____: MM

2-G: Define the following prefixes.

1. _____: hypo-
2. _____: inter-
3. _____: meta-
4. _____: cata-

5. _____: ana-
6. _____: endo-
7. _____: neo-
8. _____: a-, an-

2-H: Define the following medical terms.

1. _____: Nucleus
2. _____: Prolapse
3. _____: Evisceration
4. _____: Anabolism
5. _____: Histopathology
6. _____: Chondrosarcoma
7. _____: Abdominal cavity
8. _____: Exocrine glands

9. _____: Endocrine glands
10. _____: Urethra
11. _____: Diaphragm
12. _____: Pharynx
13. _____: Cell membrane
14. _____: Catabolism
15. _____: IVD

Answers can be found starting on page 571.

Go to www.wiley.com/go/taibo/terminology to find additional learning materials for this chapter:

- A crossword puzzle
- Flashcards
- Audio clips to show how to pronounce terms
- Case studies
- Review questions
- The figures from the chapter in PowerPoint

The Musculoskeletal System

The musculoskeletal system consists of bones, joints, cartilage, ligaments, tendons, and muscles. These different organs work together to achieve a variety of functions which include movement, protection, support, and storage.

Bones

Bone is a hard form of connective tissue that makes up most of the skeleton. It is primarily composed of collagen and minerals such as calcium and phosphorus. In the earliest stages of development, the skeleton is made up of cartilaginous tissue which is softer and more flexible. After birth, that fibrous tissue is converted into osseous tissue.

> **TECH TIP 3.1** Puppies commonly have their dewclaws removed soon after birth because they are still made of primarily cartilaginous tissue. If the owners wait too long, then the dewclaw becomes osseous tissue and the surgical procedure is far more involved. Dewclaws should be removed to avoid injuries later in the dog's life. Dogs often get their dewclaws caught on fabric and end up tearing the digit.

Table 3.1   Formation of Bone.

Osseous tissue	Another name for bone tissue.
Ossification	Process of bone formation.
Osteoblast	Bone cell that forms bone tissue. Also known as an immature bone cell.
Osteoclast	Bone cell that absorbs and removes bone tissue. Also known as a phagocyte of bone.
Osteocyte	Bone cell (Figure 3.1).

Veterinary Medical Terminology Guide and Workbook, First Edition. Angela Taibo.
© 2014 John Wiley & Sons, Inc. Published 2014 by John Wiley & Sons, Inc.
Companion website: www.wiley.com/go/taibo/terminology

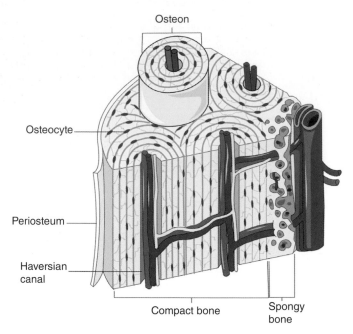

Figure 3.1   Cross section of bone. Courtesy of shutterstock/mmutlu.

Steps of Ossification

Bone formation is a constant process in that new bone tissue is continuously being formed while older bone tissue is continuously being removed. The older tissue must be removed to prevent the bone from becoming too thick or too heavy. Within the osseous tissue are cells called osteoblasts and osteoclasts. The osteoblasts are the immature bone cells that help to build bone tissue by supplying the minerals needed for bone formation. Once the osteoblasts mature, they become osteocytes, which act as part of the structural matrix of bone. Osteoclasts are responsible for removing bone tissue that is no longer needed by resorbing and digesting it. If the bone is injured, then the osteoblasts patch the break while the osteoclasts smooth it out and remove the leftover materials. Even if the body is not injured, the osteoblasts are continuously making new bone tissue and the osteoclasts are removing the older bone tissue. This constant process is what enables the bone to handle everyday stresses as well as repair itself once injured.

Anatomy of a Bone

Bones are grouped into different categories based on their shapes and functions. Regardless of the category they fall in, their basic anatomy is the same. Label the bone in Figure 3.2 using the terms in Table 3.2.

Table 3.2 Bone Anatomy.

Articular cartilage (1)	Thin layer of cartilage covering the surface of bones at a joint.
Calcium	The most abundant mineral in the body. When combined with phosphorus it forms calcium phosphate, which is the principal calcium salt and hard material found in bones and teeth.
Cancellous bone (2)	Spongy or porous bone found at the ends of long bones and in the inner portions of long bones.
Collagen	Structural protein making up the white fibrous strands found in bone.
Compact bone (3)	Hard, dense, bone tissue that forms the outer layer of bone. Also known as **cortical bone**.
Diaphysis (4)	The shaft of a long bone.
Endosteum (5)	The inner lining of bone. This forms the lining of the medullary cavity.
Epiphyseal plate (6)	Cartilaginous region of long bones where lengthwise growth takes place. This is also known as the **physis** or **growth plate**.
Epiphysis (7)	Each end of a long bone. It is composed of cancellous bone and covered with articular cartilage.
Medullary cavity (8)	Central, hollowed-out portion in the shaft of a long bone that contains yellow bone marrow.
Metaphysis (9)	The flared portion of a long bone between the epiphyseal plate and diaphysis.
Periosteum (10)	Membrane surrounding bone. This fibrous tissue contains blood vessels and nerves.
Red bone marrow (11)	Found in cancellous bone and the site of hematopoiesis.
Yellow bone marrow	Found in the diaphysis of bone and consists of fatty tissue.

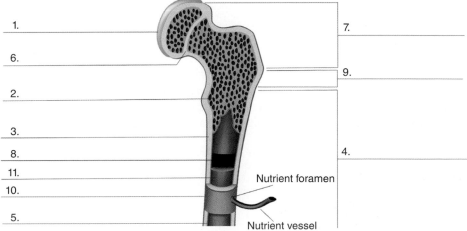

1.
6.
2.
3.
8.
11.
10.
5.
7.
9.
4.
Nutrient foramen
Nutrient vessel

Figure 3.2 Anatomy of a long bone. Courtesy of shutterstock/Alila Sao Mai.

Classifications of Bone

Bones are divided into different classifications based on their shape and function.

Long bones:	These bones are longer than they are wide. They are found in the front and rear limbs. Examples of long bones include the femur, tibia, radius, and metacarpals.
Short bones:	These bones are cuboidal (cube shaped). Examples of shorts bones include the carpals and tarsals.
Flat bones:	These bones are actually two sheets of compact bone that allow for protection. Flat bones are flat and thin. Examples include the scapula, ribs, and bones of the pelvis and skull.
Sesamoid bones:	Sesamoid bones are small bones that are embedded in tendons. They get their name because of their sesame seed shape. The patella is an example of a sesamoid bone. Horses have other sesamoid bones that will be discussed in later chapters.
Irregular bones:	These bones don't fit into the previous categories because they share traits of several categories. The best example of this classification is the vertebrae.

Related Terms and Processes

The bones of the skeleton have various protrusions and depressions that allow for structural support (Figure 3.3). They are as follows:

Table 3.3   Bone Processes.

Acetabulum	Cup-like depression in the pelvis that creates the hip joint.
Bone head	Rounded articular process separated from the shaft of the bone by a neck. The bone head is usually covered in articular cartilage. Examples include the femoral head and humeral head.
Condyle	Knuckle-like projections at the distal end of some long bones. They are usually covered by articular cartilage and articulate with other bones. Examples include the femoral and humeral condyles.
Crest	High projection or border projection of a bone. An example is the crest of the ilium (also known as the wing of the ilium).
Foramen	A hole in bone that allows for the passage of nerves and vessels. Examples include the obturator foramen and the foramen magnum.

Table 3.3   (*Continued*).

Fossa	Shallow cavity or depression in bone. An example is the trochanteric fossa which lies between the greater and lesser trochanter.
Groove	A narrow, linear depression. Also known as a **sulcus**. An example is the bicipital groove on the humerus.
Olecranon	Bony process at the proximal end of the ulna.
Sinus	A hollow space or cavity in bone. An example is the nasal sinuses.
Trochanter	Large, blunt, roughened process on the femur for attachment of muscles and tendons.
Tubercle	Rounded process on many bones for the attachment of muscles and tendons. The best example is the humeral tubercle.
Tuberosity	Small roughened process on many bones for the attachment of muscles and tendons. Examples include the tibial tuberosity and ischiatic tuberosity.

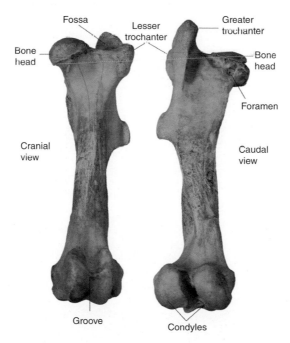

Figure 3.3   Processes on the femur of a cow.

Divisions of the Skeleton

If we look at the skeleton as a whole, we can divide it into three portions: the axial skeleton, which consists of bones along the axis (center) of the body, the appendicular skeleton, which consists of the bones of the appendages (extremities), and the visceral (splanchnic) skeleton, which consists of bones that are embedded in tissue. We will focus on small animal skeletal structure in this chapter. Large animals and exotics will be covered in later chapters.

The Axial Skeleton

Bones of the axial skeleton include the skull, vertebrae (backbones), ribs, and sternum. Notice that only bones along the axis (midline) of the body are a part of the axial skeleton. A common misconception is that the pelvis and scapula are a part of the axial skeleton. However, they don't originate from the midline and instead play a role in the function of the limbs. Therefore, they're a part of the appendicular skeleton.

The Skull

The skull is composed of several bones that surround and protect the brain (Figure 3.4).

Ethmoid bone	Bone that forms the roof of the nasal cavity and the floor of the rostral cranial cavity (orbits of the eyes).
Frontal bone	Paired bones making up the upper part of the face; the cranial aspect of the skull.
Occipital bone	The caudal aspect of the skull.
Parietal bone	Paired bones forming the sides and roof of the cranium.
Sphenoid bone	Wedge-shaped bone at the base of the skull.
Temporal bone	Paired bones forming the lower sides of the skull.

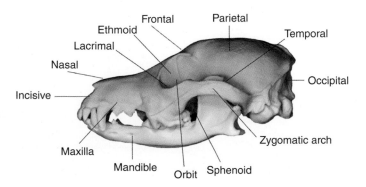

Figure 3.4   Bones of the dog's skull.

Facial bones	Facial bones make up the front of the skull. Within these facial bones are spaces of air called sinuses.
Hyoid bone	Horseshoe-shaped bone at the base of the tongue and below the thyroid cartilage.
Incisive bone	Bone bearing the incisors. Also known as the premaxilla.
Lacrimal bone	Bone forming the medial aspect of the orbit (eye socket).
Mandibular bones	Horseshoe-shaped bone forming the lower jaw.
Maxillary bones	Two identical bones that form the upper jaw.
Nasal bones	Two bones forming the bridge of the nose.
Palantine bone	Bone that forms the hard palate.
Vomer	Bone forming the base of the nasal septum. A septum is a partition.
Zygomatic bones	Bones forming the hard part of the cheek and the lower portion of the orbit (eye socket).

The Back Bones

The vertebral column, or spinal column, is composed of a series of back bones called vertebrae. They are arranged based on size and function. The vertebrae differ based on function, but the general anatomy is the same (Figure 3.5). The diagram below depicts the parts of a vertebra. Note the spinal cord, which passes through the opening in the middle, called a foramen.

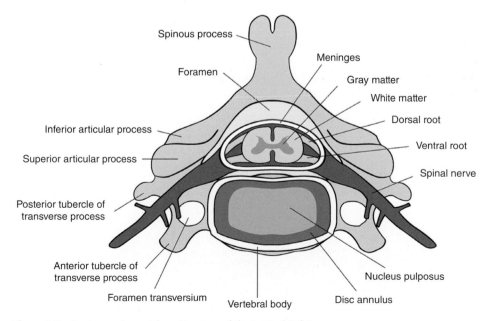

Figure 3.5   Anatomy of a vertebra. Courtesy of shutterstock/udaix.

Bones of the Thorax

The chest cavity is made up of the ribs and sternum. The number of ribs varies based on species. Each pair of ribs attaches to the thoracic vertebrae; therefore, the number of thoracic vertebrae corresponds with the number of pairs of ribs. For example, there are thirteen thoracic vertebrae in the dog; thus, there are thirteen pairs of ribs in the dog or twenty-six total.

The sternum, or breastbone, is along the midline of the chest and makes up the ventral portion of the rib cage. The sternum is made up of three portions called

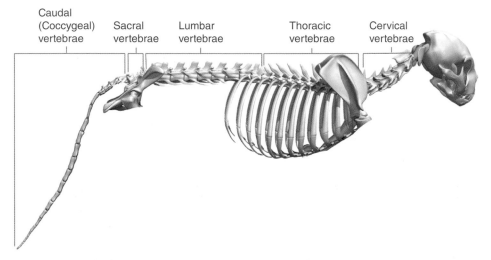

Caudal (Coccygeal) vertebrae   Sacral vertebrae   Lumbar vertebrae   Thoracic vertebrae   Cervical vertebrae

Figure 3.6   Vertebral column of the cat. Courtesy of shutterstock/Linda Bucklin.

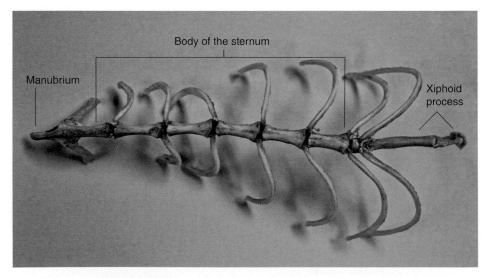

Body of the sternum

Manubrium

Xiphoid process

Figure 3.7   Parts of the sternum.

sternebrae (Figure 3.7). The upper portion of the sternum is called the manubrium, the mid-portion is called the body, and the lower portion is called the xiphoid process.

The xiphoid process is an important structure for veterinary technicians. We use the xiphoid process as a landmark when taking abdominal radiographs, and we use it to determine where to stop shaving when we are shaving an animal for abdominal surgery. Veterinarians use the xiphoid as a guide for where to incise the patient for surgery.

The Appendicular Skeleton

Bones of the appendicular skeleton include the bones of the front and rear limbs and bones of the limb girdles (pelvis and scapula).Label the thoracic limb in Figure 3.8 using Table 3.4.

Label the pelvic limb in Figure 3.9 using Table 3.5.

Table 3.4   The Thoracic Limb.

Bones	Location
Scapula (1)	A flat, triangular bone at the top of the shoulder commonly known as the shoulder blade.
Clavicle	Also known as the collarbone; some animals have a reduced (imperfect) clavicle, while other species completely lack one. Only species capable of grasping with their front limbs possess one. Examples include cats and primates.
Humerus (2)	Bone of the upper front limb between the shoulder and the elbow.
Radius (5)	One of two bones in the lower front limb between the elbow and the wrist (carpus).
Ulna (4)	One of the two bones in the lower front limb between the elbow and wrist (carpus).
Olecranon (3)	Bony process on the proximal aspect of the ulna.
Carpals(6)	Six to eight bones (depending on species) grouped together in two rows to make up the carpus.
Metacarpals (7)	A group of long bones between the carpals and phalanges.
Phalanges (8)	Commonly known as the digits. Each phalanx has three phalanges.

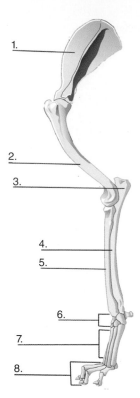

Figure 3.8 Thoracic limb of the dog. Courtesy of shutterstock/Maluson.

Table 3.5 The Pelvic Limb.

Bones	Location
Pelvis	The pelvis is made up of three pairs of bones: The **ilium** (1), **ischium** (2), and **pubis** (3).
Femur (4)	Commonly called the thigh bone. The femur is between the hip and stifle.
Patella (5)	Large sesamoid bone found in the stifle. Commonly called the kneecap.
Fabella	Sesamoid bone found in the back of the femoral condyles. Most species have two.
Tibia (7)	The larger medial bone of the lower hindlimb.
Fibula (6)	The smaller lateral bone of the lower hindlimb.
Tarsals (9)	Seven bones that make up the tarsus (hock).
Calcaneus (8)	One of the seven tarsal bones that sits in the back of the tarsus. Commonly called the heel bone.
Metatarsals (10)	Group of bones between the tarsus and the phalanges.

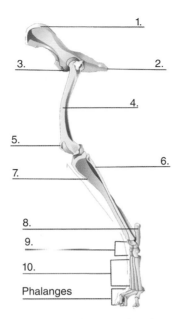

1.

3.   2.

4.

5.

6.

7.

8.

9.

10.

Phalanges

Figure 3.9   Pelvic limb of the dog. Courtesy of shutterstock/Maluson.

The Visceral Skeleton

The visceral skeleton contains bones that are embedded in tissues. This part of the skeleton helps to form an organ. Examples of bones of the visceral skeleton include the following:

Os penis   Bone found in the penis of some carnivores (Figure 3.10).
Os rostri   Bone found in the nose of pigs.
Os cordis   Bone found in the heart of ruminants.

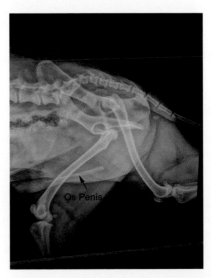

Os Penis

Figure 3.10   Radiograph showing the os penis of the dog. Courtesy of Beth Romano, CVT.

Additional Bone Pathology Terms

The following terms don't break down correctly using our rules of medical terminology.

Achondroplasia	Hereditary condition in which the bones and cartilage of limbs fail to grow to normal size. Commonly known as dwarfism, achondroplastic breeds include the dachshund and basset hound (Figure 3.11).

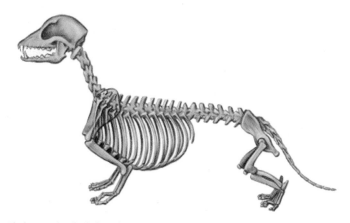

Figure 3.11   Skeleton of a dachshund. Courtesy of Getty Images/Dorling Kindersley.

TECH TIP 3.2 Achondroplasia is considered normal conformation for breeds such as basset hounds and dachshunds. In other breeds it's considered a type of chondrodystrophy or chondrodysplasia. Examples includes Alaskan Malamutes and Norwegian Elkhounds.

Amputation	Removal of a limb or other appendage.
Calcification	Deposit of calcium salts in tissue.
Callus	Bone deposit formed at the ends of a bone fracture; it is absorbed as the fracture is repaired and then replaced by true bone.
Chemonucleolysis	Procedure to dissolve a portion of the center of an intervertebral disc (IVD) to treat a herniated IVD.
Crepitation	Crackling sounds produced by the grating of broken bones. Also known as **crepitus**.
Decalcification	Loss of calcium salts in bone and teeth.
Dislocation	Displacement of a bone from its joint.
Fracture	Sudden breaking of bone (Figure 3.13).
Herniation of IVD	Abnormal protrusion of an IVD into the neural cavity or spinal nerves (Figure 3.14).

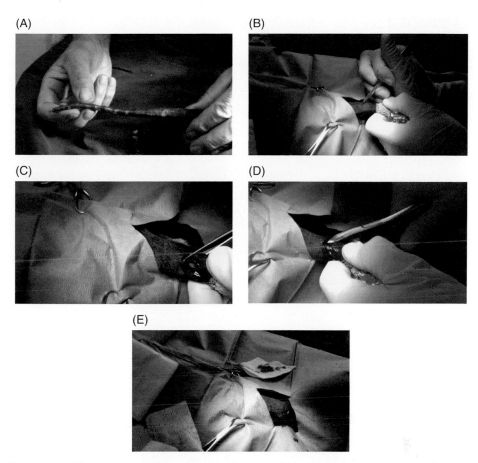

Figure 3.12   Tail amputation surgery progression. Courtesy of Greg Martinez, DVM; www.youtube.com/drgregdvm. (A) Note the skeletal appearance of the tail due to lack of blood supply. (B) An initial incision is made at the proximal aspect of the tail. (C) Scissors are used to cut soft tissue around the vertebrae. (D) Bone cutters are used to cut between the vertebrae. (E) Sutures are placed once the tail has been removed.

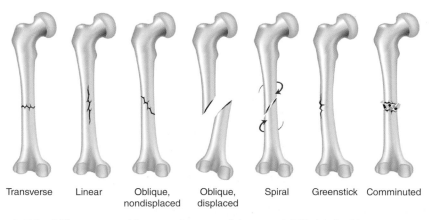

| Transverse | Linear | Oblique, nondisplaced | Oblique, displaced | Spiral | Greenstick | Comminuted |

Figure 3.13A   Different types of fractures. Courtesy of shutterstock/Alila Medical Images.

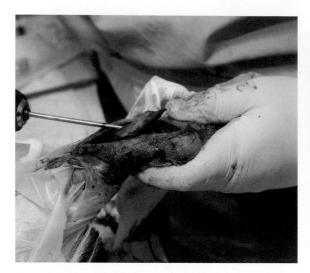

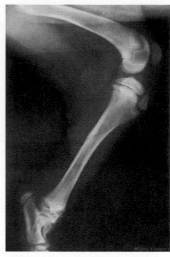

Figure 3.13B Open fracture being surgically repaired. Courtesy of shutterstock/sima.

Figure 3.13C Radiograph of a tibial fracture. Courtesy of shutterstock/olgaru79.

Spinal disc herniation

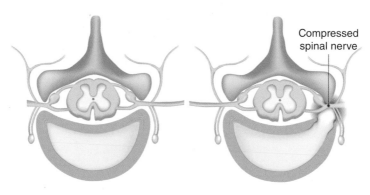

Compressed spinal nerve

Normal disc   Herniated disc

Figure 3.14 Herniation of an IVD. In many cases, the disc stays within the spinal canal and instead compresses the spinal cord. Courtesy of shutterstock/Alila Sao Mai.

Immobilization   Act of preventing a bone from being moved. Examples include sutures, bandages, and casts.

TECH TIP 3.3 The term suture has two different meanings depending on the context in which it is used. Sutures are commonly called stitches. We use sutures to close deep wounds. A suture is also a line of union that joins two bones, such as the sutures on the skull that join the skull bones together.

Kyphosis	Abnormal, increased, dorsal curvature of the spine; also known as **hunchback.**
Laminectomy	Removal of part of the vertebral arch to relieve pressure from a ruptured IVD.
Lordosis	Downward or ventral curvature of the lumbar spine; also known as **swayback.**

TECH TIP 3.4 Lordosis, or swayback, is often seen in cats in heat or in lambs born with a copper deficiency.

Orthopedic	Branch of surgery dealing with the skeletal system.
Osteoporosis	Decreased bone density due to loss of bone tissue. Bones become porous and fragile such that they can break easily. In animals, it is most often caused by malnutrition (Figure 3.15).

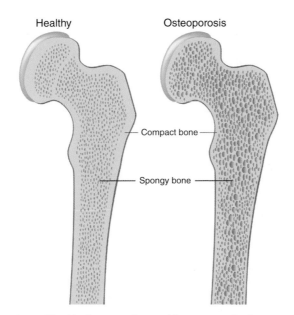

Figure 3.15   Comparison of healthy bone to a bone with osteoporosis. Courtesy of shutterstock/ Alila Sao Mai.

Reduction	Correction of a fracture. There are open reductions (after incision) and closed reductions (without incision).
Sequestrum	Piece of dead bone tissue that has separated from healthy bone tissue during necrosis (cell death).

Joints

A joint is defined as two or more bones that come together. The naming of joints is simple if you know your bone anatomy. The medical name of a joint consists of the bones that make up that joint. They are usually, not always, listed in anatomical order and are usually connected by the combining vowel of the letter "o." Below is a list of major joints with their common names.

Joints can be divided into three basic categories based on their function. Categories of joints include synarthroses (immovable joints), amphiarthroses (partially movable joints), and diarthroses (freely movable joints).

Table 3.6   Joints.

Atlanto-axial joint	Joint between the atlas and axis. Commonly known as the **"no joint."**
Atlanto-occipital joint	Joint between the atlas and occipital bone. Commonly known as the **"yes joint."** It is the only joint in which the bones are not listed in anatomical order.
Carpus	Joint consisting of the carpal bones. Commonly known as the **wrist** in small animals and the knee in horses.
Coxofemoral joint	Joint between the pelvis (os coxae) and the femur. Commonly known as the **hip**.
Femorotibial joint	Joint between the femur and the tibia. Commonly known as the **stifle**. Within the stifle is a cartilage pad, called the **meniscus**, to withstand compressive forces.
Humeroradioulnar joint	Joint where the humerus meets the radius and ulna. Commonly known as the **elbow**.
Sacroiliac joint	Joint between the sacrum and the ilium.
Scapulohumeral joint	Joint between the scapula and humerus. Commonly known as the **shoulder**.
Tarsus	Joint consisting of the tarsal bones. Commonly known as the **hock**. The **malleolus** is the rounded process on either side of the tarsus.

TECH TIP 3.5 You will commonly hear owners refer to the stifle as the knee is small animal medicine; however, it is not proper use of terminology. The only time we use the term knee in veterinary medicine is to describe the carpus in horses. Owners of dogs and cats generally don't know what a stifle is so you may need to communicate in lay terms that it is equivalent to the knee.

Table 3.7   Synovial Joints.

Ball and socket	Joint in which the rounded head of one bone fits into the socket of another. Examples include the hip and shoulder joints. Also known as **enarthroses** or **spheroid joints**.
Gliding	These joint surfaces are flat, allowing for a gliding motion. Examples include the carpus. Also known as **arthrodial joints**.
Hinge	This joint allows for movement in one plane (one direction), similar to a door hinge. Examples include the elbow and stifle. Also known as **ginglymus joints**.
Pivot	These are pulley-shaped or pivot-like joints. An example is the atlanto-axial joint. Also known as a **trochoid joint**.
Saddle	This joint can only be found in humans and non-human primates. The surfaces of both bones are concave in one plane and convex, or saddle shaped, in the other. It allows for all range of motion except an axial twist. The best example is the carpometacarpal joint of the thumb.

Examples of synarthroses (singular: synarthrosis) include the bones of the skull, which are joined together by a suture. A suture is a line of union of adjoining bones of the skull. They appear as jagged little lines (Figure 3.16A).

Examples of amphiarthroses (singular: amphiarthrosis) include the joints between the vertebrae and the symphysis between the pubic bones. A symphysis is a line of union in which two bones are united by fibrocartilage (Figure 3.16B). These types of joints allow for limited mobility.

Diarthroses, or freely movable joints, are also known as synovial joints. Examples of synovial joints include the hip, elbow, shoulder, and hock. These joints have varying degrees of mobility so they can be further divided based on their range of motions. Table 3.7 shows a list of different types of synovial joints.

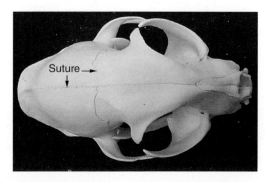

Figure 3.16A   Suture joints in the cat skull.

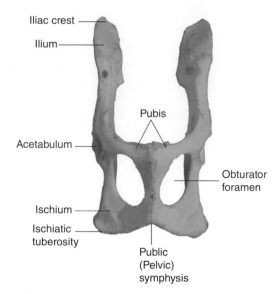

Figure 3.16B Anatomy of the pelvis showing a symphysis.

Anatomy of a Joint

The most common joint injuries involve synovial joints. Stifle injuries such as torn cranial cruciate ligaments (anterior cruciate ligaments) are very common in high-energy dogs. Below is the general anatomy of a synovial joint.

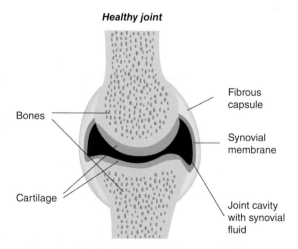

Figure 3.17 Anatomy of a synovial joint. Courtesy of shutterstock/Alila Sao Mai.

Articulation	Where two or more bones come together; also known as a joint.
Bursa	Sac of fluid near a joint that acts as a lubrication to ease friction between tissues. **Bursae** (plural form)

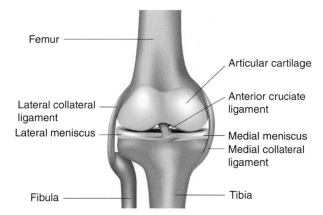

Figure 3.18A   Structures of the stifle. Courtesy of shutterstock/Alila Sao Mai.

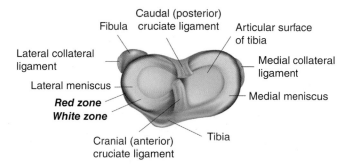

Figure 3.18B   Meniscus of the stifle. Courtesy of shutterstock/Alila Sao Mai.

can be found anywhere two types of tissue slide against one another. They can be found between bones and ligaments, skin and bones, and bones and tendons.

Ligament	Connective tissue that binds bone to bone.
Synovial cavity	Space between bones at a synovial joint which contains synovial fluid.
Synovial fluid	Viscous (sticky) fluid within the synovial cavity that acts as a lubricant between bones.
Synovial joint	A freely movable joint, Also known as diarthrosis.
Synovial membrane	Membrane lining the synovial cavity that produces synovial fluid.
Tendon	Connective tissue that binds muscle to bone.

Joint Pathology and Procedures

Anterior drawer sign	Cranial movement of the proximal tibia in relation to the distal femur to check for cranial cruciate ligament damage in the stifle.

Congenital articular rigidity (CAR)	Condition present at birth in which the joints of the limbs are fixed in position. Commonly seen in calves, limbs are fixed in strange flexed positions.
Extra capsular technique (extra cap)	Technique using nonabsorbable suture to replace the cranial cruciate ligament.
Gait	Manner of walking.
Gout	Inflammation of a joint due to the increased presence of uric acid crystals in the joint. Most commonly seen in chickens.
Lame; lameness	Incapable of normal locomotion.
Luxation	Displacement of a bone from its joint; also known as **dislocation**.
Pannus	Inflammatory fluid overlying synovial cells, commonly seen with rheumatoid arthritis.
Rheumatoid arthritis	Inflammation of joints due to an autoimmune disease. Most commonly seen in dogs.
Subluxation	Partial displacement of a bone from its joint.
Tibial plateau leveling osteotomy (TPLO)	Procedure which changes the slope of the tibial plateau to help stabilize the stifle after tearing the cranial cruciate ligament. This is a common procedure in large dog breeds.
Tibial tuberosity advancement (TTA)	Procedure to advance the tibial tuberosity to stabilize the stifle after tearing the cranial cruciate ligament.
Total hip replacement (THR)	Replacement of the femoral head and acetabulum to correct hip dysplasia.
Triple pelvic osteotomy (TPO)	Procedure in which the pelvis is cut in three different locations to change the angle in which the acetabulum meets the femoral head. This is a common procedure for correcting hip dysplasia in younger dogs.

TECH TIP 3.6 Autoimmune disease is a disease in which the immune system attacks one's own good cells. There are many examples of autoimmune disease that will be covered in later chapters.

Muscles

A muscle is an organ composed of bundles of fibers that contract to produce movement. In general, muscles are responsible for locomotion and structural support. Through movement, muscles can also assist in other functions including the functions of viscera (internal organs) and generating body heat.

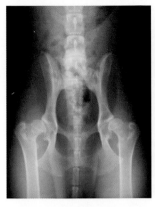 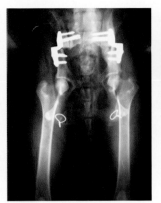 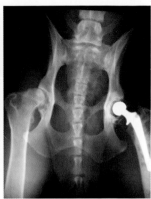

Figure 3.19A Hip dysplasia. Note that the head of the femur isn't seated firmly in the acetabulum of the pelvis.

Figure 3.19B Triple pelvic osteotomy correcting the hip dysplasia. Note that after the three incisions are made, the femoral head is now seated firmly in the acetabulum.

Figure 3.19C Total hip replacement. Note the artificial femoral head and acetabulum that have replaced the animal's femoral head and acetabulum.

Types of Muscles

Muscles can be divided into three groups based on their location and function. Table 3.8 lists the different types of muscles and their functions.

Some muscles work together to achieve a similar function. These muscles are termed synergistic. For example, the quadriceps muscle actually consists of four different muscles (heads) all working together to extend the stifle. Other muscles work against each other to achieve opposite functions. These muscles are termed antagonists. Examples of antagonists include the biceps brachii and triceps brachii. While the biceps work to flex the elbow, the triceps work to extend the elbow.

All muscles have the ability to contract and relax to produce movement. If a muscle contracts, then it's tightening, or shrinking, and drawing things together. When the muscle relaxes, it loosens its tension and returns to its original form.

Fascia is a fibrous connective tissue that envelopes, separates, and supports the muscles listed above. Within the fascia lie the muscle's blood supply, nerve supply, and lymph. Figure 3.21 shows the white fascia between the layers of skeletal muscle on the cat. Notice the spider web appearance.

Table 3.8 Muscle Types.

Cardiac muscle	Striated, involuntary muscle found in the heart.
Skeletal muscle	Striated, voluntary muscles attached to bones all over the body; responsible for movement.
Visceral muscles	Smooth, involuntary muscles responsible for the functioning of internal organs. Also known as **smooth muscle**.

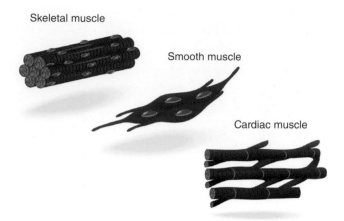

Figure 3.20   The three muscle types. Courtesy of Getty Images/Zhabaska Tetyana.

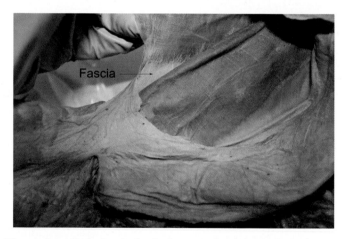

Figure 3.21   Dissected cat displaying the fasciae between the abdominal muscles.

Functions of Muscle

While some muscles are named based on their anatomical location, other muscles are named based on their point of attachment. There are two points of attachment for a muscle: a stationary bone and a movable bone. The stationary bone is considered the origin of the muscle. The origin is the point of attachment that is closest to the midline of the body. The stationary bone is held in place by other muscles. The bone that moves is considered the insertion of the muscle and is generally farthest from the midline of the body. If describing the skeletal muscles on the limbs, then the origin is generally the proximal point of attachment and the insertion is the distal point of attachment. When describing how the muscle moves we measure its range of motion using the degrees of a circle. Range of motion measures the range in which a joint can be flexed or extended. Below is a list of muscle functions and their definitions.

Abduction	Movement away from the midline of the body.
Adduction	Movement toward the midline of the body.
Dorsiflexion	Backward bending (flexion); an example is the neck.
Extension	Increasing the angle between two bones at a joint.
Flexion	Decreasing the angle between two bones at a joint.
Pronation	The act of turning the palmar or plantar surface downward.
Supination	The act of turning the palmar or plantar surface upward.
Rotation	Circular movement that turns a body part around a central point (axis).

Additional Myopathy Terms

Adhesion	Fibrous band that connects two surfaces that are normally separate. Often results from surgery in which scar tissue forms around incisions.
Ambulatory	Able to walk; also known as **ambulant** or **ambulation**.
Atrophy	No development due to a decrease from the normal cell size.
Hyperplasia	Increased development due to an increase in cell numbers.
Hypertrophy	Excessive development due to increase in cell size.
Hypoplasia	Incomplete development due to decrease in cell numbers.
Laxity	Looseness
Myasthenia	Muscle weakness.
Myasthesnia gravis	Syndrome of muscular weakness that is aggravated by activity and relieved by rest. May be inherited in dogs and cats.
Myoclonus	Repetitive contractions of skeletal muscles that persist during sleep. Sometimes seen in dogs with distemper virus.
Myotonia	Disorder in which there is a delayed relaxation of a muscle after contraction.
Tenosynovitis	Inflammation of the tendon and tendon sheath. May be seen with chronic arthritis or injuries such as paw lacerations on lawn edging.
Tetany	Continuous muscle spasms or twitching.
Tonus	Muscle tone; balanced muscle tension.

Building the Terms

Table 3.9   Chapter 3 Combining Forms.

Combining Forms	Definition	Combining Forms	Definition
Acetabul/o	Acetabulum	Kyph/o	Humpback; bent; hump
Ankyl/o	Stiff	Lacrim/o	Tear; tear duct
Arthr/o	Joint	Lamin/o	Lamina
Articul/o	Joint	Leiomy/o	Smooth (visceral) muscle
Burs/o	Bursa	Ligament/o	Ligament
Calc/o	Calcium	Lord/o	Curve; swayback; bent backward
Calcane/o	Calcaneus	Malleol/o	Malleolus
Carp/o	Carpus	Mandibul/o	Mandible;lower jaw
Chondr/o	Cartilage	Maxill/o	Maxilla; upper jaw
Clavicul/o	Clavicle	Metacarp/o	Metacarpals
Cost/o	Rib	Metatars/o	Metatarsals
Costal/o	Rib	My/o	Muscle
Crani/o	Skull	Myel/o	Bone marrow; spinal cord
Dactyl/o	Toes; digits	Myos/o	Muscle
Erg/o	Work	Necr/o	Death
Fasci/o, fasc/i	Fascia	Olecran/o	Olecranon
Femor/o	Femur	Orth/o	Bone
Fibros/o	Fibrous connective tissue	Oss/e, oss/i	Bone
Fibul/o	Fibula	Oste/o	Bone
Hem/o	Blood	Pariet/o	Side
Hemat/o	Blood	Patell/o	Patella
Humer/o	Humerus	Ped/o	Child; foot
Hydr/o	Fluid; water	Pelv/o	Pelvis; pelvic bone; hip
Ili/o	Ilium	Perone/o	Fibula
Ischi/o	Ischium	Phalang/o	Phalanges; digits
Kinesi/o	Movement	Pub/o	Pubis

Table 3.9 (*Continued*).

Combining Forms	Definition	Combining Forms	Definition
Radi/o	Radius; X-ray	**Synov/o**	Synovial membrane; tendon sheath
Rhabdomy/o	Striated (skeletal) muscle	**Tars/o**	Tarsus
Rheumat/o	Watery flow	**Ten/o**	Tendon
Sacr/o	Sacrum	**Tendin/o**	Tendon
Sarc/o	Connective tissue (flesh)	**Tibi/o**	Tibia
Scapul/o	Scapula	**Ton/o**	Tension
Sphen/o	Wedge	**Uln/o**	Ulna
Spondyl/o	Vertebra	**Vertebr/o**	Vertebra
Stern/o	Sternum		

Table 3.10 Chapter 3 Prefixes.

Prefix	Definition	Prefix	Definition
a-, an-	no; not; without	**hyper-**	above; excessive
ab-	away from	**hypo-**	deficient; below; under; less than normal
ad-	toward	**inter-**	between
amph-	around; on both sides; doubly	**meta-**	change; beyond
anti-	against	**pan-**	all
de-	lack of; down; less; removal of	**peri-**	surrounding; around
dia-	through; complete	**poly-**	many; much
dys-	bad; painful; difficult; abnormal	**sub-**	under; below
electro-	electricity	**supra-**	above; upper
endo-	in; within	**sym-**	together; with
epi-	above; upon; on	**syn-**	together; with

Table 3.11   Chapter 3 Suffixes.

Suffix	Definition	Suffix	Definition
-ac, -al, -ar, -ary, -eal, -ic, -ous	pertaining to	-metry	measurement
-algia	pain	-oma	tumor; mass; fluid collection
-blast	immature; embryonic	-osis	abnormal condition
-centesis	surgical puncture to remove fluid	-pathy	disease condition
-clast	to break	-pexy	surgical fixation; to put in place
-cyte	cell	-physis	to grow
-desis	surgical fixation; to bind; tie together	-plasia	development; formation; growth
-dynia	pain	-plasty	surgical repair
-ectomy	removal; excision; resection	-poiesis	formation
-emia	blood condition	-porosis	condition of pores (spaces)
-fication	process of making	-rrhaphy	suture
-genesis	producing; forming	-sclerosis	hardening
-graphy	process of recording	-scopy	visual examination
-ion	process	-therapy	Treatment
-itis	inflammation	-tome	instrument to cut
-kinesis	movement	-tomy	process of cutting; incision
-logy	study of	-trophy	development; nourishment
-malacia	softening	-y	condition

Now it's time to put these word parts together. This will get easier each time if you memorize the meaning of the combining forms, prefixes, and suffixes. Remember your five basic rules to medical terminology when building and defining these terms. You'll notice some word parts are repeated from the previous chapter.

Parts			Medical Term	Definition
Acetabul/o	+	-ar	= Acetabular	: _____
Ankyl/o	+	-osis	= Ankylosis	: _____
Arthr/o	+	-centesis	= Arthrocentesis	: _____
Arthr/o	+	-desis	= Arthrodesis	: _____
Arthr/o	+	-graphy	= Arthrography	: _____

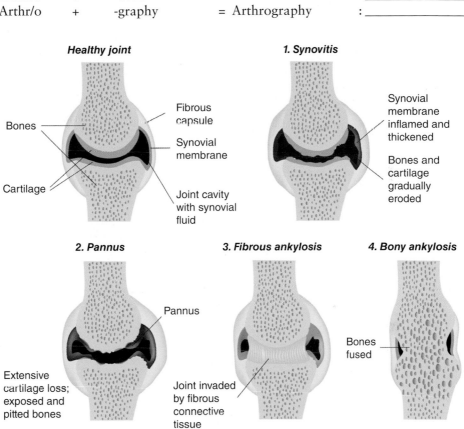

Figure 3.22 Stages of rheumatoid arthritis. Courtesy of shutterstock/Alila Sao Mai.

Arthr/o	+ -plasty		= Arthroplasty	: _____
Arthr/o	+ -scope		= Arthroscope	: _____
Arthr/o	+ -scopy		= Arthroscopy	: _____
Arthr/o	+ -tomy		= Arthrotomy	: _____
Hem/o	+ Arthr/o	+ -osis	= Hemarthrosis	: _____
Hydr/o	+ Arthr/o	+ -osis	= Hydrarthrosis	: _____
poly-	+ Arthr/o	+ -itis	= Polyarthritis	: _____
Calcane/o	+ -al		= Calcaneal	: _____
hyper-	+ Calc/o	+ -emia	= Hypercalcemia	: _____
hypo-	+ Calc/o	+ -emia	= Hypocalcemia	: _____

Carp/o	+ -al		= Carpal	: _____
Chondr/o	+ Cost/o	+ -al	= Chondrocostal	: _____
Chondr/o	+ -oma		= Chondroma	: _____
Chondr/o	+ -malacia		= Chondromalacia	: _____
Chondr/o	+ Sarc/o	+ -oma	= Chondrosarcoma	: _____
supra-	+ Clavicul/o	+ -ar	= Supraclavicular	: _____
Cost/o	+ -al		= Costal	: _____
inter-	+ Cost/o	+ -al	= Intercostal	: _____

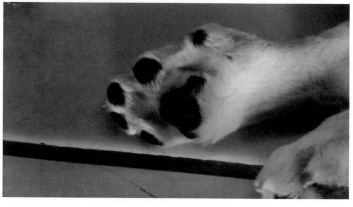

Figure 3.23   Polydactyly in a lab mix puppy. Note the extra dewclaw. Courtesy of Beth Romano, AAS, CVT.

sub-	+ Cost/o	+ -al	= Subcostal	: _____
Crani/o	+ -tome		= Craniotome	: _____
Crani/o	+ -tomy		= Craniotomy	: _____
poly-	+ Dactyl/o	+ -y	= Polydactyly	: _____
syn-	+ Dactyl/o	+ -y	= Syndactyly	: _____
dys-	+ -plasia		= Dysplasia	: _____
Fasci/o	+ -itis		= Fasciitis	: _____
Femor/o	+ -al		= Femoral	: _____
Fibr/o	+ -oma		= Fibroma	: _____
Fibul/o	+ -ar		= Fibular	: _____
Humer/o	+ -al		= Humeral	: _____
Hydr/o	+ -therapy		= Hydrotherapy	: _____
Ili/o	+ -ac		= Iliac	: _____
Ischi/o	+ -al		= Ischial	: _____
Kinesi/o	+ -logy		= Kinesiology	: _____
Leiomy/o	+ -oma		= Leiomyoma	: _____
Leiomy/o	+ Sarc/o	+ -oma	= Leiomyosarcoma	: _____
Ligament/o	+ -ous		= Ligamentous	: _____
Malleol/o	+ -ar		= Malleolar	: _____
Mandibul/o	+ -ar		= Mandibular	: _____
Maxill/o	+ -ary		= Maxillary	: _____
Metacarp/o	+ -ectomy		= Metacarpectomy	: _____
Metatars/o	+ -algia		= Metatarsalgia	: _____

Electr/o	+ My/o	+ -graphy	= Electromyography	: _____
My/o	+ -ectomy		= Myectomy	: _____
My/o	+ -pathy		= Myopathy	: _____
My/o	+ -plasty		= Myoplasty	: _____
My/o	+ -tomy		= Myotomy	: _____

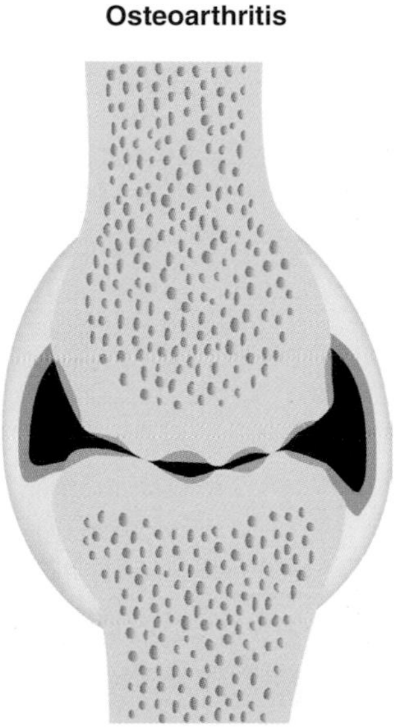

Osteoarthritis

Figure 3.24 Osteoarthritis of a synovial joint. Courtesy of shutterstock/Alila Sao Mai.

Myel/o	+ -oma	= Myeloma	: _____
Myel/o	+ -poiesis	= Myelopoiesis	: _____

TECH TIP 3.7 Myelopoiesis is often used to describe the production of white blood cells, specifically the production of a group of white blood cells called granulocytes.

Myos/o	+ -itis		= Myositis	: _____
Necr/o	+ -osis		= Necrosis	: _____
Olecran/o	+ -al		= Olecranal	: _____
Oste/o	+ -algia		= Ostealgia	: _____
Oste/o	+ -itis		= Osteitis	: _____
Oste/o	+ Arthr/o	+ -itis	= Osteoarthritis	: _____
Oste/o	+ -centesis		= Osteocentesis	: _____
Oste/o	+ Chondr/o	+ -osis	= Osteochondrosis	: _____
Oste/o	+ dys-	+ -trophy	= Osteodystrophy	: _____
Oste/o	+ -genesis		= Osteogenesis	: _____
Oste/o	+ -malacia		= Osteomalacia	: _____
Oste/o	+ Myel/o	+ -itis	= Osteomyelitis	: _____
Oste/o	+ Necr/o	+ -osis	= Osteonecrosis	: _____
Oste/o	+ -pexy		= Osteopexy	: _____
Oste/o	+ -plasty		= Osteoplasty	: _____

Oste/o	+ Sarc/o	+ -oma	= Osteosarcoma	: _____
Oste/o	+ -sclerosis		= Osteosclerosis	: _____
Oste/o	+ -tome		= Osteotome	: _____
pan-	+ Oste/o	+ -itis	= Panosteitis	: _____
peri-	+ Oste/o	+ -itis	= Periosteitis	: _____
Pelv/o	+ -metry		= Pelvimetry	: _____
Perone/o	+ -al		= Peroneal	: _____
Phalang/o	+ -eal		= Phalangeal	: _____
Pub/o	+ -ic		= Pubic	: _____
Radi/o	+ -al		= Radial	: _____
Radi/o	+ -graphy		= Radiography	: _____
Scapul/o	+ -ar		= Scapular	: _____
supra-	+ Scapul/o	+ -ar	= Suprascapular	: _____
Spondyl/o	+ -itis		= Spondylitis	: _____
Spondyl/o	+ -osis		= Spondylosis	: _____
Stern/o	+ -al		= Sternal	: _____
Patell/o	+ -ar		= Patellar	: _____
sub-	+ Patell/o	+ -ar	= Subpatellar	: _____
Synov/o	+ -itis		= Synovitis	: _____
Tars/o	+ -ectomy		= Tarsectomy	: _____
Tendin/o	+ -ectomy		= Tendinectomy	: _____

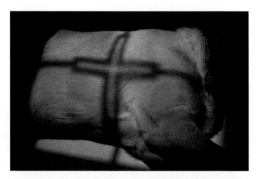

Figure 3.25A   Radiography of a dog. Courtesy of shutterstock/Kanwarjit Singh Boparai.

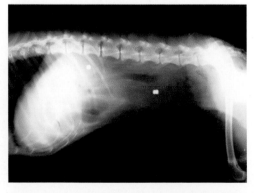

Figure 3.25B   Radiograph of a dog showing bullets from a gunshot wound (GSW). Courtesy of shutterstock/P Fabian.

TECH TIP 3.8 A tenectomy is an alternative to a declaw. A cat scratching the furniture is a common complaint of owners. Shelters are filled with cats that have been relinquished because of their scratching. Scratching posts can be purchased to try and redirect the behavior, but all too often frustrated owners will come to the clinic for a "quick fix." The options available to them include declawing, soft paws, and a tenectomy.

Declawing involves surgically removing the distal phalanx of each digit. Soft paws are caps that can be placed on the nails of the cat. A tenectomy involves cutting the tendons responsible for the control of the cat's nails. Once performed, the cat is unable to retract its nails.

Tendin/o	+ -itis	= Tendinitis	:	_____
Ten/o	+ -ectomy	= Tenectomy	:	_____
Ten/o	+ -rrhaphy	= Tenorrhaphy	:	_____
Ten/o	+ -tomy	= Tenotomy	:	_____
Tibi/o	+ -al	= Tibial	:	_____
Uln/o	+ -ar	= Ulnar	:	_____
Vertebr/o	+ -al	= Vertebral	:	_____

Abbreviations

Table 3.12   Chapter 3 Abbreviations.

Abbreviations	Definition
AAHA	American Animal Hospital Association
ACL	Anterior cruciate ligament
AVMA	American Veterinary Medical Association
Bilat.	Bilateral
CAR	Congenital articular rigidity
CCL; CrCL	Cranial cruciate ligament
CVT	Certified veterinary technician
DVM	Doctor of Veterinary Medicine
EMG	Electromyogram
Ⓛ	Left

Table 3.12   (*Continued*).

LVT	Licensed veterinary technician
NAVTA	National Association of Veterinary Technicians of America
Ortho	Orthopedic or orthopedic procedure
PDR	Physicians' Desk Reference
PROM	Passive range of motion
®	Right
ROM	Range of motion
RVT	Registered veterinary technician
THR	Total hip replacement
TPLO	Tibial plateau leveling osteotomy
TPO	Triple pelvic osteotomy
TTA	Tibial tuberosity advancement
VPB	Veterinary Pharmaceuticals and Biologicals

Case Study: Define the medical terms and abbreviations in bold print. You'll notice some terms from the previous chapter

Partner, a 2-year-old German Shepherd, comes to your clinic with **lameness**. The clinic is accredited by **AAHA**. The owners had noticed an abnormal **gait** in the past couple of weeks after a trip to the dog park. Upon **P/E** Partner wasn't ambulatory.

The doctor notes **bilat.** weakness in the rear limbs. There is slight atrophy of the rear leg muscles. To rule out an **ACL** tear the **DVM** checks **anterior drawer** signs. If there's an ACL rupture then a **TPLO** would be necessary due to the dog's size. Anterior drawer sign was normal so **PROM** is checked next. The vet notices that the ® **coxofemoral** joint has a decreased **ROM** so **radiographs** are ordered.

Osteitis is ruled out and Partner is diagnosed with hip dysplasia. The **femoral head** isn't aligned with the **acetabulum** so a **TPO** is performed to correct the problem.

Three weeks later Partner returns for **P.T.**, and he seems far more energetic. The **CVT** takes him to the back to begin his **hydrotherapy**. All the techs in the clinic are members of **NAVTA**.

Exercises

3-A: Match the combining forms with their meaning.

1.	_____ Skull	A.	Cost/o
2.	_____ Lower jaw	B.	Crani/o
3.	_____ Death	C.	Hem/o
4.	_____ Connective tissue	D.	Hydr/o
5.	_____ Tension	E.	Kinesi/o
6.	_____ Rib	F.	Leiomy/o
7.	_____ Movement	G.	Mandibul /o
8.	_____ Vertebrae	H.	Necr/o
9.	_____ Blood	I.	Sarc /o
10.	_____ Water; fluid	J.	Spondyl /o
11.	_____ Smooth muscle	K.	Ton /o
12.	_____ Ulna	L.	Uln/o

3-B: Write the correct medical term in the blank.

1. _____: Pertaining to below the ribs
2. _____: Softening of cartilage
3. _____: Inflammation of vertebrae
4. _____: Inflammation of fascia
5. _____: Pertaining to the upper jaw
6. _____: Disease condition of muscle
7. _____: Abnormal condition of bones and cartilage
8. _____: Removal of the hock
9. _____: Hardening of bone
10. _____: Study of movement
11. _____: Movement away from the midline
12. _____: Manner of walking
13. _____: Looseness
14. _____: Decrease in the angle between two bones
15. _____: Continuous muscle spasms
16. _____: Knuckle-like process at the ends of some long bones
17. _____: Membrane surrounding bone
18. _____: Shaft of a long bone
19. _____: Displacement of a bone from its joint
20. _____: Bony process on the proximal ulna

3-C: Define the following terms.

1. Hypocalcemia _____
2. Myasthenia _____
3. Rhabdomyoma _____
4. Hypertrophy _____

5. Fracture _____
6. Dysplasia _____
7. Achondroplasia _____
8. Ankylosis _____
9. Hemarthrosis _____
10. Tenorrhaphy _____

3-D: Define the following suffixes.

1.	_____: -blast	7.	_____: -emia
2.	_____: -pexy	8.	_____: -al
3.	_____: -malacia	9.	_____: -poiesis
4.	_____: -metry	10.	_____: -kinesis
5.	_____: -cyte	11.	_____: -tome
6.	_____: -desis	12.	_____: -physis

3-E: Define the following prefixes.

1.	_____: pan-	5.	_____: peri-
2.	_____: hypo-	6.	_____: dys-
3.	_____: ab-	7.	_____: endo-
4.	_____: inter-	8.	_____: supra-

3-F: Define the following abbreviations.

1.	_____: AVMA	7.	_____: TPO
2.	_____: VPB	8.	_____: TTA
3.	_____: RVT	9.	_____: CAR
4.	_____: THR	10.	_____: CCL
5.	_____: Ortho	11.	_____: PDR
6.	_____: EMG	12.	_____: TPLO

3-G: Circle the correct term in parentheses.

1. Sac of fluid near a joint that helps lubricate: (fascia, bursa)
2. Partial displacement of a bone from its joint: (subluxation, fracture)
3. Striated, voluntary muscle that controls movement: (skeletal, visceral)
4. Inflammation of muscles: (arthritis, myositis)
5. Connective tissue that binds bone to bone: (ligament, tendon)
6. Hunchback: (kyphosis, lordosis)
7. A freely movable joint: (suture, synovial)
8. Removal of a limb or other appendage: (laminectomy, amputation)
9. Crackling sounds heard due to two broken bones rubbing together: (calcification, crepitation)
10. Hole in bone that allows for the passage of nerves and vessels: (foramen, callus)

3-H: Define the following medical terms.

1. _____: Amputation
2. _____: Ossification
3. _____: Necrosis
4. _____: Fibular
5. _____: Laminectomy
6. _____: Reduction
7. _____: Articulation
8. _____: Osteoblast
9. _____: Patellar
10. _____: Phalangeal
11. _____: Pelvimetry
12. _____: Chondrosarcoma
13. _____: Subcostal
14. _____: Tenotomy
15. _____: Osteopexy

3-I: List the three types of muscle and circle the correct answers for each in the parentheses.

Types of muscle	Voluntary or involuntary	Smooth or striated
_____	(Voluntary, involuntary)	(Smooth, striated)
_____	(Voluntary, involuntary)	(Smooth, striated)
_____	(Voluntary, involuntary)	(Smooth, striated)

Answers can be found starting on page 571.

Go to www.wiley.com/go/taibo/terminology to find additional learning materials for this chapter:

- A crossword puzzle
- Flashcards
- Audio clips to show how to pronounce terms
- Case studies
- Review questions
- The figures from the chapter in PowerPoint

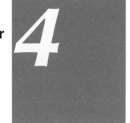
The Gastrointestinal Tract

The alimentary system, also referred to as the gastrointestinal system, has three main functions. The first function begins at the mouth, where the animal swallows the food and the food travels to the stomach to begin the process of digestion. The second function is the absorption of nutrients, which takes place in the intestines. The third function of the gastrointestinal system is the elimination of waste from the anus. In this chapter we will trace the flow of food through the gastrointestinal tract, learn about the various structures involved, and learn their individual functions.

The Pathway of Food

Figure 4.1 shows a summary of the path that food takes through the gastrointestinal tract. Keep in mind that the process of digestion is very complex. We have simplified the anatomy and physiology for introductory learning purposes.

The Oral Cavity

The pathway of food through the gastrointestinal system begins at the oral cavity, which consists of the lips, mouth, cheeks, teeth, tongue, and salivary glands.

Once food enters the mouth, the function of digestion begins. While the teeth are chewing the food, the salivary glands are releasing saliva to begin the digestive process.

The roof of the mouth is termed the palate and is actually divided into two parts, the hard palate and the soft palate. The hard palate of animals resembles that of humans in that they have ridges on their hard palate called rugae which will help increase the surface area for absorption and secretion. If you were to run your own tongue along the roof of your mouth, you'd feel the rugae. The soft

Veterinary Medical Terminology Guide and Workbook, First Edition. Angela Taibo.
© 2014 John Wiley & Sons, Inc. Published 2014 by John Wiley & Sons, Inc.
Companion website: www.wiley.com/go/taibo/terminology

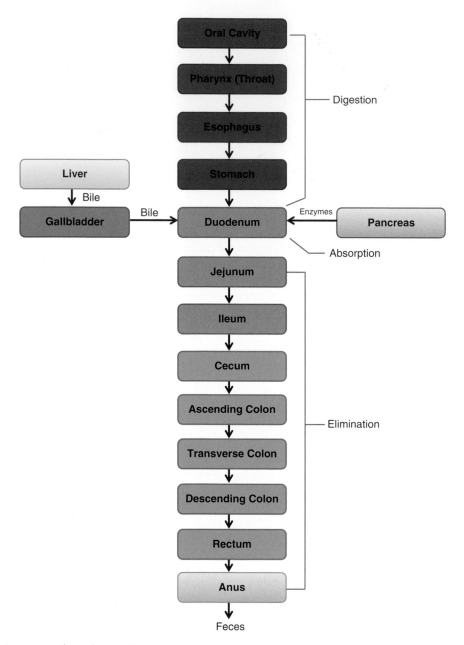

Figure 4.1   The pathway of food through the gastrointestinal tract.

palate is the smooth caudal portion of the palate. It controls the closing of the nasal passage while the animal swallows.

The muscle at the bottom of the oral cavity is the tongue. The tongue is constantly moving the food around while the animal chews and then aids in swallowing. Along

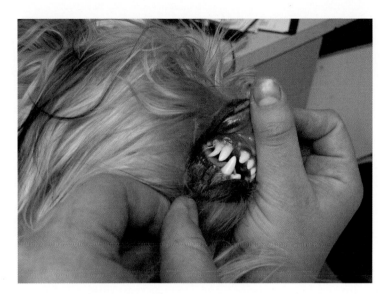

Figure 4.2   Retained deciduous canine tooth next to the permanent canine tooth.

the surface of the tongue are small raised bumps called papillae in which the taste buds can be found. In cats the papillae feel like sandpaper when they lick you.

The arrangement of the teeth in the mouth is referred to as dentition or an arcade. Just as with humans, animals have a temporary set of teeth and a permanent set of teeth. For example, in dogs think of it as having puppy teeth and adult teeth. The temporary dentition is referred to as deciduous dentition. Deciduous dentition isn't necessarily the same as the permanent dentition in some animals. When animals reach a certain age, it's important to check for any retained temporary teeth that were not shed because then they'll need to be pulled (Figure 4.2).

There are four different groups of teeth that are divided based on shape and function. The number of each group of teeth differs in each species, but the function is the same.

Incisor	Abbreviated "I," these teeth are used for shearing and grooming. They are named based on their function, which is to cut or incise.
Canine	Abbreviated "C," these teeth have a tearing function. They are commonly called fangs in some animals. In humans we commonly call them cuspids, which means tapered teeth.
Premolar	Abbreviated "P" or "PM," these teeth have a tearing and grinding function. In humans, these are called bicuspids since they have two projections.
Molar	Abbreviated "M," these teeth have a grinding function.

Once we know how many teeth are within each group in a species, we can then write the numbers into a formula. The dental formula is a shorthand method to help us remember the arrangement of teeth. To write a dental formula we first look at one side of an animal's face. Let's use a dog as an example. Start at the midline of the body and count the teeth on one side of the face. The first group of teeth you will count are the incisors. There are three incisors on top and three on the bottom. Remember, we are just counting one side of the face. Now that we've counted three on top and three on the bottom we begin writing our formula.

$$I\frac{3}{3}$$

Next we work our way lateral to the next group of teeth after the incisors, the canines. Dogs have one canine on top and one on the bottom. Let's add that to our equation.

$$I\frac{3}{3} + C\frac{1}{1}$$

Now let's move laterally to the next group of teeth, the premolars. Dogs have four on the top and four on the bottom. There are two different ways to write the premolars in a dental formula. Some people abbreviate the premolars as "P," whereas others abbreviate them using "PM." In this textbook I will use PM for the premolars. Refer to your individual instructor as to his or her preference, though both are considered correct.

$$I\frac{3}{3} + C\frac{1}{1} + PM\frac{4}{4}$$

Finally we come to the last group of teeth, the molars. Dogs have two on the top and three on the bottom. Let's add them to our equation.

$$I\frac{3}{3} + C\frac{1}{1} + PM\frac{4}{4} + M\frac{2}{3}$$

At this point you've only counted the teeth in half of the animal's mouth. To account for the other half of the face, we add a "2" in front of the equation.

$$2\left[I\frac{3}{3} + C\frac{1}{1} + PM\frac{4}{4} + M\frac{2}{3}\right]$$

If you add up the numbers inside the brackets and then multiply that number by 2, then you have the total number of teeth in the dog.

$$2\left[I\frac{3}{3} + C\frac{1}{1} + PM\frac{4}{4} + M\frac{2}{3}\right] = 42$$

Table 4.1 below shows the dental formulas for different species.

Table 4.1   Dental Formulas

Dogs	$2\left[I\dfrac{3}{3} + C\dfrac{1}{1} + PM\dfrac{4}{4} + M\dfrac{2}{3}\right] = 42$
Cats	$2\left[I\dfrac{3}{3} + C\dfrac{1}{1} + PM\dfrac{3}{2} + M\dfrac{1}{1}\right] = 30$
Horses	$2\left[I\dfrac{3}{3} + C\dfrac{1}{1} + PM\dfrac{3-4}{3} + M\dfrac{3}{3}\right] = 40-42$
Cattle, sheep, goats	$2\left[I\dfrac{0}{3} + C\dfrac{0}{1} + PM\dfrac{3}{3} + M\dfrac{3}{3}\right] = 32$
Pigs	$2\left[I\dfrac{3}{3} + C\dfrac{1}{1} + PM\dfrac{4}{4} + M\dfrac{3}{3}\right] = 44$
Humans	$2\left[I\dfrac{2}{2} + C\dfrac{1}{1} + PM\dfrac{2}{2} + M\dfrac{3}{3}\right] = 32$
Llamas	$2\left[I\dfrac{1}{3} + C\dfrac{1}{1} + PM\dfrac{2}{1} + M\dfrac{3}{2-3}\right] = 28-30$
Ferrets	$2\left[I\dfrac{3}{3} + C\dfrac{2}{2} + PM\dfrac{4}{3} + M\dfrac{1}{2}\right] = 40$
Rabbits	$2\left[I\dfrac{2}{1} + C\dfrac{0}{0} + PM\dfrac{3}{2} + M\dfrac{3}{3}\right] = 28$
Guinea pigs	$2\left[I\dfrac{1}{1} + C\dfrac{0}{0} + PM\dfrac{1}{1} + M\dfrac{3}{3}\right] = 20$
Chinchillas	$2\left[I\dfrac{1}{1} + C\dfrac{0}{0} + PM\dfrac{1}{1} + M\dfrac{3}{3}\right] = 20$
Gerbils	$2\left[I\dfrac{1}{1} + C\dfrac{0}{0} + PM\dfrac{0}{0} + M\dfrac{3}{3}\right] = 16$
Hamsters	$2\left[I\dfrac{1}{1} + C\dfrac{0}{0} + PM\dfrac{0}{0} + M\dfrac{3}{3}\right] = 16$
Mice, rats	$2\left[I\dfrac{1}{1} + C\dfrac{0}{0} + PM\dfrac{0}{0} + M\dfrac{3}{3}\right] = 16$

The dental formulas are most useful for learning the various types of teeth in each species; however, there's a different method used in dental surgeries for identifying the teeth in a patient's chart. This method is known as the triadan system (Figure 4.3). In this system each tooth is assigned a three-digit number

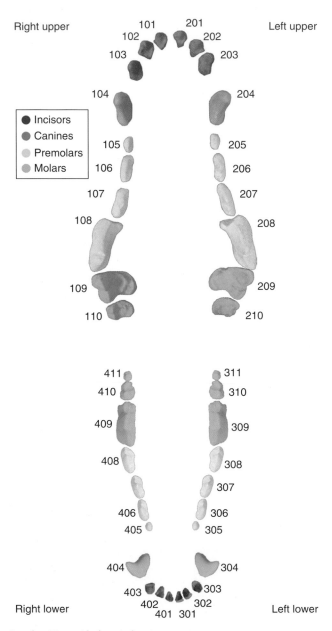

Figure 4.3   Canine dentition with the triadan system.

based on its location and type. The first number is based on the quadrant of the mouth that the tooth is in. The quadrants are numbered beginning with the right side of the maxilla and then are counted clockwise from there. The second and third numbers represent the location of the tooth when looking from rostral to caudal. This second number starts at 01 and goes up to 11, depending on the species.

Tooth anatomy is the same for all species. Label Figure 4.4 using the terms in Table 4.2.

Surrounding the oral cavity are pairs of exocrine glands called salivary glands. These glands secrete a digestive enzyme called saliva.

Table 4.2   Tooth Anatomy.

Alveolus	Tooth socket; alveolar bone.
Crown (1)	Portion of the tooth above the gum line; supragingival portion of the tooth.
Root (2)	Portion of the tooth below the gum line; subgingival portion of the tooth.
Enamel (3)	White, hard, outer covering of the tooth that protects the crown; the hardest substance in the body.
Dentin (dentine) (4)	Hard tissue of teeth between the enamel and pulp cavity.
Gingiva (gums)	Mucous membranes surrounding the teeth and lining the mouth.
Gingival sulcus	Area between the tooth and gums.
Pulp cavity	Sensitive cavity in the tooth containing blood supply and nerves.
Periodontal ligament (5)	Connective tissue that connects the tooth to the alveolar bone.
Cementum (6)	Bone-like connective tissue that covers the root.
Root canal	Portion of the pulp cavity extending from the pulp chamber to the apical foramen (opening at the distal aspect of the tooth).

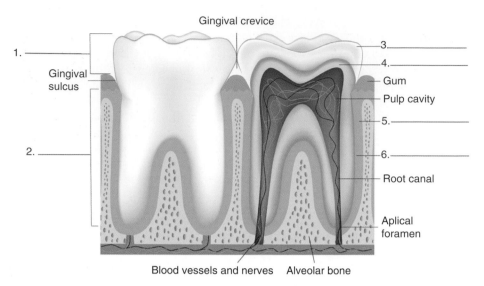

Figure 4.4 Anatomy of the tooth. Courtesy of shutterstock/Alila Sao Mai.

TECH TIP 4.1 What are Mucous Membranes?

Mucous membranes are membranes covered with epithelium that can be found lining many tubular organs of the body. These membranes produce a slimy substance called mucus.

Dental Terminology

Abscess	Localized collection of pus.
Bruxism	Grinding of teeth; common in cattle.
Deciduous teeth	Temporary teeth
Dental calculus	Also known as dental tarter, mineralized plaque that forms on the teeth (Figure 4.5).
Dental Caries	Tooth decay (Figure 4.6).
Epulis	Benign tumor arising from periodontal mucous membranes (Figure 4.8A).
Extraction	The act of pulling teeth (Figure 4.7B).
Gingival hyperplasia	Excessive development of gums due to increased cell numbers (Figure 4.8E).
Hard palate	Rostral portion of the roof of the mouth containing rugae.

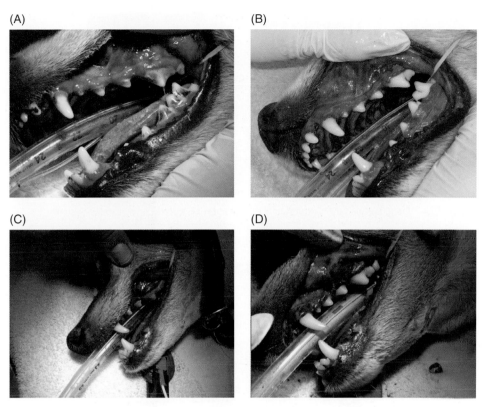

Figure 4.5   (A) Dental calculus. (B) Post dental surgery. (C) Dental calculus. (D) Post dental surgery. Courtesy of AK Traylor, DVM; Microscopy Learning Systems.

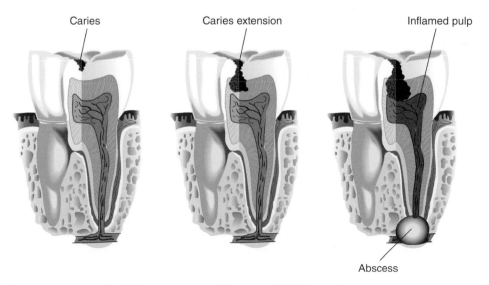

Figure 4.6   Stages of tooth decay. Courtesy of shutterstock/Alila Sao Mai.

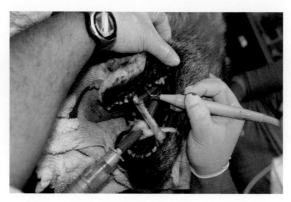

Figure 4.7A Dental procedure. Courtesy of AK Traylor, DVM; Microscopy Learning Systems.

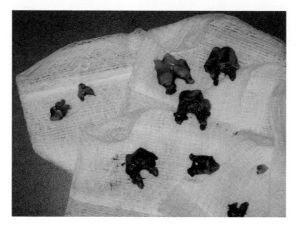

Figure 4.7B Extractions. Courtesy of AK Traylor, DVM; Microscopy Learning Systems.

Malocclusion	Abnormal position of teeth that results in faulty meeting of the teeth or jaws.
Occlusion	Relation of the teeth of both jaws during functional activity.
Oronasal fistula	Abnormal tube-like passageway between the mouth and nose. A **fistula** is an abnormal tube-like passageway that can occur anywhere on the body (Figure 4.8C).
Palate	Roof of the mouth.
Palatoschisis	Cleft palate (Figure 4.8B).
Papillae	Small, raised bumps on the tongue containing taste buds.
Periodontal disease	Inflammation and degeneration of the tissue surrounding and supporting the teeth (bone and gums); also known as **periodontitis** or **pyorrhea**.

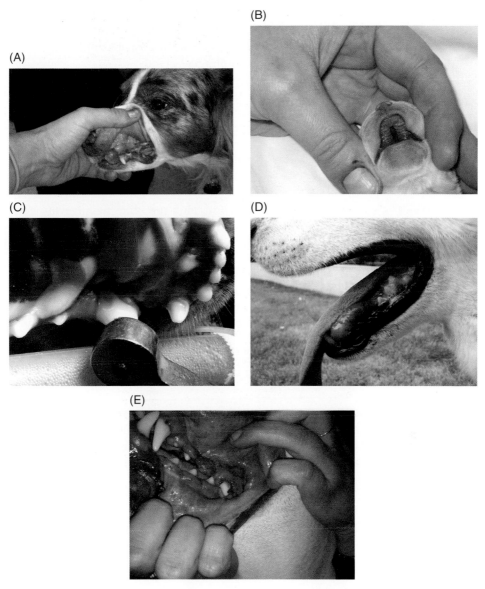

Figure 4.8   Dental pathologies. (A) Epulis. Courtesy of Amy Johnson, BS, CVT, RLATG. (B) Cleft palate in stillborn neonate. Note the rugae on the roof of the mouth. Courtesy of AK Traylor, DVM; Microscopy Learning Systems. (C) Oronasal fistula. Courtesy of A.K. Traylor, DVM; Microscopy Learning Systems. (D) Salivary mucocele. Courtesy of Amy Johnson, BS, CVT, RLATG. (E) Gingival hyperplasia. Courtesy of Amy Johnson, BS, CVT, RLATG. Courtesy of Deanna Roberts, BA, CVT.

Plaque	Collection of bacteria, salivary products, and white blood cells that adheres to the surface of the tooth.
Rugae	Ridges on the hard palate and lining the stomach to increase surface area for absorption and secretion. (Figure 4.8B).

Saliva	Digestive juice produced by salivary glands.
Salivary glands	Glands around the mouth that secrete saliva. There are three major pairs of glands called the **parotid, mandibular,** and **sublingual glands.**
Salivary mucocele	Collection of saliva that has leaked out from damaged salivary glands causing masses in the mouth. (Figure 4.8D).
Soft palate	Smooth, caudal portion of the roof of the mouth.

Pharynx

The pharynx is commonly called the throat. This tube-like passageway connects the oral cavity to the other GI tract locations. It is also responsible for joining the oral cavity to the trachea, which leads to the respiratory tract. As an animal chews its food, a leaf-like piece of cartilage called the epiglottis covers the trachea to prevent that food from "going down the wrong pipe." When the animal swallows, the epiglottis directs the food where to go. It closes over the trachea to allow the food to proceed to the next structure, the esophagus.

Esophagus

The esophagus is the tube that runs from the pharynx to the stomach. The tube is actually a muscle that contracts to move the food down toward the stomach. This process of wave-like contractions to move the food is called peristalsis (Figure 4.9). It's similar when people do the wave at a football game.

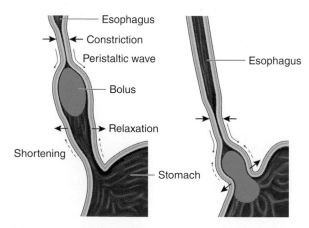

Figure 4.9   Peristalsis. Courtesy of shutterstock/blamb.

Stomach

After the food passes through the esophagus, it enters the stomach through a valve called the cardiac sphincter. Once in the stomach, the food is broken down by digestive enzymes such as hydrochloric acid. Lining the stomach are ridges called rugae that help increase the surface area for absorption and secretion. The rugae lining the stomach are the same as the rugae on the hard palate. After the food is broken down it exits the stomach through another valve called the pyloric sphincter.

In veterinary medicine there are two different types of stomachs. Most animals have what is considered a simple stomach or true stomach. Humans also have a simple stomach. The following are the parts of the simple stomach.

Body	The main portion of the stomach.
Cardiac sphincter	Valve between the esophagus and stomach.
Fundus	Cranial, rounded portion of the stomach.
Pyloric sphincter	Valve between the stomach and duodenum.
Pylorus (antrum)	Caudal portion of the stomach.
Rugae	Ridges on the hard palate and in the stomach to increase surface area for absorption and secretion.

Figure 4.10 shows the parts of a simple stomach.

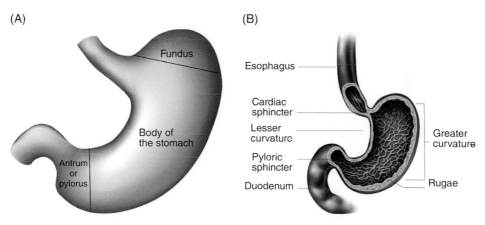

Figure 4.10   Anatomy of the simple stomach. (A) External stomach anatomy. Courtesy of shutterstock/Alila Sao Mai. (B) Internal stomach anatomy and upper GI. Courtesy of shutterstock/Lightspring.

Other animals, ruminants, have a more specialized stomach that contains four compartments. Examples of ruminants include cattle, sheep, and goats. These animals regurgitate their food, chew it, and then swallow it again. By regurgitating and chewing their food, they're breaking it down further for digestion. That regurgitated food is referred to as cud and the process of regurgitating, re-chewing, and re-swallowing is known as ruminating.

Each compartment of the ruminant stomach has a specific function (Figure 4.11).

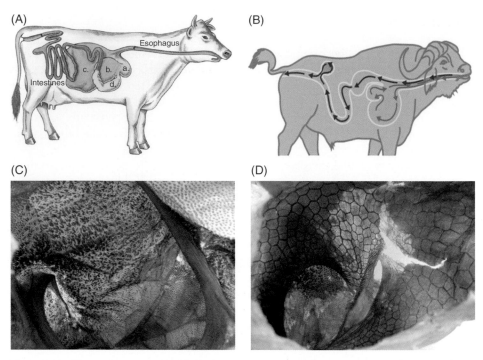

Figure 4.11   The ruminant stomach. (A) The four compartments of the ruminant stomach: (a) reticulum, (b) omasum, (c) rumen, and (d) abomasum. Courtesy of Getty Images/John Woodcock. (B) The flow of food through the ruminant GI tract. Courtesy of Getty Images/Dorling Kindersley/The Agency Collection. (C) Lining of the rumen. (D) Lining of the reticulum.

Rumen	This is the largest compartment of the ruminant stomach, where fermentation takes place. **Fermentation** is the process of breaking down organic compounds into simpler substances. Larger ingesta is broken down in the rumen.
Reticulum	This small, most cranial portion of the ruminant stomach is lined with mucous membranes in a hexagon pattern. It is commonly called the honeycomb because of its internal appearance. Smaller food particles are collected in the reticulum to be transferred to the omasum.
Omasum	The third and smallest of the compartments. Inside are folds of tightly packed papillae used for grinding food. It's commonly called the **bible** because the folds resemble pages in a book. The folds help to increase surface area for absorption of water.
Abomasum	The fourth and final compartment, which is considered the true stomach. Its function and anatomy resemble that of the true stomach in other mammals. Like small animals and humans, this portion of the stomach contains digestive enzymes and hydrochloric acid to break down food.

Small Intestine

The small intestine is divided into three portions: the duodenum, the jejunum, and the ileum. Lining the inside of the small intestine are small finger-like projections called villi (Figure 4.12). These projections are used to absorb nutrients into the bloodstream.

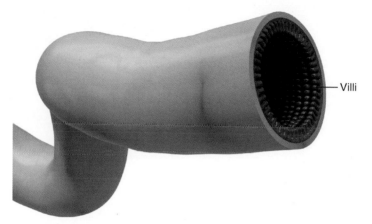

Villi

Figure 4.12   Small intestine villi. Courtesy of shutterstock/blamb.

TECH TIP 4.2 Watch your spelling on ileum. It looks very similar to the ilium of the pelvis.

The first part of the small intestine is the duodenum. Once food enters the duodenum, the pancreas releases digestive enzymes that further digest the food. Simultaneously, the liver and gallbladder send bile to the duodenum to aid in the break down of the food. Once the food has been digested further and the nutrients have been absorbed, the remaining material passes to the second part of the small intestine, the jejunum. Following the jejunum is the third part of the small intestine called the ileum.

The small intestines are anchored to the abdominal wall by a membranous sheet called mesentery (Figure 4.13). The mesentery contains blood vessels, lymph nodes, and nerves that supply the organs of the digestive tract. The mesentery prevents the intestines from entangling.

TECH TIP 4.3 Where's the Appendix?

The appendix is a blind pouch that hangs from the cecum. Most mammals lack an appendix with the exception of humans, apes, and rabbits.

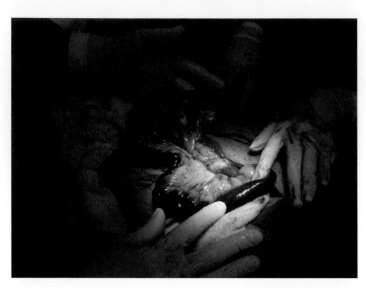

Figure 4.13   Mesentery. Courtesy of AK Traylor, DVM; Microscopy Learning Systems.

Large Intestine

The large intestine doesn't get its name because of its length, but rather its width. Its diameter is nearly three times that of the small intestine. It consists of the cecum, ascending colon, transverse colon, descending colon, rectum, and anus. Although the large intestine is used for elimination in all species, it has additional functions in herbivores due to their plant-based diets.

The cecum is a small, blind sac where the small and large intestine meet. In horses and rabbits, the cecum plays a major role in digestion. Fermentation takes place in the cecum of horses and rabbits because they have a simple stomach. Because of the significant role that the cecum plays in the horse and rabbit, its size is considerably larger than that of other mammals.

The large intestine, or colon, consists of three portions. They are arranged in the animal's body similar to a question mark. The ascending colon would be the portion of the question mark going towards the head, the transverse colon is the portion that goes across, and the descending colon is in the caudal direction.

In horses, ruminants, and pigs, the colon is slightly different. Horses have a large colon and small colon in which fermentation takes place and water is reabsorbed. Because of the colon's long length, there's an increased chance that it will become twisted and cause colic. The colon also has a series of sharp twists and turns which divide it into further portions.

Ruminants and pigs have an ascending, transverse, and descending colon; however, their ascending colon takes on a spiral arrangement, giving it the name spiral colon.

After passing through the colon, the remaining waste then passes through the anus to the outside of the body.

Prebiotics and probiotics are often used to ensure colon health in animals. In large animals, plant material can be difficult to digest; therefore, prebiotics and probiotics are given to aid in digestion. A prebiotic is a plant fiber that the stomach is unable to digest. Once ingested, this fiber goes to the intestines and nourishes the normal bacteria, or normal flora, in the intestines. A healthy environment of "good bacteria" ensures proper digestion. Probiotics are actually living bacteria administered to increase the population of normal flora.

These two substances can be very helpful in large animal medicine, and they are becoming increasingly popular in small animal medicine. Many veterinarians recommend probiotics to animals with diarrhea depending on the cause. Animals taking antibiotics risk destroying their normal flora with the medication so probiotics might be recommended to prevent this.

Liver and Gallbladder

The liver is the largest organ in the body and has many important functions. Anatomically, the liver is caudal to the diaphragm. Below is a list of the functions of the liver.

1. Synthesizes (produces) bile.
2. Maintains blood sugar by storing excess glucose in the form of glycogen.
3. Synthesizes proteins, including clotting proteins.
4. Conjugates bilirubin.
5. Detoxifies the blood.
6. Metabolizes drugs.
7. Synthesizes cholesterol.

In this chapter, we will focus on the functions of the liver that pertain to the alimentary system. The remaining functions will be discussed in later chapters.

Bile is composed of bilirubin, cholesterol, and bile acids (bile salts). While animals get cholesterol from their diets, their liver also produces cholesterol. The cholesterol is then stored to help produce bile. Once produced, the bile travels from the liver to the gallbladder to be stored. When food reaches the duodenum, the bile in the gallbladder travels to the duodenum via the common bile duct to assist in digestion (Figure 4.14).

Bilirubin is a metabolite of hemoglobin breakdown. Bilirubin travels to liver to become conjugated (water soluble) and is then stored by the liver to be added to bile. Bile salts are used for emulsification (fat breakdown) and are then reabsorbed by the body to be recycled and used again in the future. The bile salts travel back to the liver via the portal vein. The bilirubin and remaining bile are passed in the feces and are what give feces its color.

If bilirubin doesn't leave the body, then it builds up in the blood and tissues, causing a yellowish coloration of the skin and mucous membranes called jaundice.

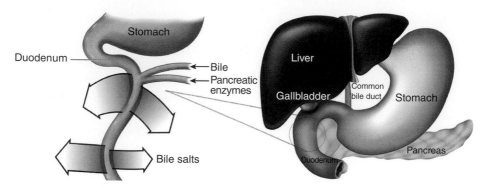

Figure 4.14 The flow of bile and digestive enzymes between the liver, stomach, and pancreas. Courtesy of shutterstock/blamb.

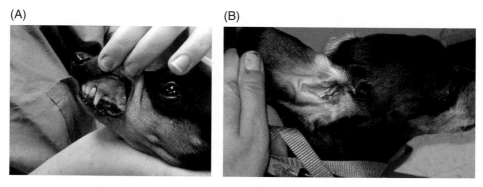

Figure 4.15 (A and B) Dachshund with jaundice on gingiva and ears. Courtesy of AK Traylor, DVM; Microscopy Learning Systems.

Jaundice is synonymous with the term icterus, which is the yellowish coloration of the plasma. Many practicing veterinarians and technicians use these two terms interchangeably (Figure 4.15).

Pancreas

The pancreas is both an endocrine and an exocrine organ. It's outward appearance resembles chewed gum. We will discuss the endocrine functions of the pancreas in a later chapter. This chapter will focus on its exocrine functions. The pancreas produces the digestive enzymes amylase, lipase, and trypsin. Amylase is a digestive enzyme that breaks down starch, lipase is an enzyme produced to digest fat, and trypsin is an enzyme that digests protein.

Related Terms

Absorption	Passage of materials through the walls of the intestine into the bloodstream.
Abdominal cavity	Space below, or caudal to, the diaphragm containing organs such as the liver, stomach, and intestines; also known as the **abdomen**.
Alimentary tract	All organs associated with the passage of food from the mouth to the anus; also known as the **gastrointestinal tract**.
Amino acids	"Building blocks" of proteins that are produced with the ingestion of protein.
Anal sacs	Pair of sacs between the internal and external anal sphincters. The walls of these sacs are lined with glands that secrete a malodorous material. Normal animals express their anal sacs during defecation for the purposes of territorial marking. Fear may also cause an animal to express its anal sacs (Figure 4.16).

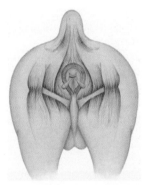

Figure 4.16A   Diagram of the location of anal glands in a dog. Courtesy of Getty Images/Dorling Kindersley.

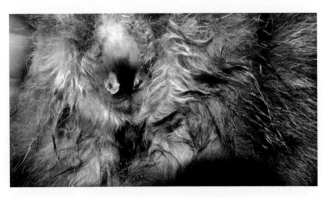

Figure 4.16B   Anal gland secretion from a dog. Courtesy of Greg Martinez, DVM; www.youtube. com/drgregdvm.

Anus	Opening from the GI tract to the outside of the body.
Bile	Digestive juice produced in the liver and stored in the gallbladder. Aids in the breakdown of fat (emulsification).
Bilirubin	Metabolite of hemoglobin breakdown; pigment released by the liver in bile.
Bolus	Rounded mass of food. In the case of pharmaceuticals, it refers to the preparation ready to be swallowed.
Bowel	Intestine.
Cardiac sphincter	Ring of muscle fibers at the proximal aspect of the stomach where it joins the esophagus.
Cecum	Small, blind sac where the small and large intestines meet; site of fermentation in horses and rabbits.
Colon	Large intestine; cecum, ascending colon, transverse colon, descending colon, and rectum.
Common bile duct	Carries bile from the liver and gallbladder to the duodenum.
Defecation	Passage of feces from the anus to the outside of the body; **elimination**.
Deglutition	Swallowing.
Diaphragm	Thin, muscular partition separating the thoracic and abdominal cavities.
Diverticulum	Pouch occurring on the wall of tubular organs of the GI tract.
Duodenum	First part of the small intestine where absorption takes place.
Emulsification	Breakdown of large fat globules into smaller globules.
Enzymes	Chemicals that speed up a reaction.

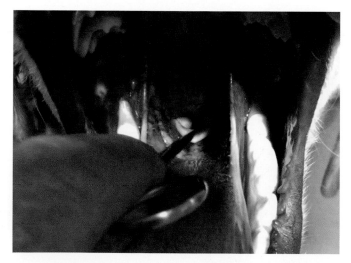

Figure 4.17   Hemostats pulling down the epiglottis. Note the vocal folds behind the epiglottis. Courtesy of Greg Martinez, DVM; www.youtube.com/drgregdvm.

Epiglottis	Leaf-like piece of cartilage over the trachea (windpipe) to prevent aspiration of food.
Esophagus	Tube connecting the throat to the stomach.
Feces	Stool; solid wastes.
Flatulence	Presence of gas in the stomach and intestines; flatus.
Gallbladder	Sac under the liver that stores bile.
Glucose	Simple sugar.
Gluconeogenesis	Production of glucose in the liver using fats and proteins.
Glycogen	Form of glucose stored in the liver; starch.
Glycogenolysis	Glycogen is converted back into glucose in the liver when the patient becomes hypoglycemic.
Hydrochloric acid	Produced in the stomach to digest food.
Jejunum	Second part of the small intestine.

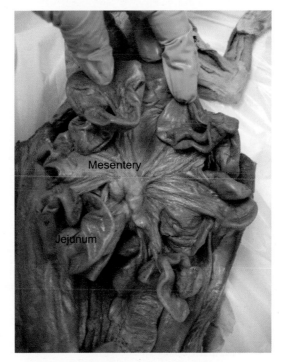

Figure 4.18   Mesentery and jejunum in a dissected cat. Mesenteric vessels are a landmark for identifying jejunum.

Labia	Lips; singular is **labium**.
Liver	Largest organ in the abdomen; responsible for synthesizing protein and bile, maintaining blood sugar, and detoxifying blood.
Mastication	Chewing.
Mesentery	Membranous sheet that holds the organs of the abdominal cavity in place. Contains blood vessels and lymph nodes.

Mucosa	Mucous membrane (i.e., intestinal mucosa is defined as mucous membranes of the intestine).
Nutrients	Substances that are necessary for normal body function.
Omentum	Fold of peritoneum extending from the greater curvature of the stomach to the other organs in the abdominal cavity. Absorbs excess fluid and adheres to wounds to act as the body's natural band-aid (Figure 4.19).

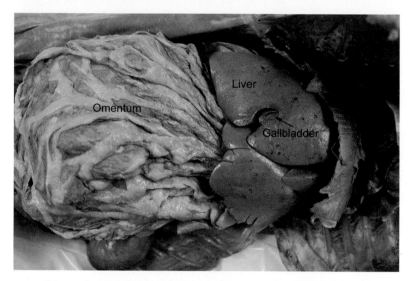

Figure 4.19   Abdominal cavity of a dissected cat showing the omentum, liver, and gallbladder.

Pancreas	Organ under the stomach that produces digestive enzymes, insulin, and glucagon.
Parenchyma	Tissue composed of the essential cells of any organ (i.e., liver parenchyma is liver tissue).
Peristalsis	Wave-like contractions of the tubes of the GI tract.
Peritoneum	Membrane surrounding the organs of the abdomen.
Pharynx	Throat.
Pyloric sphincter	Ring of muscle fibers at the distal end of the stomach where it joins the duodenum.
Rectum	Last portion of the colon.
Rugae	Ridges on the hard palate and in the stomach to increase surface area for absorption and secretion.
Ruminant stomach	Specialized four-compartment stomach consisting of the rumen, reticulum, omasum, and abomasum.
Sphincter	Group of ring-like muscles that can contract in diameter.
Trachea	Windpipe.
Tongue	Muscular organ on the floor of the mouth.
Villi	Microscopic, finger-like projections in the walls of the small intestine that absorb nutrients into the bloodstream.

Pathology and Procedures

Achalasia	Inability to relax the smooth muscles of the GI tract; most often associated with the esophagus.
Activated charcoal	Substance administered orally after accidental ingestion of a toxic substance. After inducing vomiting, activated charcoal is administered to coat the lining of the GI tract to prevent further absorption of any remaining toxins (Figure 4.20).

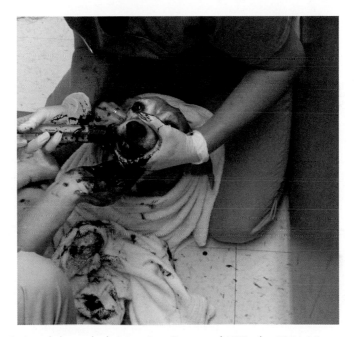

Figure 4.20   Activated charcoal administration. Courtesy of AK Traylor, DVM; Microscopy Learning Systems.

Anal sacculitis	Inflammation of the anal sacs. These sacs are prone to abscesses, blockage, and infections (Figure 4.21).
Anastomosis	Surgical connection between two tubes.
Anorexia	Lack of appetite.
Antidiarrheal	A substance given to counteract diarrhea.
Antiemetic	Substance given to counteract vomiting.
Ascites	Abnormal accumulation of fluid in the abdomen. (Figure 4.22).
Atresia	Closure of a normal body opening (i.e., esophageal atresia).

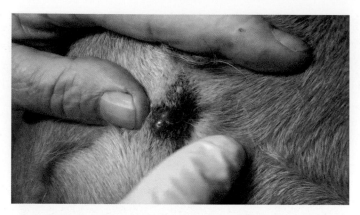

Figure 4.21   Anal gland abscess. Courtesy of Greg Martinez, DVM; www.youtube.com/drgregdvm.

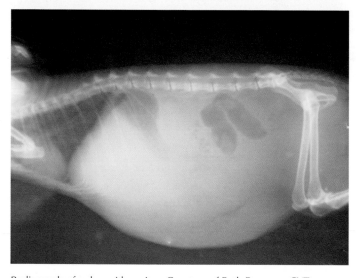

Figure 4.22   Radiograph of a dog with ascites. Courtesy of Beth Romano, CVT.

Barium study	Barium test; introduction of contrast material used to evaluate the GI tract. A series of radiographs is then taken to isolate GI tract disorders (Figure 4.23).
Biopsy	Removal of tissue for microscopic examination.
Body condition score	A method to assess an animal's weight based on outward appearance.
Borborygmus	Rumbling noises caused by the movement of gas or fluid through the GI tract.
Cachexia	General ill health and malnutrition (Figure 4.26A).

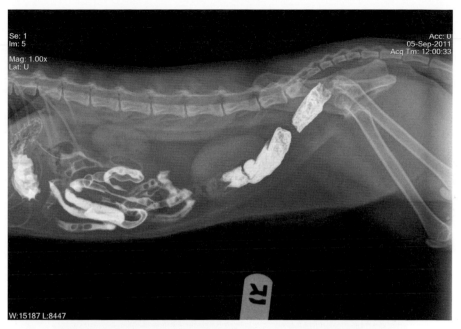

Figure 4.23   Barium study to locate an obstruction. Courtesy of Beth Romano, CVT.

TECH TIP 4.4 Emaciation vs. Cachexia

In both emaciation and cachexia, the patient is wasting away; however, the causes are different. Emaciation is caused by malnutrition and starvation. In general, emaciation can be corrected with nutrition. Cachexia is caused by an underlying pathology such as cancer, which means nutrition cannot fix the loss of body mass. No matter how much the patient eats, he or she will continue to lose weight.

Carcinoma   Malignant tumor arising from epithelial tissue.

TECH TIP 4.5 The definition for carcinoma is very similar to sarcoma at first glance, so be careful.

The rules for carcinoma are the same as the rules in Chapter 2 for sarcoma. You insert the organ of issue into the definition of carcinoma. For example, a gastric carcinoma is a malignant tumor of the stomach arising from epithelial tissue.

Remember to use this format: malignant tumor of _____ arising from epithelial tissue.

Cirrhosis   Degenerative disease in which the liver cells are
                                 replaced with scar tissue (Figure 4.24).
Colic   Acute abdominal pain.

TECH TIP 4.6 **Acute vs. Chronic**

Acute = sudden onset.
Chronic = existing over a long period of time.

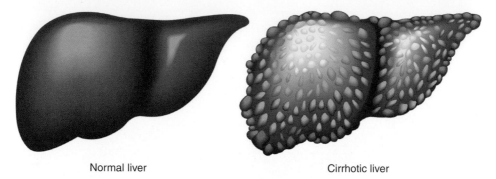

Normal liver   Cirrhotic liver

Figure 4.24   Healthy liver vs. cirrhosis. Courtesy of shutterstock/Rob3000.

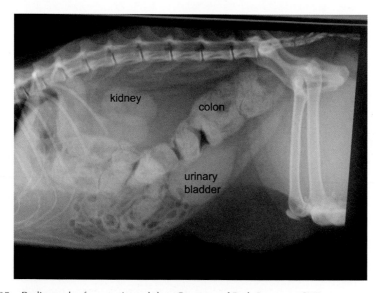

kidney   colon

urinary
bladder

Figure 4.25   Radiograph of a constipated dog. Courtesy of Beth Romano, CVT.

Constipation	Difficulty passing feces (Figure 4.25).
Coprophagia	Ingestion of feces.
Diarrhea	Rapid movement of feces through the GI tract; loose, watery stool.
Displaced abomasum	Condition in which the abomasum becomes trapped under the rumen. Displacement may be to the left or right side.

Diverticulitis	Inflammation of the diverticulum.
Drench	To give medication in liquid form by mouth and forcing the animal to drink.
Emaciation	Marked wasting or excessive leanness. (Figure 4.26B).

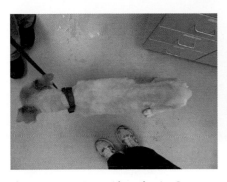

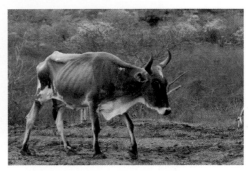

Figure 4.26A   Dog with cachexia. Courtesy of Deanna Roberts BA, AAS, CVT.

Figure 4.26B   Emaciation. Courtesy of shutter-stock/GlobetrotterJ.

Emesis	Vomiting; forceable expulsion of stomach contents through the mouth. The material vomited is termed **vomitus**.
Emetic	Substance given to produce vomiting.
Enema	Introduction of fluid into the rectum to promote defecation.
Eructation	Gas expelled from the stomach out of the mouth; a belch.
Esophageal atresia	Closure of the opening of the esophagus. The suffix -tresia means opening. When combined with the prefix a-, which means no or not, its meaning is reversed to a closure.
Esophageal reflux	A backward or return flow of stomach contents into the esophagus; also known as **GERD** (**gastroesophageal reflux disease**).
Etiology	Study of the cause of disease.
Fecal exam	Group of tests used to detect parasites in feces.
Gastric dilatation	Abnormal condition in which the stomach fills with air and expands. This is a common problem in large breed dogs, particularly the deep-chested breeds.
Gastric dilatation volvulus	Abnormal condition in which the stomach fills with air, expands, and then twist on itself. This is a common problem in large breed dogs, particularly the deep-chested breeds. Commonly called "bloat" (Figure 4.27).

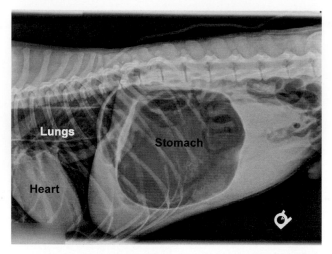

Figure 4.27   Radiograph of gastric dilatation volvulus in a dog. Courtesy of Beth Romano, CVT.

Gavage	Forced feeding or irrigation through a tube passed into the stomach.
Hematochezia	Bright, red, fresh blood from the rectum.
Hemorrhagic gastroenteritis	Acute condition in dogs causing vomiting and bloody diarrhea leading to dehydration, heart failure, and eventually death.
Hepatic lipidosis	Accumulation of fat in the liver that leads to liver damage. Disease typically occurs in cats after a period of anorexia (Figure 4.28).

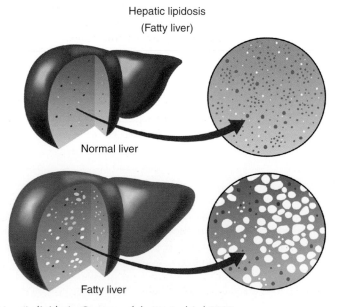

Figure 4.28   Hepatic lipidosis. Courtesy of shutterstock/rob3000.

Hiatal hernia   Protrusion of a structure, usually the stomach,
                                     through the esophageal opening in the
                                     diaphragm (Figure 4.29).

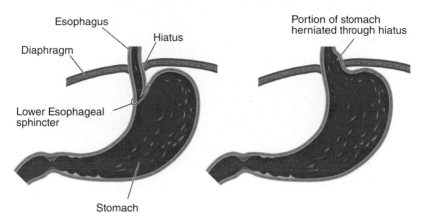

Esophagus

Hiatus

Diaphragm

Portion of stomach
herniated through hiatus

Lower Esophageal
sphincter

Stomach

Figure 4.29   Hiatal hernia. Courtesy of shutterstock/blamb.

Idiopathic   When the cause of disease is neither known nor
                                     understood.
Ileus   Failure of peristalsis with obstruction of the
                                     intestines.
Inappetence   Lack of appetite.
Incontinence   Inability to control excretory functions
                                     (defecation or urination).
Intussusception   Telescoping of the intestines.
Jaundice   Yellowish-orange coloration of the skin and
                                     mucous membranes due to excessive bilirubin in
                                     the blood; synonymous with **icterus**.
Lethargy   Condition of drowsiness or indifference.
Malabsorption   Impaired absorption of nutrients in the
                                     duodenum.

TECH TIP 4.7 Jaundice vs. Icterus

These two terms are often used interchangeably. There is a difference between the
two terms, though. Both terms are used to describe a yellowish coloration; the
difference is in where the yellow color is.

In jaundice, the yellow color is on the skin and mucous membranes. In icterus,
the yellow color is in the plasma of the blood.

Both are caused by excessive levels of bilirubin.

Maldigestion	Inability to digest food due to lack of digestive enzymes. Also known as **exocrine pancreatic insufficiency.**
Malaise	A vague feeling of bodily discomfort.
Megaesophagus	Enlargement of the esophagus (Figure 4.30).
Megacolon	Enlargement of the colon (Figure 4.30).

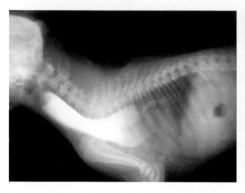

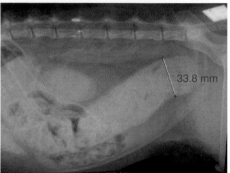

Figure 4.30A Radiograph of megaesophagus. Courtesy of shutterstock/P Fabian.

Figure 4.30B Radiograph of megacolon. Courtesy of Beth Romano, CVT.

TECH TIP 4.8 Melena vs. Hematochezia

Both melena and hematochezia involve blood in the feces. The appearance of the blood is what separates these two terms. If the blood is bright, red, and fresh, then it came from the lower GI tract. If the blood is black and tarry in appearance, then it has been digested in the stomach and duodenum. Using the appropriate term can therefore isolate where in the GI tract the problem may be.

Melena	Black tarry stool; blood in feces.
Nasogastric intubation	Placement of a tube from the nose to the stomach (Figure 4.31).
Nausea	Upset stomach and a tendency to vomit.
Obese	Excessive fat accumulation in the body (Figure 4.32).
Obstipation	Inability to eliminate.
Obstruction	Complete stoppage or impairment of passage.
Orogastric intubation	Placement of a tube from the mouth to the stomach.
Palpation	Method of examining the internal body by touching and feeling.
Parenteral	Route of administration other than oral.
Pica	Eating or licking abnormal substances; a depraved appetite (Figure 4.33).

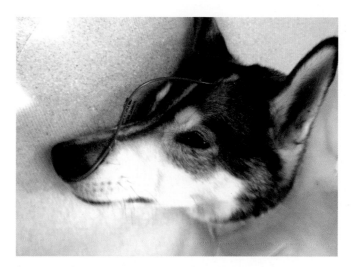

Figure 4.31   Nasogastric tube in a Husky. Courtesy of AK Traylor, DVM; Microscopy Learning Systems.

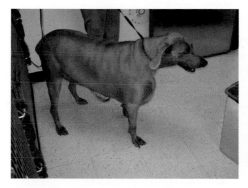

Figure 4.32A   Overweight Weimaraner. Courtesy of AK Traylor, DVM; Microscopy Learning Systems.

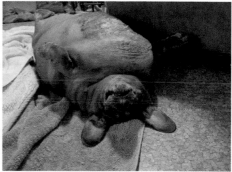

Figure 4.32B   Seventy-seven-pound Dachshund named Obie. Courtesy of Nora Vanatta.

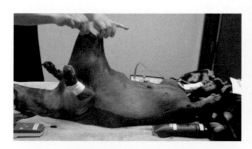

Figure 4.32C   Obie being prepped for surgery to remove excess skin after losing 40 pounds. Courtesy of Nora Vanatta.

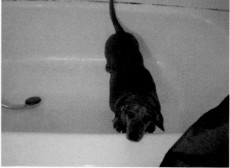

Figure 4.32D   Obie 40 pounds lighter after a proper diet and exercise. Courtesy of Nora Vanatta.

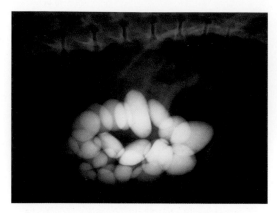

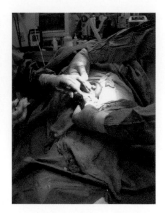

Figure 4.33A Radiograph of a canine abdomen showing rocks in the stomach.

Figure 4.33B Surgery to remove a GI foreign body. Courtesy of AK Traylor, DVM; Microscopy Learning Systems.

Pneumocolon	Air in the colon; procedure that places air in the colon as a means of diagnosis (Figure 4.34A).
Portosystemic shunt	Condition in which the blood vessels bypass the liver and the blood is not detoxified.
Regurgitate	Passive event in which swallowed food is returned to the oral cavity.
Rumen fistula	Procedure in which a canula is placed on the side of a cow for access to digestive contents in the rumen. This method allows for ingesta and the cow's digestive tract to be studied (Figure 4.34B).

(A)

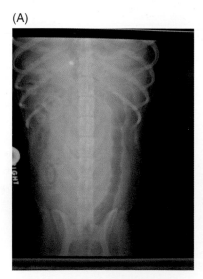

(B)

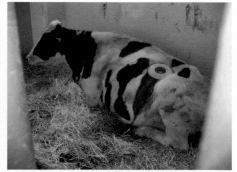

Figure 4.34A (A) Radiograph of pneumocolon.

Figure 4.34B Rumen fistula. Courtesy of Deanna Roberts, BA, CVT.

TECH TIP 4.9 **Vomiting vs. Regurgitation**

Vomiting is a forcible event, whereas regurgitation is a passive event. My students will often think of newborn babies when trying to distinguish these two terms. Newborn babies regurgitate often. They don't even realize that it's happening. It just comes up!

(A)   (B)

(C)

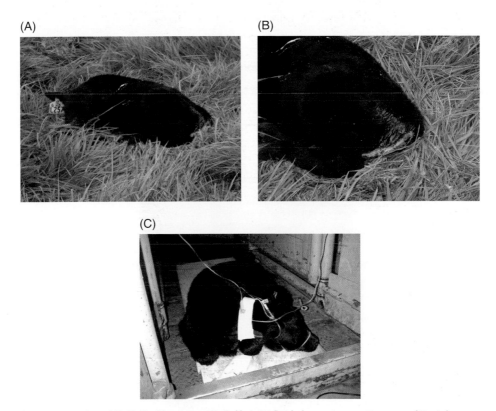

Figure 4.35   (A and B) Calf with scours. (C) Calf on IV fluids for treatment. Courtesy of Patrick Hemming, DVM.

Scours	Diarrhea in livestock (Figure 4.35).
Shunt	To bypass or divert.
Spasm	Sudden, involuntary contraction.
Stasis	Stopping or controlling.
Steatorrhea	Fat in feces.
Stenosis	Tightening, narrowing, or stricture.
Stoma	An incised opening that is kept open for drainage and other purposes.

> **TECH TIP 4.10 Suffixes Used as Terms**
>
> Some suffixes can be used as separate terms. Examples include:
> * Emesis
> * Spasm
> * Stasis
> * Stenosis
>
> Their meanings are still the same as when they are used as suffixes.

Tenesmus	Ineffectual and painful straining at defecation and urination.
Torsion	Axial twist; twisting around the long axis of the gut.
Trichobezoar	Hairball.
Ulcer	Erosion of the skin and mucous membranes (Figure 4.36).

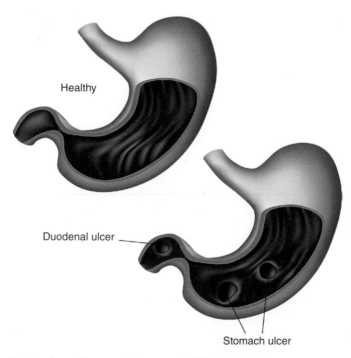

Healthy

Duodenal ulcer

Stomach ulcer

Figure 4.36   Gastric ulcers. Courtesy of shutterstock/Alila Sao Mai.

Ultrasound	Diagnostic technique using ultrasound waves to produce an image of an organ or tissue (Figure 4.37).
Volvulus	Twisting on itself.

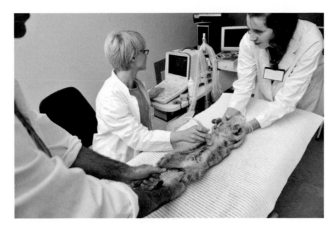

Figure 4.37   Ultrasound of a cat. Courtesy of shutterstock/shock.

Building the Terms

Table 4.3   Chapter 4 Combining Forms.

Combining Forms	Definition	Combining Forms	Definition
Abdomin/o	Abdomen	Cheil/o	Lip
Acu/o	Sudden; sharp; severe	Chol/e	Bile; gall
Adip/o	Fat	Cholangi/o	Bile vessel; bile duct
Aliment/o	To nourish	Cholecyst/o	Gallbladder
Amyl/o	Starch	Choledoch/o	Common bile duct
An/o	Anus	Chron/o	Time
Bi/o	Life	Cib/o	Meals
Bil/i	Bile; gall	Col/o, Colon/o	Large intestine; colon
Bilirubin/o	Bilirubin	Copr/o	Feces
Bucc/o	Cheek	Cyst/o	Urinary bladder; cyst; sac of fluid
Carcin/o	Cancerous; cancer	Decidu/o	Shedding
Cec/o	Cecum	Dent/o, Dent/i	Tooth
Celi/o	Belly; abdomen	Dips/o	Thirst

(Continued)

Table 4.3   (Continued).

Combining Forms	Definition	Combining Forms	Definition
Duoden/o, Duoden/i	Duodenum	**Mandibul/o**	Mandible; lower jaw
Enter/o	Small Intestine	**Muc/o**	Mucus
Esophag/o	Esophagus	**Nas/o**	Nose
Faci/o	Face	**Necr/o**	Death
Gastr/o	Stomach	**Odont/o**	Tooth
Gingiv/o	Gums	**Or/o**	Mouth
Gloss/o	Tongue	**Palat/o**	Palate; roof of the mouth
Gluc/o	Sugar	**Pancreat/o**	Pancreas
Glyc/o	Sugar	**Peritone/o**	Peritoneum
Glycogen/o	Glycogen	**Phag/o**	Eat; swallow
Gnath/o	Jaw	**Pharyng/o**	Throat; pharynx
Hem/o	Blood	**Proct/o**	Anus and rectum
Hemat/o	Blood	**Prote/o**	Protein
Hepat/o	Liver	**Py/o**	Pus
Herni/o	Hernia	**Pylor/o**	Pyloric sphincter; pylorus
Hydr/o	Fluid; water	**Radi/o**	X-ray; radius; radioactivity
Ile/o	Ileum	**Rect/o**	Rectum
Inguin/o	Groin	**Rug/o**	Wrinkle or fold
Jejun/o	Jejunum	**Sial/o**	Saliva; salivary
Labi/o	Lips	**Sialaden/o**	Salivary gland
Lapar/o	Abdomen	**Steat/o**	Fat; sebum
Lingu/o	Tongue	**Stomat/o**	Mouth
Lip/o	Fat	**Trich/o**	Hair
Lith/o	Stone	**Vill/i**	Tuft of hair; thread-like projection from membrane

Table 4.4 Chapter 4 Prefixes.

Prefix	Definition	Prefix	Definition
a-, an-	no; not; without	**mega-**	large
ante-	before; forward	**meta-**	change; beyond
anti-	against	**neo-**	new
brachy-	short	**para-**	near; beside; abnormal; apart from; along the side of
de-	lack of; down; less; removal of	**peri-**	surrounding; around
dys-	bad; painful; difficult; abnormal	**poly-**	many; much
endo-	in; within	**post-**	after; behind
hyper-	above; excessive	**pre-**	before; in front of
hypo-	deficient; below; under; less than normal	**pro-**	before; forward
mal-	bad	**sub-**	under; below

Table 4.5 Chaapter 4 Suffixes.

Suffix	Definition	Suffix	Definition
-al, -ar, -ary, -eal, -ic, -ous	pertaining to	**-emic**	pertaining to a blood condition
-ase	enzyme	**-gen**	producing; forming
-ation	process; condition	**-genesis**	producing; forming
-blast	immature; embryonic	**-graph**	instrument for recording
-cele	hernia	**-graphy**	process of recording
-centesis	surgical puncture to remove fluid	**-ia**	condition
-chezia	defecation; elimation of waste	**-iasis**	abnormal condition
-cyte	cell	**-ion**	process
-ectasis, -ectasia	stretching; dilation; dilatation	**-ism**	process; condition
-ectomy	removal; excision; resection	**-itis**	inflammation
-emesis	vomiting	**-lithiasis**	abnormal condition of stones
-emia	blood condition	**-logy**	study of

(Continued)

Table 4.5   (*Continued*).

Suffix	Definition	Suffix	Definition
-lysis	breakdown; separation; destruction; loosening	**-ptysis**	spitting
-megaly	enlargement	**-rrhaphy**	suture
-oma	tumor; mass; fluid collection	**-rrhea**	flow; discharge
-opsy	view of	**-scope**	instrument for visual examination
-orexia	appetite	**-scopy**	visual examination
-ose	full of; pertaining to; sugar	**-spasm**	sudden involuntary contraction of muscles
-osis	abnormal condition	**-stalsis**	contraction
-otic	pertaining to the abnormal condition	**-stasis**	stopping; controlling
-pepsia	digestion	**-stenosis**	tightening; narrowing; stricture
-pexy	surgical fixation; to put in place	**-stomy**	new opening to the outside of the body
-phagia	eating; swallowing	**-tomy**	incision; process of cutting
-plasty	surgical repair	**-tresia**	opening
-prandial	meal	**-um**	structure; tissue; thing; pertaining to
-ptyalo	spit; saliva		

TECH TIP 4.11 Rules for Using the Suffix "-stomy"

Rule 1: If "–stomy" is attached to just one combining form, then its definition is a new opening to the outside of the body. You insert the combining form into the definition of "–stomy." For example, a gastrostomy is a new opening from the stomach to the outside of the body. Just remember to use this format: a new opening from the _____ to the outside of the body.

Rule 2: If "–stomy" is attached to more than one combining form, then its meaning changes to a surgical fixation or an anastomosis. For example, a gastrojejunostomy is a surgical connection between the stomach and jejunum. Or you could say an anastomosis between the stomach and jejunum. Remember your basic rules to medical terminology. Combining forms must be listed in anatomical order.

Now it's time to put these word parts together. If you memorize the meaning of the combining forms, prefixes, and suffixes, then this will get easier each time. Remember your five basic rules to medical terminology when building and defining these terms. You'll notice some word parts are repeated from the previous chapter.

Parts			Medical Term	Definition
Abdomin/o	+ -al		= Abdominal	: _____
Abdomin/o	+ -centesis		= Abdominocentesis	: _____
			Also called a paracentesis.	
Adip/o	+ -ose		= Adipose	: _____
Amyl/o	+ -ase		= Amylase	: _____
An/o	+ -al		= Anal	: _____
peri-	+ An/o	+ -al	= Perianal	: _____
An/o	+ -plasty		= Anoplasty	: _____
An/o	+ Rect/o	+ -al	= Anorectal	: _____
anti-	+ -emesis	+ -ic	= Antiemetic	: _____
Bi/o	+ -logy		= Biology	: _____
Bil/i	+ -ary		= Biliary	: _____
hyper-	+ Bilirubin/o	+ -emia	= Hyperbilirubinemia	: _____
Bucc/o	+ -al		= Buccal	: _____
Carcin/o	+ -gen		= Carcinogen	: _____
Cec/o	+ -al		= Cecal	: _____
Celi/o	+ -ac		= Celiac	: _____
Cheil/o	+ -osis		= Cheilosis	: _____
Cholangi/o	+ -ectasia		= Cholangiectasia	: _____
Cholangi/o	+ -stomy		= Cholangiostomy	: _____
Cholangi/o	+ Carcin/o	+ -oma	= Cholangiocarcinoma	: _____
Cholangi/o	+ Hepat/o	+ -itis	= Cholangiohepatitis	: _____
Cholangi/o	+ Gastr/o	+ -stomy	= Cholangiogastrostomy	: _____
Cholangi/o	+ Enter/o	+ -stomy	= Cholangioenterostomy	: _____
Chol/e	+ -stasis		= Cholestasis	: _____
Cholecyst/o	+ -ic		= Cholecystic	: _____
Cholecyst/o	+ -ectomy		= Cholecystectomy	: _____
Cholecyst/o	+ -itis		= Cholecystitis	: _____
Cholecyst/o	+ -lithiasis		= Cholecystolithiasis	: _____
Cholecyst/o	+ Jejun/o	+ -stomy	= Cholecystojejunostomy	: _____
Choledoch/o	+ -al		= Choledochal	: _____
Choledoch/o	+ -lithiasis		= Choledocholithiasis	: _____
Choledoch/o	+ Jejun/o	+ -stomy	= Choledochojejunostomy	: _____
Choledoch/o	+ -tomy		= Choledochotomy	: _____
ante-	+ Cib/o	+ -um	= Antecibum	: _____
post-	+ Cib/o	+ -um	= Postcibum	: _____
Colon/o	+ -ic		= Colonic	: _____
Col/o	+ -itis		= Colitis	: _____
			Also called colonitis.	

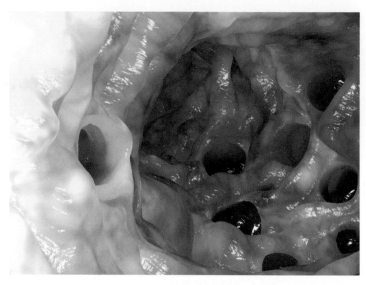

Figure 4.38   Colonoscopy showing diverticulitis. Courtesy of shutterstock/Juan Gaertner.

Colon/o	+ -scopy		= Colonoscopy	: _____
Col/o	+ -stomy		= Colostomy	: _____

Also called colonostomy.

Col/o	+ -tomy		= Colotomy	: _____
Copr/o	+ -phagia		= Coprophagia	: _____
Copr/o	+ Phag/o	+ -ic	= Coprophagic	: _____
Duoden/o	+ -al		= Duodenal	: _____
dys-	+ -chezia		= Dyschezia	: _____
dys-	+ -pepsia		= Dyspepsia	: _____
dys-	+ -phagia		= Dysphagia	: _____
Enter/o	+ -itis		= Enteritis	: _____
Enter/o	+ -tomy		= Enterotomy	: _____
Enter/o	+ -stomy		= Enterostomy	: _____
Enter/o	+ -ic		= Enteric	: _____
Enter/o	+ -ic Carcin/o + -oma		= Enteric carcinoma	: _____
Enter/o	+ Col/o	+ -stomy	= Enterocolostomy	: _____
Enter/o	+ Col/o	+ -itis	= Enterocolitis	: _____
Esophag/o	+ -eal		= Esophageal	: _____
Esophag/o	+ -eal	+ Spasm	= Esophageal spasm	: _____
Esophag/o	+ -plasty		= Esophagoplasty	: _____
Esophag/o	+ -itis		= Esophagitis	: _____
Faci/o	+ -al		= Facial	: _____
Gastr/o	+ -ic		= Gastric	: _____
Gastr/o	+ -tomy		= Gastrotomy	: _____
Gastr/o	+ -ectomy		= Gastrectomy	: _____
Gastr/o	+ -stomy		= Gastrostomy	: _____

Gastr/o   +   Jejun/o   + -stomy   = Gastrojejunstomy   : _____
Gastr/o   +   Enter/o   + -itis   = Gastroenteritis   : _____
Gastr/o   +   Duoden/o + -stomy   = Gastroduodenostomy   : _____
Gastr/o   +   -pexy   = Gastropexy   : _____

This is the procedure
used to correct bloat.

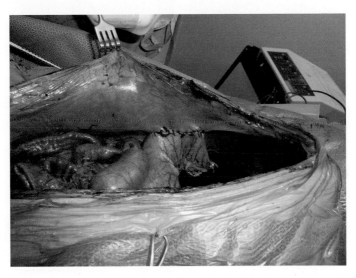

Figure 4.39   Gastropexy to correct a gastric dilatation volvulus. Courtesy of Deanna Roberts, BA, AAS, CVT.

Gingiv/o   +   -al   = Gingival   : _____
Gingiv/o   +   -itis   = Gingivitis   : _____
Gingiv/o   +   -ectomy   = Gingivectomy   : _____
Gloss/o   +   -al   = Glossal   : _____
Gloss/o   +   -itis   = Glossitis   : _____
hypo-   +   Gloss/o   + -al   = Hypoglossal   : _____
Glyc/o   +   -emic   = Glycemic   : _____
hyper-   +   Glyc/o   + -emia   = Hyperglycemia   : _____
hypo-   +   Glyc/o   + -emia   = Hypoglycemia   : _____
hyper-   +   Glyc/o   + -emic   = Hyperglycemic   : _____
hypo-   +   Glyc/o   + -emic   = Hypoglycemic   : _____
brachy-   +   Gnath/o   + -ia   = Brachygnathia   : _____
pro-   +   Gnath/o   + -ia   = Prognathia   : _____
Gnath/o   +   -ism   = Gnathism   : _____

Condition can affect the
mandible or the maxilla.

Hemat/o   +   -emesis   = Hematemesis   : _____
Hemat/o   +   -chezia   = Hematochezia   : _____
Hem/o   +   peritoneum   = Hemoperitoneum   : _____

(A)   (B)

(C)   (D)

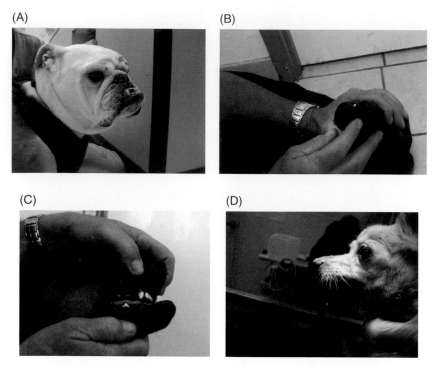

Figure 4.40 Mandibular deformities. (A) Elongated mandible. Courtesy of AK Traylor, DVM; Microscopy Learning Systems. (B and C) Elongated mandible. Courtesy of Greg Martinez, DVM; www.youtube.com/drgregdvm. (D) Chihuahua with mandibular brachygnathism. Courtesy of Deanna Roberts, BA, AAS, CVT.

Hem/o	+ -ptysis		= Hemopytsis	:_____
Hepat/o	+ -megaly		= Hepatomegaly	:_____
Hepat/o	+ -itis		= Hepatitis	:_____
Hepat/o	+ -oma		= Hepatoma	:_____
Hepat/o	+ -tomy		= Hepatotomy	:_____
Hepat/o	+ -cyte		= Hepatocyte	:_____
Herni/o	+ -rrhaphy		= Herniorrhaphy	:_____
de-	+ Hydr/o	+ -ation	= Dehydration	:_____
Ile/o	+ -itis		= Ileitis	:_____
Ile/o	+ -stomy		= Ileostomy	:_____
Ile/o	+ Cec/o	+ -al	= Ileocecal	:_____
Inguin/o	+ -al		= Inguinal	:_____
Jejun/o	+ -stomy		= Jejunostomy	:_____
Labi/o	+ -al		= Labial	:_____
Lapar/o	+ -tomy		= Laparotomy	:_____

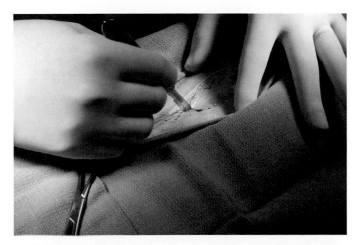

Figure 4.41   Laparotomy incision. Courtesy of shutterstock/Kanwarjit Singh Boparai.

Lingu/o	+ -al		= Lingual	:	_____
sub-	+ Lingu/o	+ -al	= Sublingual	:	_____
Lip/o	+ -ase		= Lipase	:	_____
Lip/o	+ -oma		= Lipoma	:	_____
Mandibul/o	+ -ar		= Mandibular	:	_____
sub-	+ Mandibul/o	+ -ar	= Submandibular	:	_____
Muc/o	+ -ous		= Mucous	:	_____
Necr/o	+ -opsy		= Necropsy	:	_____
Necr/o	+ -osis		= Necrosis	:	_____
Nas/o	+ -al		= Nasal	:	_____
Nas/o	+ Gastr/o	+ -ic	= Nasogastric	:	_____
Or/o	+ -al		= Oral	:	_____

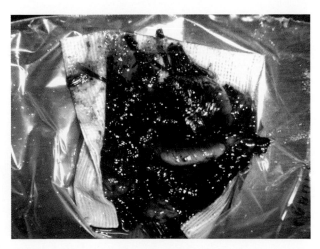

Figure 4.42   Intestine necrosis. Courtesy of AK Traylor, DVM; Microscopy Learning Systems.

Or/o	+	Gastr/o	+ -ic	= Orogastric	: _____
Or/o	+	Nas/o	+ -al	= Oronasal	: _____
Palat/o	+	-plasty		= Palatoplasty	: _____
Pancreat/o	+	-itis		= Pancreatitis	: _____
Pancreat/o	+	-ic		= Pancreatic	: _____
Peritone/o	+	-itis		= Peritonitis	: _____

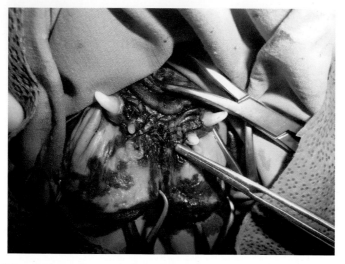

Figure 4.43　Palatoplasty in a dog in which the hard palate separated from the bone plate. Courtesy of Deanna Roberts BA, AAS, CVT.

| Peritone/o | + | -al | = Peritoneal | : _____ |
| Pharyng/o | + | -eal | = Pharyngeal | : _____ |

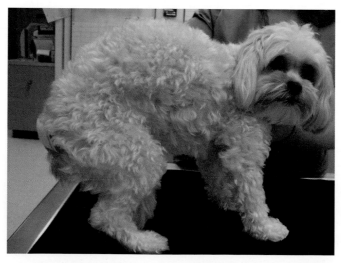

Figure 4.44　Dog with pancreatitis. Note the hunched appearance due to abdominal pain. Courtesy of AK Traylor, DVM; Microscopy Learning Systems.

Pharyng/o   +   -itis   = Pharyngitis   :_____

poly-   +   Dips/o   + -ia   = Polydipsia   :_____

poly-   +   -phagia   = Polyphagia   :_____

pre-   +   -prandial   = Preprandial   :_____

post-   +   -prandial   = Postprandial   :_____

Proct/o   +   -logy   = Proctology   :_____

Proct/o   +   -plasty   = Proctoplasty   :_____

Prote/o   +   -ase   = Protease   :_____

Py/o   +   -rrhea   = Pyorrhea   :_____

Pylor/o   +   -ic   = Pyloric   :_____

Pylor/o   +   -plasty   = Pyloroplasty   :_____

Pylor/o   +   -ic   + Stenosis   = Pyloric stenosis   :_____

Pylor/o   +   -spasm   = Pylorospasm   :_____

Radi/o   +   -graph   = Radiograph   :_____

Radi/o   +   -logy   = Radiology   :_____

Rect/o   +   -al   = Rectal   :_____

Rect/o   +   -cele   = Rectocele   :_____

Sialaden/o +   -itis   = Sialadenitis   :_____

Sialaden/o +   -osis   = Sialadenosis   :_____

Sial/o   +   -cele   = Sialocele   :_____

Steat/o   +   -oma   = Steatoma   :_____

Also called lipoma.

Steat/o   +   -lysis   = Steatolysis   :_____

Also called emulsification.

Steat/o   +   -itis   = Steatitis   :_____

Stomat/o   +   -itis   = Stomatitis   :_____

Stomat/o   +   Gastr/o   + -ic   = Stomatogastric   :_____

Stomat/o   +   -logy   = Stomatology   :_____

Abbreviations

Table 4.6   Chapter 4 Abbreviations.

Abbreviation	Definition
ac	Before meals (ante cibum)
Alk. phos.	Alkaline phosphatase (liver enzyme)
ALT	Alanine aminotransferase (liver enzyme)
cc	cubic centimeter
GDV	Gastric dilatation volvulus

(Continued)

Table 4.6 *(Continued).*

Abbreviation	Definition
GI	Gastrointestinal
g or gm	Gram
gr	Grain
gtt	Drop
HGE	Hemorrhagic gastroenteritis
IC	Intracardiac
ID	Intradermal
IM	Intramuscular
IV	Intravenous
IVC	Intravenous catheter
inj	Injection
L (l)	Liter
LDA/RDA	Left displaced abomasum/right displaced abomasum; condition in which the abomasum becomes trapped under the rumen.
meq	Milliequivalents
mg	Milligram
ml	Milliliter
mm	Millimeter
NG tube	Nasogastric tube
NPO	Nothing by mouth (nil per os)
oz	Ounce
pc	After meals (post cibum)
PO	By mouth (per os)
SQ or SC	Subcutaneous (sub Q)
# or lbs	Pounds
kg	Kilograms

Case Study: Give the medical terms and abbreviations for definitions in bold print. You'll notice some terms from the previous chapter

Maverick, a 3-year-old Shetland Sheepdog, presents to your clinic with **blood in the feces** and **vomiting blood**. On exam you notice a **condition of drowsiness**. Abdominal palpation is difficult because Maverick has hunched posture. He also appears to have a **condition of lack of fluid**. A **group of tests is performed to check for parasites**. After the tests come back negative a **diagnostic procedure using ultrasound waves** is performed. **Inflammation of the pancreas** is noted and a slight **enlargement of the liver** is seen.

An **IVC** is placed and Maverick is given **IV** fluids. He was **NPO** for 24 hours. A **substance is given to counteract the vomiting**. Blood work is performed and the lab results show that Maverick has a **blood condition of excessive sugar**. His **ALT** and **Alk. Phos.** are also elevated.

Maverick's owner asks that we give him eye drops that he usually gets each night. The directions are to give 2 **gtts** in each eye at night. Maverick is also given an **inj.** for the pain.

After 2 days of hospitalization, Maverick improves and is allowed to go home.

Exercises

4-A: Give the definition for the following:

1. adip/o, lip/o, and steat/o: _____
2. dent/i and odont/o: _____
3. -osis and -iasis: _____
4. or/o and stomat/o: _____
5. chol/e and bil/i _____
6. gloss/o and lingu/o: _____
7. labi/o and cheil/o: _____
8. lapar/o and celi/o: _____
9. hem/o and hemat/o: _____
10. gluc/o and glyc/o: _____

4-B: Give the structure for the following definitions.

1. _____: Throat
2. _____: Proximal small intestine
3. _____: Small blind sac between small and large intestine
4. _____: Distal large intestine
5. _____: Opening from the GI to outside of the body
6. _____: Organ that synthesizes protein and bile
7. _____: Tube from the throat to the stomach
8. _____: Sac that stores bile
9. _____: Large intestine
10. _____: Exocrine and endocrine organ

11. _____: Produces digestive enzymes and insulin
12. _____: Second part of small intestine
13. _____: Leaf-like piece of cartilage over the trachea
    to prevent aspiration of food
14. _____: Windpipe

4-C: Define the following terms.

1. Anorexia _____
2. Steatorrhea _____
3. Colostomy _____
4. Gastrectomy _____
5. Ascites _____
6. Dysphagia _____
7. Hepatitis _____
8. Fistula _____
9. Peristalsis _____
10. Scours _____

4-D: Give the term for the following definitions.

1. Surgical connection between two tubes _____
2. Ring-like muscles between the esophagus and stomach _____
3. Stricture of the ring-like muscles between the stomach
   and duodenum _____
4. Inflammation of the membrane surrounding the organs of the
   abdomen _____
5. Ridges on the roof of the mouth and in the stomach that increase
   surface area for absorption _____
6. Thin, muscular partition between the thoracic and abdominal
   cavities _____
7. Passage of feces through the anus to the outside of the
   body _____
8. Vomiting _____
9. Removal of tissue for microscopic exam _____
10. Ingestion of feces _____
11. Yellowish-orange coloration of the skin and mucous
    membranes _____
12. Enlargement of the esophagus _____
13. To bypass or divert _____
14. Condition of a shortened jaw _____
15. Hairball _____

4-E: Define the following terms.

1. Laparoscopy _____
2. Enterocolostomy _____
3. Glossitis _____

4. Hypoglycemia _____
5. Submandibular _____
6. Gingivitis _____
7. Cholecystectomy _____
8. Palatoplasty _____
9. Hyperbilirubinemia _____
10. Buccal _____

4-F: Define the following abbreviations.

1. _____: cc
2. _____: gr
3. _____: HGE
4. _____: GDV
5. _____: mg
6. _____: gm
7. _____: gtt
8. _____: ID
9. _____: IM
10. _____: IVC
11. _____: ml
12. _____: LDA
13. _____: pc
14. _____: meq
15. _____: PO

4-G: Circle the correct term in parentheses.

1. Route of administration other than oral: (parenteral, peritoneum)
2. Erosion of the skin and mucous membranes: (ulcer, mucocele)
3. Passive event in which swallowed food is returned to oral cavity: (vomit, regurgitation)
4. Intestines: (bowel, colon)
5. Telescoping of intestines: (obstipation, intussusception)
6. Acute abdominal pain: (ascites, colic)
7. Surgical fixation of the stomach: (gastropexy, gastrostomy)
8. Anastomosis of the stomach and second part of the small intestine: (gastroduodenostomy, gastrojejunostomy)
9. Swallowing: (mastication, deglutition)
10. Excessive thirst: (polydipsia, polyphagia)

4-H: Answer the following.

1. What is the dental formula for the dog? _____
2. How many incisors does a horse have? _____
3. Which organ stores glucose in the form of glycogen? _____
4. List the four parts of the ruminant stomach in order of occurrence. _____

5. The medical name for "puppy teeth" is _____.
6. Where does food go after leaving the cecum? _____
7. T or F: The correct spelling for chewing is mastification _____.
8. When the cause of disease is neither known nor understood, it is termed _____.
9. The synonymous term for jaundice is _____.
10. T or F: Unpleasant sensation and tendency to vomit defines flatus _____.
11. T or F: GERD results from a failure of the muscles of the esophagus to relax _____.
12. If a patient is jaundiced, what organ is of concern? _____.

4-I: Match the following terms with their descriptions.

1. _____ Twist on itself
2. _____ Incision of the common bile duct
3. _____ Formation of new sugar from proteins and fats
4. _____ Finger-like projections in the small intestines
5. _____ Hard, outermost layer of the crown of the tooth
6. _____ Tooth decay
7. _____ Chemical that speeds up a reaction
8. _____ Breakdown of fat
9. _____ Tissue composed of essential cells of any organ
10. _____ Small, raised bumps on the tongue

A. Choledochotomy
B. Dental caries
C. Emulsification
D. Enamel
E. Enzyme
F. Gluconeogenesis
G. Papillae
H. Parenchyma
I. Villi
J. Volvulus

Answers can be found starting on page 571.

Go to www.wiley.com/go/taibo/terminology to find additional learning materials for this chapter:

- A crossword puzzle
- Flashcards
- Audio clips to show how to pronounce terms
- Case studies
- Review questions
- The figures from the chapter in PowerPoint

5

The Reproductive System

Animal reproduction is a broad area of study. The foundation of reproduction is similar to that of humans–it takes two to tango. The union of sperm (male sex cell) and ovum (female sex cell) is required to produce offspring. We use the term theriogenology to describe the study of animal reproduction. This area includes obstetrics, gynecology, neonatology (study of newborns), artificial insemination, and embryo transfer.

The Male Reproductive System

The goal of both the male and female reproductive systems is to create life. Because the male reproductive system is the less complex of the two, this chapter will discuss the males first. The male reproductive organs produce and transport sperm out of the body and they produce hormones such as testosterone. Please note that the male reproductive system differs between species because some animals don't possess all of the organs discussed.

Spermatozoon

A spermatozoon (sperm cell) is the male gamete or sex cell (Figure 5.1). Its anatomy is simplistic, consisting of a head, midpiece, and tail. The head of the sperm contains the DNA material (chromosomes), as well as an acrosome, which allows the sperm cell to penetrate the ovum during fertilization. The midpiece contains the mitochondria of the cell, which provides energy. The tail consists of a single flagellum that is used for motility (movement). Approximately 300 million to 2 billion sperm are released from the dog during ejaculation (ejection of sperm and fluid from the urethra). Sperm concentrations vary depending on species. Only one sperm can fertilize an ovum. If there are multiple ova released during ovulation, then multiple ova will be fertilized.

Veterinary Medical Terminology Guide and Workbook, First Edition. Angela Taibo.
© 2014 John Wiley & Sons, Inc. Published 2014 by John Wiley & Sons, Inc.
Companion website: www.wiley.com/go/taibo/terminology

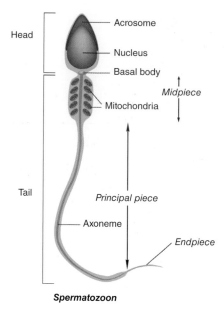

Head

Acrosome

Nucleus

Basal body

Midpiece

Mitochondria

Tail

Principal piece

Axoneme

Endpiece

Spermatozoon

Figure 5.1A   Anatomy of a sperm cell. Courtesy of shutterstock/Alila Sao Mai.

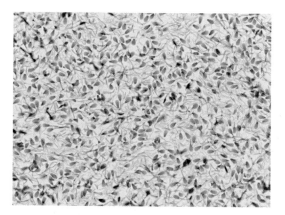

Figure 5.1B   Stained slide of spermatozoan from a bull. Courtesy of shutterstock/vetpathologist.

Anatomy and Physiology

The male gonads (sex organs) are the testicles, or testes (singular: testis). The testes develop in the abdomen of the male fetus and then descend into the scrotum before birth. If the testes fail to descend, it is termed cryptorchism.

The scrotum is a sac that encloses and supports the testes on the outside of the body. It provides an environment with a lower temperature than that of the normal body temperature. The lower temperature is necessary for the formation of sperm (spermatogenesis).

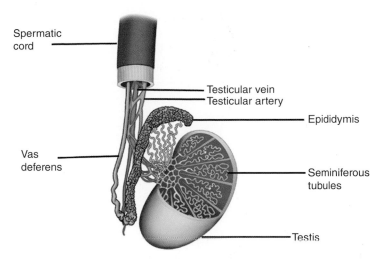

Figure 5.2   Structures of the testicle. Courtesy of shutterstock/Alex Luengo.

The area between the anus and genital organs is termed the perineum. Because we're describing the perineum in males, its meaning changes to the area between the anus and scrotum.

Throughout the testes are sections of coiled tubes called seminiferous tubules, which are the site of spermatogenesis. The seminiferous tubules are surrounded by two groups of interstitial cells (cells between spaces). The Sertoli cells line the inside of the tubules and provide nourishment to the developing sperm cells. Leydig's cells are those outside of the tubules and they produce the hormone testosterone.

Once sperm cells are produced, they move to the next structure of the male reproductive system, the epididymis. The epididymis is a large tube where sperm cells mature, become motile, and are stored before ejaculation. The epididymis runs the length of the testicle, eventually turning upward where it becomes a more narrow tube called the vas deferens, or ductus deferens (Figure 5.2).

The vas deferens carries sperm from the epididymis to the urethra (tube from the urinary bladder to the outside of the body). It is encased in a structure called the spermatic cord, which also contains nerves and blood vessels. The vas deferens merges with the seminal vesicles to form the ejaculatory duct. Seminal vesicles are two glands at the base of the urinary bladder. These two glands produce a thick, yellowish substance that nourishes the sperm and adds volume to the ejaculated fluid (semen). Semen is the combination of sperm and fluid.

The prostate gland is a single gland that encircles the urethra and secretes a thick fluid that aids in the motility of the sperm. Below, or caudal to, the prostate gland is a pair of glands called the bulbourethral glands which also secrete fluid into the urethra.

The urethra is a tube that extends from the urinary bladder, through the penis, to the outside of the body. This tube acts as both a reproductive organ (transports semen) and a urinary organ (transports urine).

The penis consists of the gland penis (sensitive tip), the prepuce (cutaneous sheath or foreskin), and erectile tissue (Figure 5.3). When an animal is sexually stimulated, the erectile tissue fills with blood, causing an erection. Some carnivores, such as dogs, also have a bone in their penis called the os penis. Figure 5.4 shows the passage of sperm through the male reproductive system.

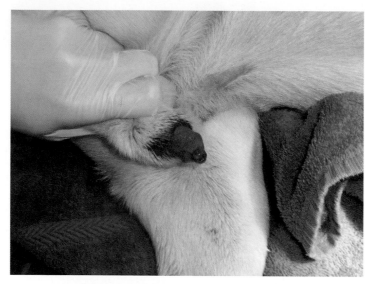

Figure 5.3   The prepuce and the glans penis of a dog. Courtesy of Deanna Roberts, BA, AAS, CVT.

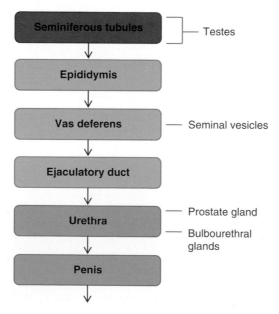

Figure 5.4   The passage of sperm through the male reproductive system.

Terms for the Male Reproductive System

Bulbourethral glands	Pair of glands below the prostate that secrete fluid into the urethra.
Ejaculation	Ejection of sperm and fluid from the male urethra.
Ejaculatory duct	Tube through which semen enters the urethra.
Epididymis	One of a pair of tightly coiled tubes lying on top of each testicle. They carry sperm from the seminiferous tubules to the vas deferens.
Flagellum	Hair-like projection on a sperm cell that makes it motile.
Gametes	Sex cell; sperm in males and ova in females.
Genitalia	Reproductive organs such as the ovaries, uterus, and vagina in females; the testes, penis, and vas deferens in males. Also called **genitals**.
Glans penis	Sensitive tip of the penis.
Gonads	Sex organs that produce gametes (sex cells). Testes in males and ovaries in females.
Intact	Male that has not been neutered; male that still has its reproductive capability.
Os penis	Bone found in the penis of some carnivores (Figure 5.5).
Perineum	In males, the area between the anus and scrotum.

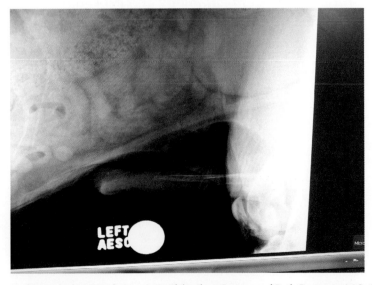

Figure 5.5   Radiograph showing the os penis of the dog. Courtesy of Beth Romano, AAS, CVT.

Prostate gland	Gland in males that surrounds the urethra. Depending on the species, it may be well defined or diffuse. It secretes a thick fluid that aids the motility of sperm.
Scrotum	External sac that contains the testes.
Semen	Spermatozoa and fluid.
Seminal vesicles	Pair of glands that secrete a fluid into the vas deferens.
Seminiferous tubules	Narrow, coiled tubules that produce sperm in the testes.
Spermatozoon (Plural: spermatozoa)	Sperm cell.
Sterility	Inability to reproduce.
Testes (Singular: testis)	Male gonads that produce spermatozoa and the hormone testosterone.
Testosterone	Hormone produced by the testes and responsible for male sex characteristics.
Urethra	In males, tube that carries urine and semen to the outside of the body. The tube extends from the urinary bladder, through the penis, to the outside of the body.
Vas deferens	Narrow tube that carries sperm from the epididymis toward the urethra. Also called the ductus deferens.

Male Reproductive System Pathology and Procedures

Azoospermia	Lack of spermatozoa in the semen.
Castration	Removal of gonads (sex organs).

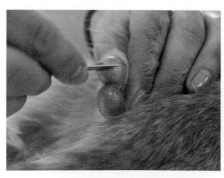

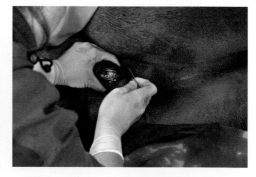

Figure 5.6A   Castration of a cat. Courtesy of shutterstock/Henk Vrieselaar.

Figure 5.6B   Equine castration. Courtesy of shutterstock/kiep.

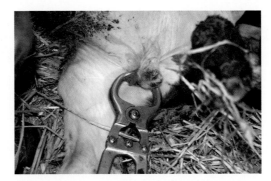

Figure 5.6C   Castration in a calf using Burdizzo forceps. This instrument crushes the blood vessels leading to the testicle so eventually they shrink and necrose. Courtesy of shutterstock/ Claudia Otte.

TECH TIP 5.1 Castration

Because the definition of castration is the removal of gonads, can females be castrated? The answer is yes. Castration is a generalized term; however, in veterinary medicine, it is most commonly used to describe the removal of male gonads.

Cryptorchism   Condition in which one or both testicles in undescended. Also called **cryptorchidism**. If only one testicle is undescended, then it is termed **monorchid**. If both are undescended, then the condition is termed **bilateral cryptorchism** (Figure 5.7).

(A)   (B)

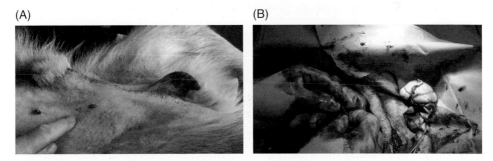

Figure 5.7   Cryptorchism. Courtesy of Greg Martinez, DVM; www.youtube.com/drgregdvm. (A) Monorchid. Note the absence of one testicle. (B) Monorchid. Testicle has been found in the abdominal cavity.

Electroejaculation   Method used for the collection of semen for artificial insemination or for examination. Electrical stimulation is provided by electrodes to the nerves to promote ejaculation. The rectal probe used is called an electroejaculator (Figure 5.8).

(A)

(B)

(C)

(D)

(E)

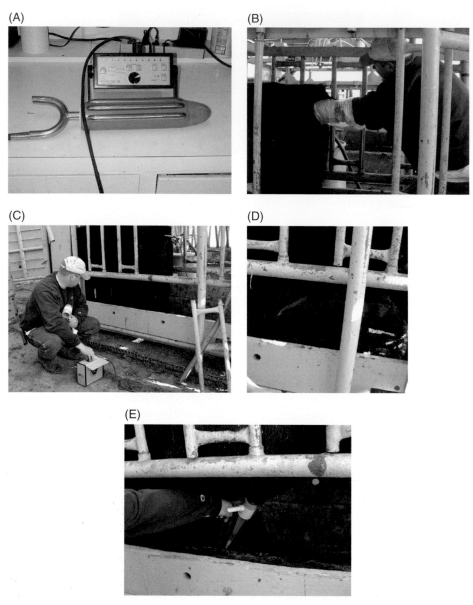

Figure 5.8 Electroejaculation. Courtesy of Patrick Hemming, DVM. (A) Lane electroejaculator probe. (B) Electroejaculator probe insertion. (C) Adjusting the power on the electroejaculator. (D) Erection caused by the probe. (E) Collection of semen.

Neuter	Removal of male gonads; orchiectomy (Figure 5.6).
Paraphimosis	Inability to retract the penis due to its swollen state or due to the constriction of the preputial orifice.
Persistent frenulum	Incomplete separation of the penis and prepuce which causes an inability to breed.

Phimosis	Constriction of the orifice of the prepuce preventing it from drawing back over the glans penis.
Priapism	Persistent erection of the penis due to injury or disease. Causes include injuries to the spinal cord or penis.
Scrotal hydrocele	Swelling of the scrotum due to a collection of fluid in the testes or along the spermatic cord.
Semen analysis	Testing done to evaluate a male as a potential breeder. Examinations include evaluation of motility, morphology, and concentration of sperm cells.

Building the Terms

Table 5.1   Chapter 5 Male Combining Forms.

Combining Forms	Definition	Combining Forms	Definition
Balan/o	Glans penis	**Priap/o**	Penis
Crypt/o	Hidden	**Prostat/o**	Prostate gland
Epididym/o	Epididymis	**Semin/i**	Semen; seed
Gen/o	Producing	**Sperm/o**	Spermatozoa; semen
Hydr/o	Fluid; water	**Spermat/o**	Spermatozoa; semen
Later/o	Side	**Test/o**	Testis; testicles
Orch/o	Testis; testicles	**Theri/o**	Beast
Orchi/o	Testis; testicles	**Urethr/o**	Urethra
Orchid/o	Testis; testicles	**Vas/o**	Vessel; vas deferens
Pen/i	Penis	**Zo/o**	Animal life

Table 5.2   Chapter 5 Male Prefixes.

Prefix	Definition	Prefix	Definition
a-, an-	no; not; without	**mono-**	one; single
bi-	two; both	**oligo-**	scanty

Table 5.3 Chapter 5 Male Suffixes.

Suffix	Definition	Suffix	Definition
-al, -ar	pertaining to	**-logy**	study of
-cele	hernia	**-lytic**	to reduce; to destroy; separate; breakdown
-ectomy	removal; excision; resection	**-megaly**	enlargement
-genesis	producing; forming	**-one**	hormone
-ia	condition	**-pexy**	surgical fixation; to put in place
-ism	process; condition	**-stomy**	new opening; anastomosis
-itis	inflammation	**-tomy**	incision; process of cutting

Note: Remember your rules for the use of the suffix "-stomy."

Now it's time to put these word parts together. If you memorize the meaning of the combining forms, prefixes, and suffixes, then this will get easier each time. Remember your five basic rules to medical terminology when building and defining these terms. You'll notice some word parts are repeated from the previous chapters.

Parts			Medical Term	Definition
Balan/o	+ -itis	=	Balanitis	: _____
Epididym/o	+ -itis	=	Epididymitis	: _____
an-	+ Orch/o + -ism	=	Anorchism	: _____
Orch/o	+ -itis	=	Orchitis	: _____
Orchi/o	+ -pexy	=	Orchiopexy	: _____
Orchi/o	+ -ectomy	=	Orchiectomy	: _____
				This is the medical term for a neuter.
Prostat/o	+ -ectomy	=	Prostatectomy	: _____
Prostat/o	+ -itis	=	Prostatitis	: _____

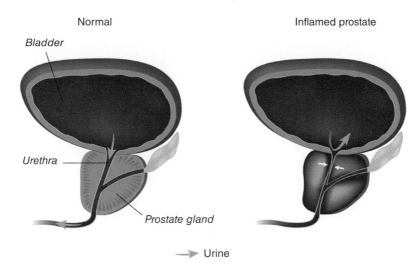

Normal

Inflamed prostate

Bladder

Urethra

Prostate gland

→ Urine

Figure 5.9   Comparison of a normal prostate gland with prostatitis. Courtesy of shutterstock/Alila Medical Images.

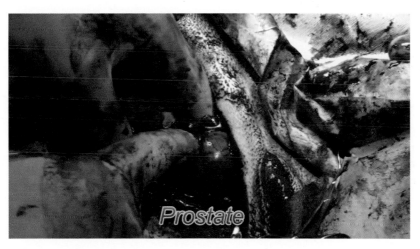

Prostate

Figure 5.10   Inflamed prostate. Courtesy of Greg Martinez, DVM; www.youtube.com/drgregdvm.

Prostat/o   + -megaly   =   Prostatomegaly   : _____

a-   + Sperm/o + -ia =   Aspermia   : _____

oligo-   + Sperm/o + -ia =   Oligospermia   : _____

Sperm/o   + -lytic   =   Spermolytic   : _____

Spermat/o   + -genesis   =   Spermatogenesis   : _____

Testicul/o   + -ar   =   Testicular   : _____

Vas/o   + -ectomy   =   Vasectomy   : _____

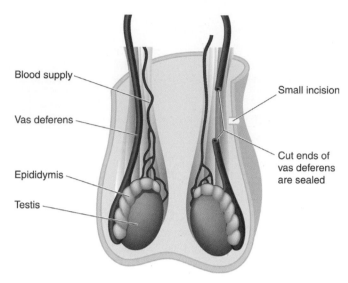

Blood supply

Vas deferens

Epididymis

Testis

Small incision

Cut ends of
vas deferens
are sealed

Figure 5.11   Diagram of a vasectomy procedure. Courtesy of shutterstock/blamb.

Vas/o + Vas/o + -stomy   =   Vasovasostomy   : _____

This is the reversal of a vasectomy. "-stomy" means anastomosis in this term because it is attached to two structures. In this case it is the anastomosis of the ends of the severed vas deferens.

The Female Reproductive System

While the goal of both reproductive systems is to create life, the female reproductive system must also support life.

Ovaries

The ovaries are a pair of female gonads (sex organs) on each side of the pelvis. They produce ova (eggs) and the hormones estrogen and progesterone. Within the ovary are small sacs called follicles that contain the ova and their encasing cells. There are different kinds of follicles within the ovary that are named based on the age of the ovum they contain (Figure 5.12).

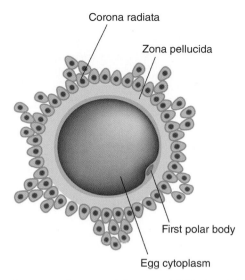

Figure 5.12A   Anatomy of an ovum. Courtesy of shutterstock/Alila Sao Mai.

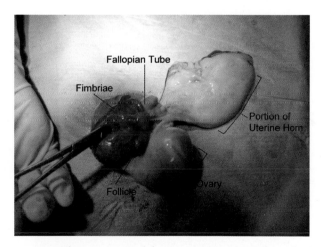

Figure 5.12B   Equine ovary. This was removed during a necropsy. Note the multiple follicles at various stages of development.

Uterine Tubes

Once the ovum has matured in the ovary, it passes into the uterine tubes. These tubes are equivalent to the fallopian tubes in humans. They are sometimes referred to as fallopian tubes or oviducts. On the ends of the uterine tubes are finger-like projections called fimbriae, which "catch" the ovum once it is released from the ovary. The ovum then travels through the uterine tubes to the uterine horns. The uterine tubes are also used for the passage of sperm and are the site of fertilization (union of sperm and ovum).

Uterus

The uterus is a hollow, muscular organ in females which includes two uterine horns (cornus), a uterine body (corpus), and the cervix (neck). Uterine horns are a pair of tubes extending from the uterine tubes to the body of the uterus. It is the uterine horns that make animals adapted for litter bearing. The uterine horns are larger in species that bear multiple offspring. These animals are referred to as bicornuate.

The body of the uterus is the mid-portion of the uterus (Figure 5.13).

The caudal aspect of the uterus is called the cervix. It extends from the uterine body to the vagina. The cervix remains closed unless the animal is in heat (estrus). Estrus is the time of sexual receptivity. When the animal goes into heat, the cervix relaxes its sphincters to allow for the passage of sperm. When the heat cycle ends, the sphincters close. If the animal becomes pregnant, the cervix is closed with a mucous plug. The mucous plug breaks off when an animal is about to give birth to allow for the passage of the offspring.

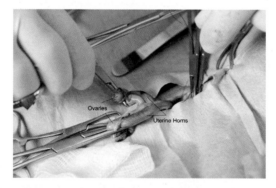

Figure 5.13A   Routine spay surgery showing the uterine horns and ovaries about to be removed. Courtesy of shutterstock/CREATISTA.

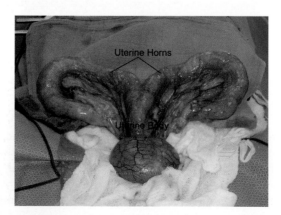

Figure 5.13B   Pyometra in a dog. Note the swollen uterine horns filled with pus. Courtesy of Deanna Roberts, BA, AAS, CVT.

All three portions of the uterus have three layers of tissue. The endometrium is the inner lining of the uterus and is lined with mucous membranes. The myometrium is the muscular lining of the uterus and the perimetrium is the membrane surrounding the uterus (Figure 5.14).

> **TECH TIP 5.2 Rules for the Prefixes "endo-," "myo-," and "peri-"**
>
> When "endo-," "myo-," and "peri-" are attached to organs, their meanings change. "Endo-" means the inner lining of that organ, "myo-" means the muscle lining of that organ, and "peri-" means the membrane surrounding that organ.

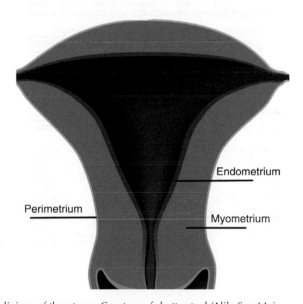

Figure 5.14   The linings of the uterus. Courtesy of shutterstock/Alila Sao Mai.

The Vagina and Vulva

The vagina is the tube that extends from the cervix to the outside of the body. Cattle, sheep, and cats have a pair of glands on either side of their vaginal orifice (opening) called Bartholin glands which produce a mucous secretion that helps lubricate the vaginal orifice during copulation (sexual intercourse) and birth.

There is a membranous fold that partially or completely closes the vaginal orifice in some species, called the hymen; however, it is different than what is thought of in humans. In general, most domestic animals lack a true hymen.

The external genitalia of the female is called the vulva. Primates have two pairs of skin folds that protect the vaginal orifice, whereas carnivores have one pair.

These skin folds are called labia (lips). On the ventral aspect of the vulva is a small, elongated, erectile portion of tissue called a clitoris. The clitoris in females is homologous to the glans penis in males.

The area between the anus and genital organs is called the perineum. Because we're describing the perineum in a female, its meaning changes to the area between the anus and vagina. This area is sometimes torn during parturition (giving birth) so veterinarians may elect to cut the perineum before the female gives birth and then suture the area after delivery. This procedure is called an episiotomy.

Mammary Glands

The milk-producing glands of females are called mammary glands. The term breast isn't used in veterinary medicine. In large animals, the mammary glands are referred to as udders. Males of each species have rudimentary (imperfect) mammary glands.

The number of mammary glands varies with each species. Horses, goats, sheep, and guinea pigs have two mammary glands. Cattle have four mammary glands. Litter-bearing species have four or more pairs of mammary glands.

The location of the mammary glands also varies with each species. Some species have mammary glands in their inguinal region, whereas others have them along their ventral abdomen and thorax.

The fleshy projection on each mammary gland is called the nipple. After milk has been produced by the mammary gland, it exits through the nipple. In ruminants, they are called teats (Figure 5.15).

Mammary glands are made up of alveolar tissue (glandular tissue), adipose tissue, fibrous connective tissue, lactiferous ducts, and sinuses. Alveolar tissue consists of milk-secreting glands called alveoli. When an animal becomes pregnant,

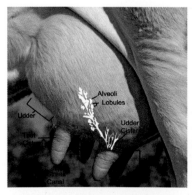

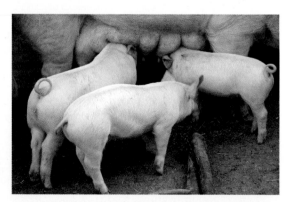

Figure 5.15A   Anatomy of a cow's mammary gland. Internal structures have been superimposed on the actual image. Courtesy of shutterstock/smereka.

Figure 5.15B   Piglets nursing. Courtesy of shutterstock/InavanHateren.

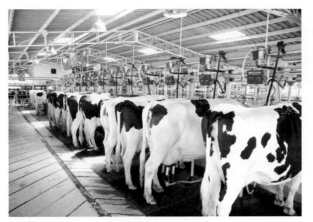

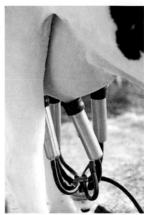

Figure 5.15C   Milking facility. Courtesy of shutterstock/basketman23.

Figure 5.15D   Cow milking tubes. Courtesy of shutterstock/2bears.

hormones from the ovaries and placenta stimulate the alveolar tissue of the mammary glands to further development. After parturition, hormone changes cause the mammary glands to produce milk (lactation).

Once produced, the milk travels towards the nipple (teat) through lactiferous ducts and lactiferous sinuses (cavities). Another name for the lactiferous sinus is the gland cistern. Milk travels from the lactiferous sinus, which is at the base of the teat, to the teat sinus (teat cistern). When an animal becomes pregnant, hormones from the ovaries and placenta stimulate the alveolar tissue of the mammary glands.

Estrous Cycle

The estrous cycle is comprised of four phases: proestrus, estrus, diestrus, and anestrus. The common name of the estrous cycle is a heat cycle. During this cycle, males are attracted to females and females are receptive to the males. In most cases ovulation has just occurred or is about to occur. Besides behavior, some species display changes to their external genitalia. While the behavior and external changes vary from species to species, the basic physiology of the cycle is the same.

Proestrus

The anterior pituitary gland releases a hormone called follicle-stimulating hormone (FSH) which has two effects on the ovaries. FSH stimulates the maturation of ova in the Gratian follicles. It also causes the ovaries to release estrogen in anticipation of a possible pregnancy. The estrogen causes the cells in the vagina to become cornified. Behaviorally the males are attracted to the females, but the

TECH TIP 5.3 **Types of Estrous Cycles**

Different species have different frequencies of estrous cycles. Below is a list of different types of estrous cycles.

Induced ovulators	Animal that releases ovum after copulation. Examples include cats, camelids (alpacas and llamas), rabbits, and ferrets.
Monestrous	Animal has one estrous cycle per year.
Polyestrous	Animal has multiple estrous cycles per year.
Seasonal	Animal has an estrous cycle at a specific time of year. For example, cats are polyestrous from February to October. Horses are polyestrous as well, but their cycle centers around the length of daylight. Their breeding season runs from April to September.
Spontaneous ovulators	Animal in which estrus occurs cyclically.

females do not accept them. Animals may have a serosanguineous (thin, light red) to bloody discharge.

Estrus

Estrus is the time of sexual receptivity. During estrus, luteinizing hormone (LH) is released by the anterior pituitary, causing the Graafian follicle to rupture and release the ovum from the ovary. This process is known as ovulation (Figure 5.16).

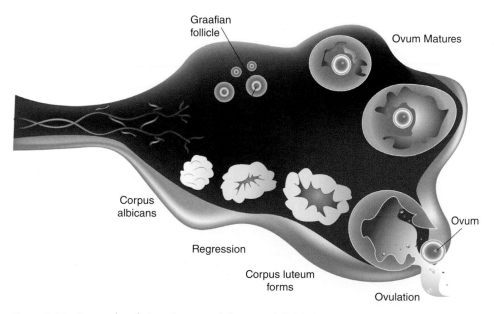

Figure 5.16   Stages of ovulation. Courtesy of shutterstock/GRei.

> **TECH TIP 5.4   Estrous or Estrus?**
>
> Be careful with the spelling of these two terms because the meaning changes with the addition of the letter "o." Estrous with the "o" is the term for the entire cycle. Estrus without the "o" is a stage within the cycle. Therefore, estrus is one of several stages of estrous.

Once ovulation occurs, the ovum moves into the uterine tubes. If sperm is present at that point then the ovum will be fertilized.

LH also plays a role in the formation of the corpus luteum. When the follicle ruptures, it fills with a yellow substance and begins secreting progesterone. This yellow secreting mass of the ovary is the corpus luteum. The progesterone that's secreted prepares the lining of the uterus for implantation.

If an animal fails to conceive, then the corpus luteum will regress and reduce its secretion of progesterone. As the corpus luteum shrinks, it is replaced with white fibrous tissue and becomes a corpus albicans. If the animal does conceive, the corpus luteum will continue to secrete progesterone to prevent future estrus cycles.

Behaviorally males are attracted to the female and she's accepting of them.

Diestrus

Diestrus is the resting period that follows estrus. Estrogen levels decrease and the females begin rejecting the males. The cornified cells quickly disappear. This is why vaginal cytologies can be so useful in determining stages of heat. Progesterone levels may still be increased in anticipation of possible fetal implantation and development. Ultimately the levels should eventually decrease if fertilization does not occur.

In some cases, hormone levels fail to decrease and the body develops all of the signs of pregnancy, even though the animal isn't pregnant. This condition is known as pseudocyesis or false pregnancy. Pseudocyesis can be seen in any species, but is most commonly seen in dogs. There are different theories as to the exact cause of pseudocyesis. In fact, there is also a disagreement on whether it is breed specific. Some journals believe Pointers, Dalmatians, and Basset Hounds are more susceptible.

Anestrus

Anestrus is the time of the estrous cycle in which the female is not sexually receptive.

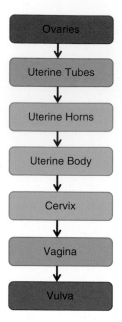

Figure 5.17 The path of ovum during ovulation.

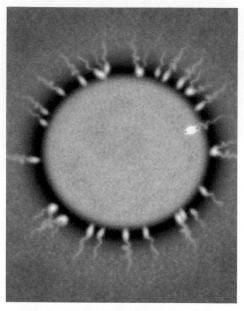

Figure 5.18 Sperm fertilizing an ovum. Courtesy of Getty Images/Chad Baker/Photodisk.

Pregnancy

Fertilization is the union of sperm and ovum (Figure 5.18). If fertilization succeeds, then the fertilized egg will implant in the endometrium. The condition of having a developing fetus in the uterus is termed gestation (pregnancy).

The endometrium and chorion (outermost membrane surrounding the embryo) form a vascular organ called the placenta (Figure 5.19). The placenta is the site of communication between the maternal and fetal bloodstreams. The bloodstreams never mix; instead, various soluble substances are transferred from the maternal blood to the fetal blood in the placenta (Figure 5.20).

Once the fetal blood receives vital nutrients from the maternal blood, it travels from the placenta back to the fetus via the umbilical cord. The umbilical cord extends from the placenta to the umbilicus (navel) of the developing embryo.

The developing embryo is surrounded by a series of membranes called fetal membranes. The innermost membrane is called the amnion, or amniotic sac (Figure 5.19). The amnion contains fluid in which the embryo is suspended, called amniotic fluid.

If the fetus is capable of living outside the mother, then it is termed viable. The time at which a fetus becomes viable depends on the species because the length of gestation varies in different species.

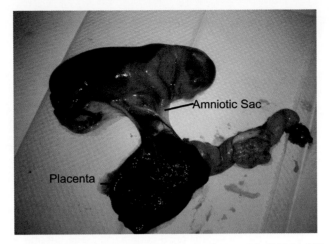

Figure 5.19 Canine fetus with placenta. Courtesy of Amy Johnson, BS, CVT, RLATG.

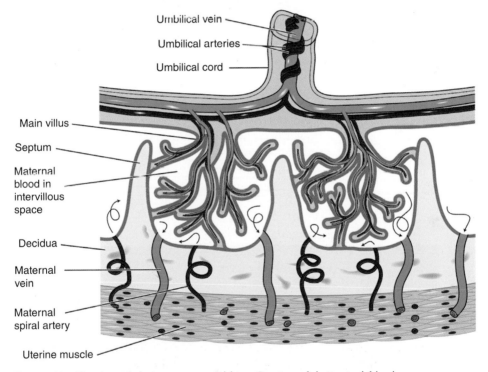

Figure 5.20 Blood supply between mom and fetus. Courtesy of shutterstock/blamb.

TECH TIP 5.5 The Ruminant Placenta

The anatomy is slightly different in ruminants. A pregnant cow develops fleshy masses on the wall of her uterus called caruncles. The ruminant placenta develops elevations called cotyledons, which adhere to the maternal caruncles. When the caruncle and cotyledon unite, they form a placentome.

TECH TIP 5.6 **Different Types of Placentation**

Placentation refers to the structure and formation of the placenta. Placentation can vary among different species. There are three types of placentation: endotheliochorial placentation, epitheliochorial placentation, and hemochorial placentation. The different types of placentation are based on the number of tissue layers separating the maternal and fetal blood supplies.

Endotheliochorial placentation is seen in dogs and cats. In this instance, the uterine endothelium is in contact with the chorion of the embryo. With epitheliochorial placentation, which is most often seen in horses and cattle, there are three tissue layers in contact with the chorion: maternal connective tissue, uterine endothelium, and endometrial epithelium. Hemochorial placentation is seen in most lab animals and humans. In this type of placentation, the maternal blood is in direct contact with the chorion of the embryo.

Terms for the Female Reproductive System

Amnion	Innermost membrane around the developing embryo; **amniotic sac.**
Amniotic fluid	Fluid contained within the amnion.
Cervix	Lower neck-like portion of the uterus.
Chorion	Outermost membrane surrounding the embryo.
Clitoris	Small, elongated, erectile portion of tissue on the ventral aspect of the vulva.
Coitus	Sexual intercourse; also called **copulation** (Figure 5.21).

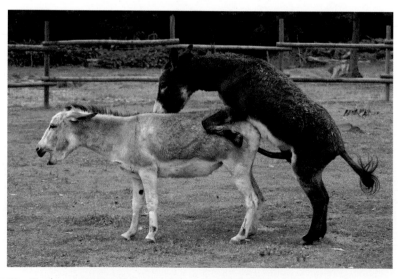

Figure 5.21 Donkey mounting. Courtesy of shutterstock/Four Oaks.

| Colostrum | First milk-like substance produced by the female after parturition (birth); high in protein and antibodies (Figure 5.22). |

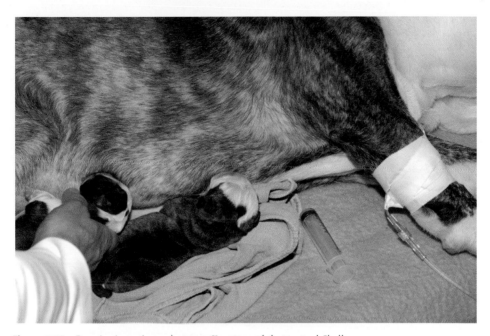

Figure 5.22   Puppies ingesting colostrum. Courtesy of shutterstock/jkelly.

Conception	The onset of pregnancy.
Embryo	Early stage of development from fertilization to when major structures begin to develop.
Endometrium	Inner lining of the uterus.
Estrogen	Hormone produced by the ovaries and responsible for the female secondary sex characteristics.
Estrus	Time of sexual receptivity; also known as **heat**.
Fertilization	The union of sperm and ovum; **conception**.
Fetus	Later stages of development after major structures have developed.
Fimbriae	Finger-like projections at the ends of the uterine tubes (fallopian tubes).
Follicle-stimulating hormone (FSH)	Hormone produced by the pituitary to stimulate the maturation of ovum.
Gestation	Length of pregnancy.
Genital lock	Male and female canine become locked together during coitus due to erectile tissue. Commonly called a **"tie."**

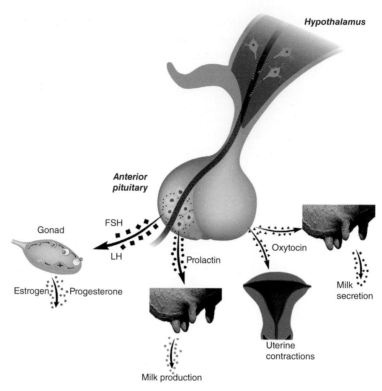

Figure 5.23 The effects of the pituitary on the female reproductive system. Courtesy of shutterstock/ Alila Sao Mai.

TECH TIP 5.7 Length of Gestation

Please note that these are averages.

Dogs and cats	62–65 days
Cattle	283 days
Ferret	42 days
Gerbils	24 days
Guinea pigs	63–68 days
Horses	330 days
Hamsters	15–18 days
Llamas and alpacas	344 days
Mice	20 days
Pigs	114 days
Rabbits	30 days
Sheep and goats	150 days

Hymen	Membranous fold that partially or completely closes the vaginal orifice.
Implantation	Attachment of the fertilized egg (**zygote**) to the uterus.
Involution of the uterus	The uterus returns to its normal non-pregnant size.
Lactation	The normal secretion of milk.
Litter	Group of offspring born during the same labor.
Luteinizing hormone (LH)	Hormone produced by the pituitary to promote ovulation.
Meconium	First feces of the newborn.
Mount	Preparatory step to mating of animals.
Myometrium	Muscle lining of the uterus.
Neonate	Newborn.
Ovaries	Pair of female organs on either side of the pelvis that produce estrogen and progesterone.

TECH TIP 5.8 Can an Animal Have Both Sex Organs?

Animals may be born with both ovaries and testes. These animals are referred to as hermaphrodites. In most cases, the sex organs are nonfunctional. Hermaphrodites may have tissue from both sets of sex organs or the full organs themselves.

Ovulation	Release of ovum from the ovary.
Ovum (Plural: ova)	Female gamete (sex cell).
Oxytocin	Hormone produced by the pituitary to stimulate the uterus to contract as well as milk secretion.
Parturition	The act of giving birth (Figure 5.24).

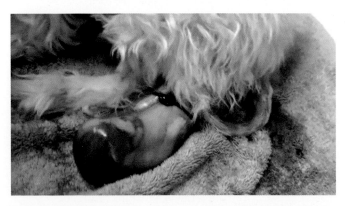

Figure 5.24   Shih Tzu giving birth. Courtesy of Greg Martinez, DVM; www.youtube.com/drgregdvm.

Perineum	In females, the area between the anus and vagina.
Pituitary gland	Endocrine gland at the base of the brain that produces FSH and LH; also called the **master gland** or **hypophysis.**
Placenta	Vascular organ that develops in the uterine wall during pregnancy. Used for communication between maternal and fetal blood.
Pregnancy	Condition of having a developing embryo or fetus in the body. (Figure 5.25).

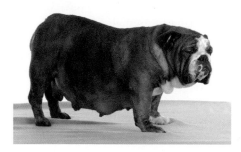

Figure 5.25A   Pregnant bulldog, 59 days along. Courtesy of shutterstock/WilleeCole.

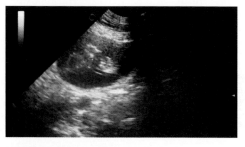

Figure 5.25B   Fetal ultrasound. Courtesy of Greg Martinez, DVM; www.youtube.com/drgregdvm.

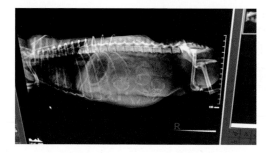

Figure 5.25C   Radiograph to determine how many puppies the bitch will have.

TECH TIP 5.9 Types of Pregnancies

Multipara (multiparous)	Female having two or more pregnancies resulting in viable offspring.
Multigravida	Female has been pregnant at least twice.
Nullipara (nulliparous)	Female has never had a pregnancy resulting in viable offspring.
Nulligravida	Female has never been pregnant.
Primipara (primiparous)	Female has had one pregnancy resulting in viable offspring.
Primigravida	Female is pregnant for the first time.

Presentation	Orientation of the fetus before delivery.
Progesterone	Hormone produced by the ovaries during pregnancy to protect the embryo and stimulate lactation.
Umbilicus	Navel.
Urethra	Tube that carries urine from the urinary bladder to the outside of the body.
Uterine horns	Pair of tubes extending from the uterine tubes to the body of the uterus. Makes animals adapted for litter bearing.
Uterine tubes	Pair of ducts through which the ovum travels to the uterine horns. Also called the **fallopian tubes**.
Uterus	The womb. Consists of three sections: the uterine horns, uterine body, and cervix.
Vagina	Tube extending from the uterus to the outside of the body.
Vaginal orifice	Opening of the vagina.
Viable	Capable of living outside the uterus.
Vulva	External genitalia of the female (Figure 5.26).
Wean	Remove the young from the mother so that they no longer nurse.

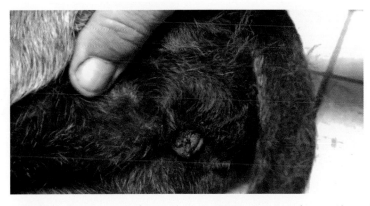

Figure 5.26   Inverted vulva. Courtesy of Greg Martinez, DVM; www.youtube.com/drgregdvm.

Female Reproductive System Pathology and Procedures

Abortion	Spontaneous or induced termination of pregnancy before the fetus is viable.
Artificial insemination	Implanting of live sperm into the female genital tract.
Assisted delivery	Aiding delivery of a fetus through use of equipment or hands (Figure 5.27).

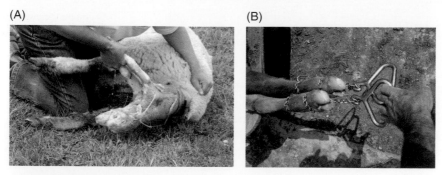

Figure 5.27 Examples of assisted delivery. A. Assisting in delivery of a lamb. Courtesy of shutterstock/Margo Harrison. B. Assisted delivery of a calf using chains and handles. Courtesy of Patrick Hemming, DVM.

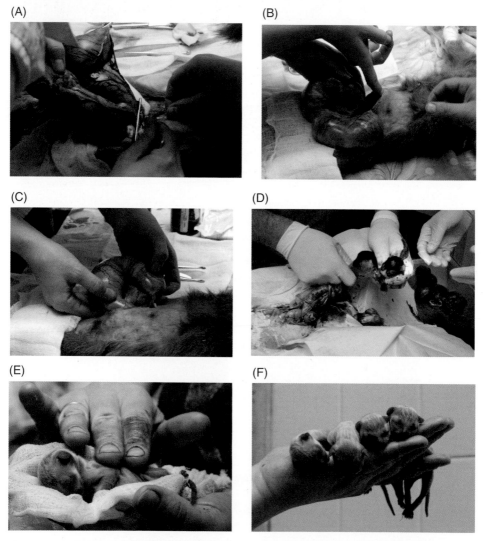

Figure 5.28 Cesarean section (C-section) of kittens. C-sections should always be performed using sterile technique which includes sterile gloves. This particular surgery was performed in a small clinic in Russia where doctors would sometimes perform a pre-surgical scrub and then perform routine surgeries with ungloved hands. Courtesy of shutterstock/kotomiti. (A-C) Uterine horns containing kittens. (D) Removal of the kittens. (E) Stimulating the newborn to breathe. (F) Four healthy kittens.

| Cesarean section | Removal of the fetus by abdominal incision; also spelled **caesarean section** (Figure 5.28). |
| Congenital anomaly | Malformation present at or existing from birth (Figure 5.29). **Congenital** means present at or existing from birth. An **anomaly** is a defect or malformation. |

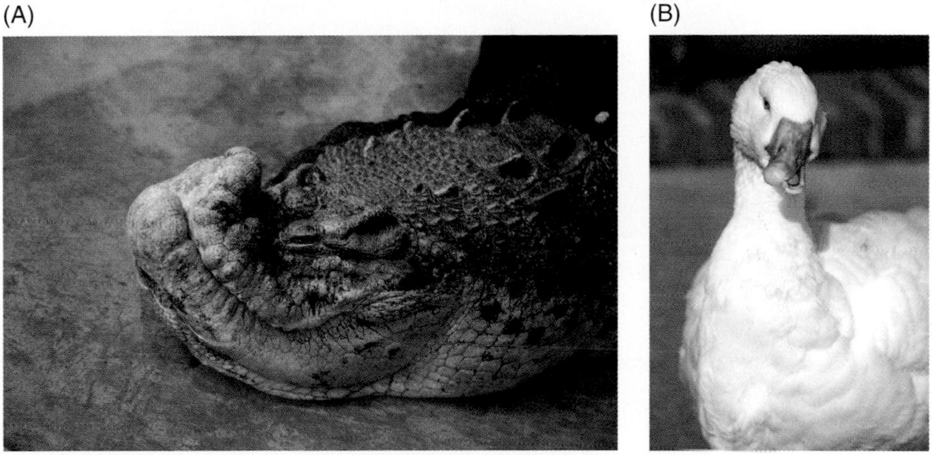

(A)   (B)

Figure 5.29   Examples of congenital anomalies. (A) Deformed mouth on a crocodile. Courtesy of shutterstock/Shunsho. (B) Deformed beak on a goose. Courtesy of shutterstock/chris2766.

Eclampsia	Decreased calcium during lactation causing convulsions and coma; commonly called **milk fever** in most species. Cattle have a similar disorder called **periparturient hypocalcemia**.
Ectopic pregnancy	Fertilized ovum becomes implanted outside the uterus.
Embryo transfer	Transfer of fertilized ova from one female to another. Typically done with cattle.
Episiotomy	Incision through the skin of the perineum to enlarge the vaginal opening for delivery.
Fetotomy	Surgical excision of a fetus; also known as **embryotomy** or **abortion**.
Galactorrhea	Abnormal, persistent discharge of milk.
Hydrocephalus	Abnormal accumulation of fluid in the spaces of the brain. Commonly called water on the brain.
Leukorrhea	Sticky, white discharge from the vagina indicative of a disease elsewhere in the reproductive system.
Malpresentation	Faulty fetal presentation.
Pneumovagina	Involuntary aspiration of air into the vagina due to a conformational defect. Seen in cattle and horses. Animals are commonly referred to as **windsuckers**.
Pyometra	Pus in the uterus (Figure 5.30).

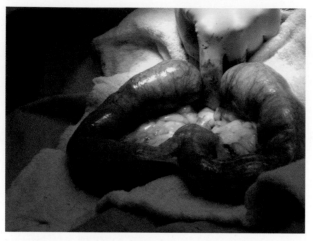

Figure 5.30   Pyometra in a dog. Courtesy of AK Traylor, DVM; Microscopy Learning Systems.

TECH TIP 5.10 What is pus?

Pus is a protein-rich inflammatory product which consists of white blood cells, thin fluid, and cellular debris.

Retained placenta	Failure to pass the placenta after delivery of the fetus. Causes metritis and eventually infertility.
Ultrasound	Diagnostic technique using ultrasound waves to produce an image of an organ or tissue.
Uterine prolapse	Displacement of the uterus through the vaginal orifice (Figure 5.31).

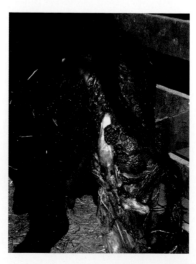

Figure 5.31   Uterine prolapse in a cow. Note the caruncles from the endometrium.

Vaginal cytology   Study of cells from the vagina to determine stage of heat.
Vaginal prolapse   Displacement of the vagina through the vaginal orifice.

Building the Terms

Table 5.4   Chapter 5 Female Combining Forms.

Combining Forms	Definition	Combining Forms	Definition
Amni/o	Amnion (amniotic sac)	**Nat/i**	Birth
Cervic/o	Cervix; neck	**O/o**	Egg
Colp/o	Vagina	**Obstetr/o**	Midwife; one who receives
Cyt/o	Cell	**Oophor/o**	Ovary
Episi/o	Vulva	**Ov/i**	Egg
Galact/o	Milk	**Ov/o**	Egg
Genit/o	Related to birth; reproductive organs	**Ovari/o**	Ovary
Gest/o	Pregnancy	**Ovul/o**	Egg
Gestat/o	Pregnancy	**Part/o**	Birth; labor
Gester/o	Pregnancy	**Parturit/o**	Birth; labor
Gynec/o	Woman	**Perine/o**	Perineum
Hyster/o	Uterus; womb	**Py/o**	Pus
Lact/o	Milk	**Radi/o**	X-rays; radius; radioactivity
Later/o	Side	**Salping/o**	Fallopian tubes; uterine tubes; auditory (Eustachian) tubes
Mamm/o	Mammary glands	**Umbilic/o**	Umbilicus; navel
Mast/o	Mammary glands	**Uter/o**	Uterus; womb
Metr/o	Uterus; womb; measure	**Vagin/o**	Vagina
Metri/o	Uterus; womb	**Viv/o**	Life
My/o	Muscle	**Vulv/o**	Vulva

Table 5.5   Chapter 5 Female Prefixes.

Prefix	Definition	Prefix	Definition
a-, an-	no; not; without	**nulli-**	none
ante-	before; forward	**oxy-**	sharp; swift; rapid; acid; oxygen; quick
bi-	two; both	**peri-**	surrounding
di-	twice	**post-**	after; behind
dys-	bad; painful; difficult; abnormal	**pre-**	before
in-	in; into; not	**primi-**	first
intra	within; into	**pro-**	before; forward
multi-	many	**pseudo-**	false
neo-	new	**vivi-**	live; life

Table 5.6   Chapter 5 Female Suffixes.

Suffixes	Definition	Suffixes	Definition
-al, -an, -ary	pertaining to	**-mortem**	death
-ation	process; condition	**-osis**	abnormal condition
-centesis	surgical puncture to remove fluid	**-para**	to bear; bring forth (live births)
-cyesis	pregnancy	**-parous**	to bear; bring forth
-cyte	cell	**-partum**	birth; labor
-ectomy	removal; excision; resection	**-plasty**	surgical repair
-genesis	producing; forming	**-rrhaphy**	suture
-graphy	process or recording	**-rrhea**	flow; discharge
-gravida	pregnancy	**-scopy**	visual examination
-itis	inflammation	**-tocia**	labor; birth
-ium	structure; tissue	**-tomy**	incision; process of cutting
-logy	study of	**-version**	to turn

Now it's time to put these word parts together. If you memorize the meaning of the combining forms, prefixes, and suffixes, then this will get easier each time. Remember your five basic rules to medical terminology when building and defining these terms. You'll notice some word parts are repeated from the previous chapter.

Parts			Medical Term	Definition
Amni/o	+ -centesis		= Amniocentesis	: _____
Cervic/o	+ -itis		= Cervicitis	: _____
Cervic/o	+ -al		= Cervical	: _____
endo-	+ Cervic/o	+ -itis	= Endocervicitis	: _____

Remember your rules for the prefix "endo-."

Parts			Medical Term	Definition
Colp/o	+ -scopy		= Colposcopy	: _____
Colp/o	+ -rrhaphy		= Colporrhaphy	: _____
Cyt/o	+ -logy		= Cytology	: _____
a-	+ Galact/o	+ -ia	= Agalactia	: _____
Hyster/o	+ -ectomy		= Hysterectomy	: _____
Hyster/o	+ -scopy		= Hysteroscopy	: _____
Lact/o	+ -genesis		= Lactogenesis	: _____
Mamm/o	+ -ary		= Mammary	: _____
Mamm/o	+ -ary		= Mammary	
	+ Carcin/o	+-oma	carcinoma	: _____

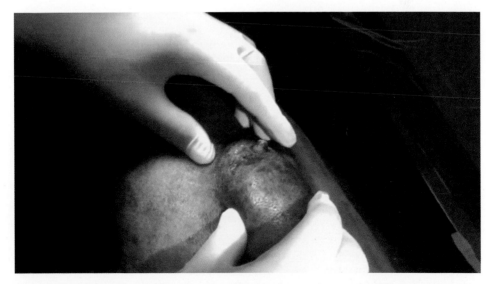

Figure 5.32A   Mammary carcinoma in a dog. Chances of cancer increase by 10% each time a female goes into heat. Courtesy of Greg Martinez, DVM; www.youtube.com/drgregdvm.

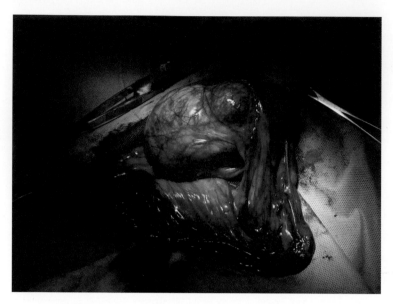

Figure 5.32B   Ovarian carcinoma in a dog. Courtesy of shutterstock/P Fabian.

Mamm/o	+ -plasty		= Mammoplasty	:	_____
Mast/o	+ -itis		= Mastitis	:	_____
Mast/o	+ -ectomy		= Mastectomy	:	_____
Metr/o	+ -itis		= Metritis	:	_____
endo-	+ Metr/o	+ -itis	= Endometritis	:	_____
endo-	+ Metri/o	+ -osis	= Endometriosis	:	_____
Py/o	+ Metr/o	+ -itis	= Pyometritis	:	_____
neo-	+ Nat/i	+ -al	= Neonatal	:	_____
neo-	+ Nat/i	+ -logy	= Neonatology	:	_____
O/o	+ -genesis		= Oogenesis	:	_____
O/o	+ -cyte		= Oocyte	:	_____
Oophor/o	+ -ectomy		= Oophorectomy	:	_____
bi-	+ Later/o	+ -al	= Bilateral		_____
	+ Oophor/o	+ -ectomy	oophorectomy	:	
Ovari/o	+ -an		= Ovarian	:	_____
Ovari/o	+ Hyster/o	+ -ectomy	= Ovario-		
			hysterectomy	:	_____
an-	+ Ovul/o	+ -ation	= Anovulation	:	_____
ante-	+ -partum		= Antepartum	:	_____
post-	+ -mortem		= Postmortem	:	_____
post-	+ -partum		= Postpartum	:	_____
Perine/o	+ -rrhaphy		= Perineorrhaphy	:	_____
pseudo-	+ -cyesis		= Pseudocyesis	:	_____
Py/o	+-rrhea		= Pyorrhea	:	_____
Radi/o	+-graphy		= Radiography	:	_____

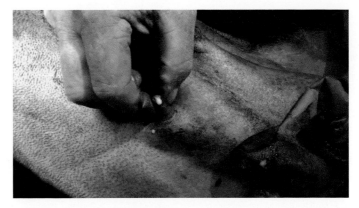

Figure 5.33   Pseudocyesis in a dog showing lactation. The dog was spayed shortly afterward. Courtesy of Greg Martinez, DVM; www.youtube.com/drgregdvm.

oxy-	+-tocia	=	Oxytocia	:	_____
dys-	+-tocia	=	Dystocia	:	_____
Umbilic/o	+-al	=	Umbilical	:	_____
Vagin/o	+-itis	=	Vaginitis	:	_____
Vulv/o	+Vagin/o + -itis	=	Vulvovaginitis	:	_____

Abbreviations

Table 5.7   Chapter 5 Abbreviations

Abbreviation	Definition
AB	Abortion
AI	Artificial insemination
C-Sect	Cesarean section (**C-Section**)
DES	Diethylstilbestrol
GU	Genitourinary
Gyn	Gynecology
OB	Obstetrics
PG	Pregnant

(Continued)

Table 5.7   (*Continued*).

Abbreviation	Definition
SC	Scrotal circumference
OHE	Spay (**OVH**)
SF (F/S)	Spayed female
NM (M/N)	Neutered male
CM	Castrated male
FSH	Follicle-stimulating hormone
LH	Luteinizing hormone
ad. lib.	As desired
prn	As needed
qn	Every night
qh	Every hour
qd	Every day
SID	Once daily; q24h
BID	Twice daily; q12h
TID	Three times daily; q8h
QID	Four times daily; q6h
EOD	Every other day

Case Study: You'll notice some terms from the previous chapters

Sassy, an intact 9-year-old female Newfoundland, comes to your clinic after the owner notices a vaginal discharge. On P/E, Sassy is panting excessively and has leukorrhea. There is an odiferous smell coming from Sassy and she keeps licking her vulva. Her abdomen is distended and she has an elevated temperature. After restraining Sassy for the veterinarian, the doctor notes vulvitis.

After a thorough examination, radiographs, and blood work, the veterinarian diagnoses Sassy with pyometra. An immediate OHE is recommended and Sassy is placed on antibiotics PO BID. The owner wonders if Sassy's previous history of dystocia and multiple pregnancies may have contributed to her current condition. The OHE goes well and Sassy has a routine recovery.

Case Study Questions

1. Which of the following describes Sassy's clinical signs?
   a. Bloody discharge from the vagina
   b. Vomiting a white thick substance
   c. White thick discharge from the vagina
2. Which of the following structures was inflamed?
   a. Tube from the uterus to the outside of the body
   b. Womb
   c. External genitalia
3. Why is surgery necessary?
   a. Inflammation of the uterus
   b. Pus in the uterus
   c. Inflammation of the inner lining of the uterus
4. What kind of surgery was recommended?
   a. Neuter
   b. Mastectomy
   c. Spay
5. How were the antibiotics given?
   a. By mouth, once daily
   b. By mouth, twice daily
   c. By mouth, three times daily
6. The owner had two concerns about Sassy's history. What were they?
   a. Difficult labor and abortions
   b. Rapid labor and nulliparous
   c. Difficult labor and multigravida

Exercises

5-A: Give the definition for the following:

1. hyster/o, metri/o, and uter/o:_____
2. ovari/o and oophor/o:_____
3. lact/o and galact/o:_____
4. colp/o and vagin/o:_____
5. ov/o and o/o:_____
6. episi/o and vulv/o:_____
7. -cyesis and -gravida:_____
8. -partum and -tocia:_____
9. test/o and orch/o:_____
10. pen/i and priap/o:_____

5-B: Give the structure for the following definitions.

1. —————————————: External female genitalia
2. —————————————: Male gamete
3. —————————————: Tube from ovary to uterine horns
4. —————————————: Site of spermatogenesis
5. —————————————: Sac containing the testes
6. —————————————: Sperm and fluid
7. —————————————: Sensitive tip of the penis
8. —————————————: Inner lining of the uterus
9. —————————————: Lower, neck-like portion of uterus
10. ————————————: Tube from the urinary bladder to the outside of the body
11. ————————————: Bone found in the penis of some carnivores
12. ————————————: Tube carrying sperm from seminiferous tubules to the vas deferens
13. ————————————: The womb
14. ————————————: Inner membrane surrounding the embryo

5-C: Define the following terms.

1. Monorchid ————————————————————
2. Coitus ——————————————————————
3. Vasectomy ————————————————————
4. Orchiectomy————————————————————
5. Ovarian ——————————————————————
6. Fetotomy —————————————————————
7. Fetus ——————————————————————
8. Castration————————————————————
9. Meconium —————————————————————
10. Colostrum ————————————————————

5-D: Define the following:

1. ——————————: Cervic/o   7. ——————————: oligo-
2. ——————————: Semin/i   8. ——————————: -cele
3. ——————————: -megaly   9. ——————————: -pexy
4. ——————————: primi-   10. ——————————: -parous
5. ——————————: Balan/o   11. ——————————: -oxy
6. ——————————: nulli-   12. ——————————: Py/o

5-E: Define the following terms.

1. Balanitis————————————————————
2. Spermatogenesis——————————————————
3. Cytology—————————————————————
4. Mastectomy————————————————————
5. Postpartum————————————————————

6. Orchiopexy————————————————
7. Prostatectomy—————————————————
8. Endometriosis—————————————————
9. Pseudocyesis——————————————————
10. Amniocentesis——————————————————

5-F: Define the following abbreviations.

1. ———————————: qn   9. ———————————: AI
2. ———————————: OHE   10. ———————————: q6h
3. ———————————: C-sect   11. ———————————: MN
4. ———————————: FS   12. ———————————: qd
5. ———————————: CM   13. ———————————: q8h
6. ———————————: q24h   14. ———————————: eod
7. ———————————: PRN   15. ———————————: PG
8. ———————————: AB

5-G: Circle the correct term in parentheses.

1. Animal that gives birth to live young: (oviparous, viviparous)
2. Area between the anus and scrotum: (peritoneum, perineum)
3. Termination of pregnancy: (OHE, AB)
4. Fertilized ovum outside the uterus: (ectopic, hermaphroditic)
5. Study of cells to determine stage of heat: (semen analysis, vaginal cytology)
6. The act of giving birth: (gestation, parturition)
7. Sex cell: (gamete, genitalia)
8. Time of sexual receptivity: (proestrus, estrus)
9. Normal secretion of milk: (lactorrhea, lactation)
10. Newborn: (neonate, meconium)

5-H: Match the following terms with their descriptions.

1. _____Discharge of pus   A. Agalactia
2. _____Inflammation of the vagina   B. Anorchism
3. _____False pregnancy   C. Bilateral oophorectomy
4. _____Visual exam of the vagina   D. Colposcopy
5. _____Condition of no testes   E. Fimbriae
6. _____Condition of no milk   F. Perineorrhaphy
7. _____Removal of both ovaries   G. Pseudocyesis
8. _____Suture of the area between   H. Pyorrhea
        the anus and vagina
9. _____Uterus returns to normal,   I. Uterine involution
        non-pregnant size
10. _____Finger-like projections on   J. Vaginitis
        uterine tubes

Answers can be found starting on page 571.

Go to www.wiley.com/go/taibo/terminology to find additional learning materials for this chapter:

- A crossword puzzle
- Flashcards
- Audio clips to show how to pronounce terms
- Case studies
- Review questions
- The figures from the chapter in PowerPoint

Chapter 6

The Cardiovascular System

The cardiovascular system consists of the heart and blood vessels. The goal of these structures is to circulate blood—which is made up of cells, water, nutrients, gases, and much more—to tissues throughout the body. This chapter focuses on the heart and blood vessels.

Blood Vessels

Before discussing the anatomy of the heart, we must first introduce blood vessels. There are three major types of blood vessels in the body: arteries, veins, and capillaries (Figure 6.1).

Arteries are the largest of the blood vessels and always carry blood away from the heart. They have an inner lining called endothelium, which is a layer of epithelial cells that can be found lining the heart cavities and blood vessels. The endothelial cells in the arteries are able to increase and decrease the size of the artery itself which then affects the blood flow. The layer surrounding the endothelial cells is smooth muscle. Arteries pump a large volume of blood from the heart so they need the strength to carry that blood to the rest of the body without rupturing. Arteries eventually branch out to various organs and the extremities of the body. These smaller branches of arteries are called arterioles, and they carry blood to the capillaries.

Capillaries are the smallest of all the blood vessels. They are lined with a single layer of endothelial cells. The capillaries are where systemic gas exchange occurs. The oxygenated blood that was brought to the capillaries crosses the lining of the capillaries into the tissues. Simultaneously, as the tissue is receiving oxygen, it's releasing carbon dioxide and other waste products into the capillaries. The newly deoxygenated blood then begins traveling back to the heart by entering smaller veins called venules. These venules then branch out and enlarge into veins.

Veterinary Medical Terminology Guide and Workbook, First Edition. Angela Taibo.
© 2014 John Wiley & Sons, Inc. Published 2014 by John Wiley & Sons, Inc.
Companion website: www.wiley.com/go/taibo/terminology

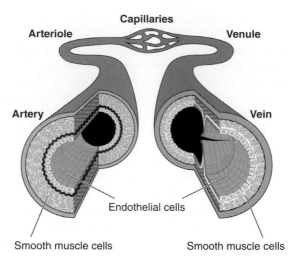

Figure 6.1   Anatomy of blood vessels. Courtesy of shutterstock/blamb.

Veins always carry blood toward the heart. As with arteries, a common mistake is to think that all veins are blue and carry deoxygenated (oxygen-poor) blood. That is not always the case. Veins are smaller than arteries because the volume of blood they carry is considerably smaller. Unlike arteries and capillaries, veins contain interior valves that prevent the blood from flowing in the opposite direction. These valves are required due to the veins' lack of muscle strength. If a patient has hypertension (high blood pressure), then the valves are unable to work due to the increased volume of blood, which causes the veins to swell.

A common misconception is that all arteries carry oxygenated (oxygen-rich) blood and are red in color. The pulmonary arteries carry deoxygenated blood from the heart to the lungs.

TECH TIP 6.1 Venous Valves

When performing venipuncture on animals, sometimes the blood stops flowing into your syringe. The animal didn't necessarily move. When this happens, it's usually due to the valves within the veins that have closed in response to your needle. Rotating the needle slightly within the vessel should get the blood flowing into your syringe again.

Anatomy of the Heart

External Anatomy

The heart lies in the thoracic cavity, underneath the body of the sternum between the lungs. The space between the lungs is called the mediastinum. If one were to look at the cardiovascular system as a symphony, then the heart would be its conductor and the blood vessels, its players.

There are three layers of the heart.

Endocardium	Inner lining of the heart. This layer of endothelial cells lines the chambers and valves within the heart.
Myocardium	Muscle layer of the heart. This is literally the heart muscle and gives the heart the power to push the blood throughout the body.
Pericardium	Membrane surrounding the heart. This membrane is actually a two-layer sac made up of the **visceral pericardium** and **parietal pericardium**. The visceral layer adheres to the heart, whereas the parietal layer lines the fibrous outer portion of the pericardium. The space between the heart and the pericardium is termed the **pericardial space.** Within this pericardial space is a fluid that acts as a lubricant for the membranes as the heart beats. This fluid is called **pericardial fluid.**

TECH TIP 6.2 Remember Your Rules

When "peri-," "endo-," or "myo-" are attached to organs, then their meanings change. "Peri-" becomes a membrane surrounding that organ. "Endo-" becomes the inner lining of that organ. "Myo-" becomes the muscle layer of that organ.

From the outside, the heart has a "top" and a "bottom" where it comes to a point. In fact, the heart is a bit of an oxymoron in how these two parts are named. The top of the heart, where major vessels enter, is called the base. The bottom of the heart, where it comes to a point, is called the apex. On the surface of the heart are small blood vessels which solely supply the heart. The red vessels are coronary arteries and they supply blood and oxygen to the myocardium. The blue vessels on the surface of the heart are the coronary veins. The coronary veins remove the heart's waste products. If the blood supply within these vessels is interrupted, then the heart can no longer function.

Internal Anatomy–The Flow of Blood

Use Figure 6.2 to follow the flow of blood in Figure 6.3.

Deoxygenated blood enters the heart through the vena cavae. These two veins are the largest veins in the body. The cranial, or anterior, vena cava carries deoxygenated blood from the upper body to the heart. The caudal, or posterior, vena cava carries blood from the lower body to the heart.

The first chamber the blood enters is the right atrium, which is the chamber on the upper right side of the heart. From the right atrium, the blood then passes through the first of several heart valves, the tricuspid valve. The tricuspid valve is also known as the right atrioventricular (AV) valve. The valve is named based

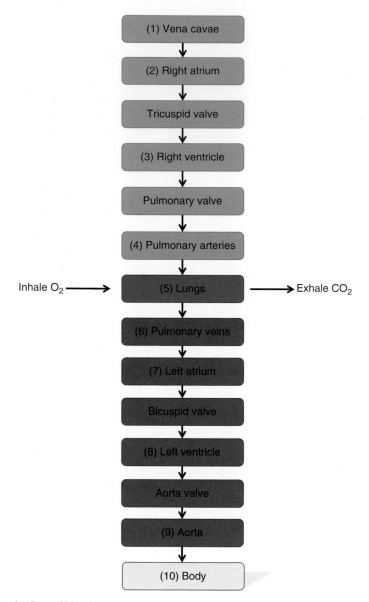

Figure 6.2   The flow of blood through the heart.

on the number of cusps, or flaps, that are on the valve. After passing through the tricuspid valve, the blood enters the right ventricle, which is on the bottom right side of the heart. The blood moves from the right ventricle through the pulmonary valve and into the pulmonary arteries. Remember that arteries always carry blood away from the heart. The pulmonary arteries carry blood from the heart to the lungs. The blood is still deoxygenated at this point so these arteries are blue in color.

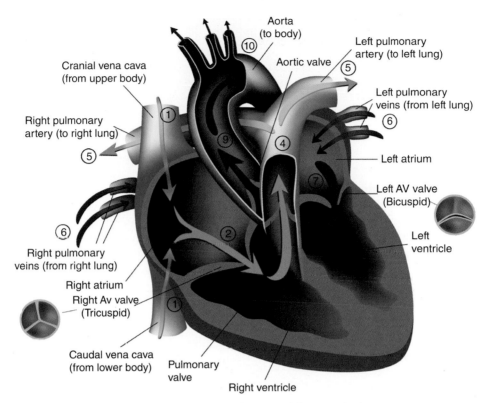

Figure 6.3   The path of blood through the heart. Courtesy of shutterstock/Alila Sao Mai.

The pulmonary arteries branch into smaller vessels, arterioles, which branch further into capillaries. These capillaries are where gas exchange occurs. The blood loses its carbon dioxide and gains fresh oxygen. As the animal inhales oxygen, it crosses from the lungs into the blood. When the animal exhales, the carbon dioxide in the blood crosses into the lungs. The newly oxygenated blood moves from the capillaries to venules and then to the pulmonary veins. Veins always carry blood toward the heart, so these veins carry blood from the lungs to the heart. Pulmonary veins are red in color because they're carrying oxygenated blood.

Blood enters the heart again through the left atrium in the upper left side of the heart. From the left atrium, the blood passes through the bicuspid valve to the left ventricle. The bicuspid valve is also known as the left AV valve or the mitral valve. The left ventricle is the largest and thickest of all the heart chambers. The heart muscle of the left ventricle is almost three times as thick as that of the right ventricle because of where it has to pump the blood to. While the right ventricle has to pump blood to the lungs, the left ventricle has to pump blood to the rest of the body. From the left ventricle, the blood passes through the aortic valve and into the aorta, the largest artery in the body. The aorta branches out to carry blood to the rest of the body.

TECH TIP 6.3 **Heart Valves: Helpful Reminders**

When memorizing the flow of blood through the heart, remember that the blood must go through a valve before it leaves the heart. The valves are named based on the structures that follow them.

  If you are having difficulty remembering the order of the AV valves, use this sentence to help: You TRY something before you BUY it. In other words, the tricuspid is before the bicuspid.

The deoxygenated blood never mixes with the oxygenated blood in a healthy heart because of partitions within the heart called septa (singular: septum). The upper two chambers of the heart are separated by the interatrial septum. The lower two chambers of the heart are separated by the interventricular septum. If an animal has a septal defect, then a hole in one or both of the partitions is allowing the two kinds of blood to mix. In that case the deoxygenated blood would be pumped to the rest of the body.

Please note that fetal circulation differs from the blood flow described above. This chapter focuses on normal circulation after birth.

The Heartbeat

The heartbeat is created through a series of electrical impulses that travel through the myocardium (Figure 6.4). The electrical impulses are created through a collection of specialized muscle fibers called the sinoatrial node (SA node). The rhythm of the heart's contraction is established through the SA node, which is why it is commonly called the pacemaker of the heart. The impulse produced by the SA node causes the atria to contract and thereby causes the blood to move to the ventricles.

The electrical impulse then travels from the SA node to the next collection of muscle fibers called the atrioventricular node (AV node), which resides in the interatrial septum. The function of the AV node is to carry the electrical impulse from the SA node to the walls of the ventricles. The impulse moves from the AV nodes through a bundle of specialized muscle fibers called the atrioventricular bundle or bundle of His. The bundle runs through the interventricular septum to the walls of the ventricles and branches further into small muscle fibers called Purkinje fibers. The bundle of His and Purkinje fibers cause the ventricles to contract.

The contraction phase of the heartbeat is termed systole. When systole occurs, both the pulmonary and aortic valves are open and blood is pumped to the lungs and body. The tricuspid and bicuspid valves are closed.

The relaxation phase of the heartbeat is termed diastole. Diastole occurs when both the tricuspid and bicuspid valves are open and blood is pumped to both ventricles. The pulmonary and aortic valves are closed.

To summarize, the heart is pumping during systole and then filling during diastole (Figure 6.5).

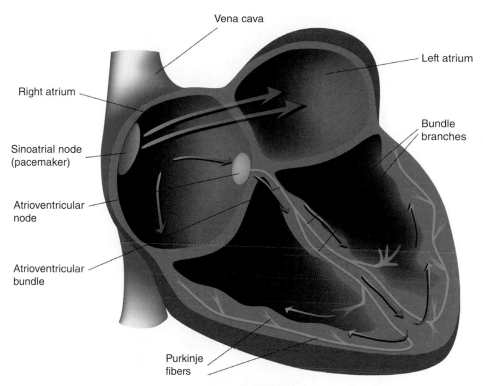

Vena cava

Left atrium

Right atrium

Bundle branches

Sinoatrial node (pacemaker)

Atrioventricular node

Atrioventricular bundle

Purkinje fibers

Figure 6.4   The conduction system of the heart. Courtesy of shutterstock/Alila Sao Mai.

When listening to the heart with a stethoscope, the sounds heard are described as a "lub-dub" sound. The sounds are created when the heart valves close. The first sound, the lub, can be heard when both the tricuspid and bicuspid valves close. This is the beginning of systole. The second sound, the dub, can be heard when the aortic and pulmonary valves close at the end of systole. If an extra heart sound is heard, then it is referred to as a murmur.

Heart murmurs can be caused by abnormal thickness of vessels, abnormal diameter of vessels, and abnormal blood flow. There are many causes of abnormal blood flow. Murmurs are typically assigned a grade depending on their severity. For example, a grade-I heart murmur is softest. Grade-VI murmurs are so loud they can be heard without a stethoscope. Listening to where the murmur is heard during the lub-dub can isolate where the cause may lie.

Electrocardiogram

The electrocardiogram (ECG or EKG) is the record of electricity in the heart, or more specifically, the heart muscle (Figure 6.6). The procedure of an EKG involves using colored wires (conductors) called leads that are connected from the patient to the EKG machine. Each lead is connected to a specific area of the body (Figure 6.7).

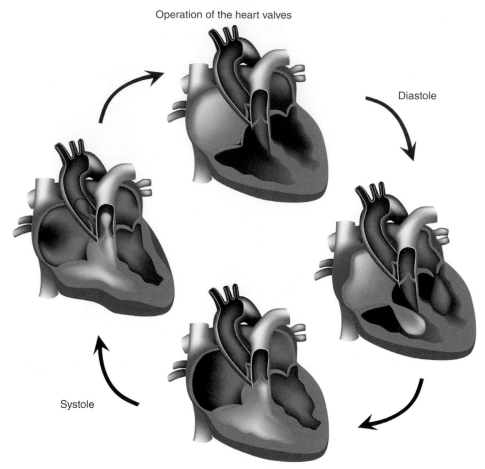

Operation of the heart valves

Diastole

Systole

Figure 6.5   The flow of blood during systole and diastole. Note that the valves that are open and closed during each cycle. In systole, the ventricles pump blood and the AV valves remain closed. In diastole, the ventricles fill with blood and the AV valves remain open, and both atria and ventricles are at rest. Courtesy of shutterstock/Alila Sao Mai.

The animal is usually placed in right lateral recumbency. The placement of the leads is as follows:

White lead	Right front
Green lead	Right rear
Black lead	Left front
Red lead	Left rear

There is sometimes a fifth lead (brown lead) that acts as a ground. A mnemonic to help remember the placement of the leads is "snow (white) over grass (green), smoke (black) over fire (red). "White" rhymes with "right" to help get things started.

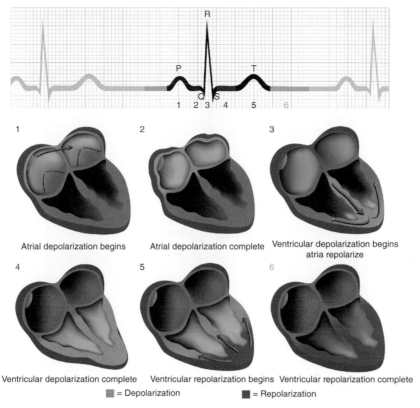

Atrial depolarization begins   Atrial depolarization complete   Ventricular depolarization begins atria repolarize

Ventricular depolarization complete   Ventricular repolarization begins   Ventricular repolarization complete

■ = Depolarization   ■ = Repolarization

Figure 6.6   Comparison of the electrical activity of the myocardium with an EKG tracing. Courtesy of shutterstock/Alila Sao Mai.

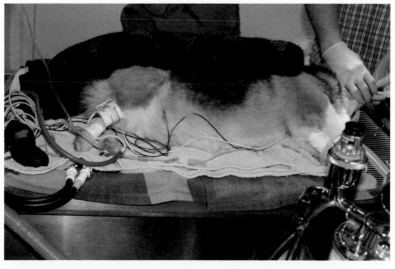

Figure 6.7   EKG leads on an older Corgi during dental surgery. Note the sphygmomanometer attached to her right rear leg.

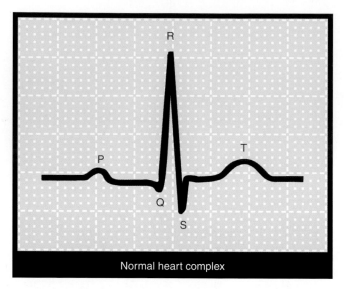

Figure 6.8 Waves of a typical EKG. The P wave represents atrial function, the QRS wave represents ventricular function, and the T wave represents the relaxation phase of the contraction. Courtesy of shutterstock/sfam_photo.

    The EKG machine measures the electrical changes in the heart muscle by tracing the changes in polarity. The machine then prints this activity in a series of waves (deflections) called tracings (Figure 6.8).

P wave	Represents atrial function, specifically depolarization or excitation of the atria.
PR segment	Represents conduction through the AV valve.
QRS wave	Represents ventricular function, specifically the excitation of the ventricles.
ST segment	Represents the end of ventricular depolarization and the onset of ventricular repolarization.
T wave	Represents the relaxation phase from the contraction. This is the recovery (repolarization) of the ventricles.

    If an animal has a normal heart rhythm, then it is called sinus rhythm (Figure 6.9).

Blood Pressure

Blood pressure is the pressure of the blood against the walls of the blood vessels. The force of the blood flow is determined by the pumping of the heart, blood volume, resistance of blood flow through arterioles, elasticity of the arteries, and

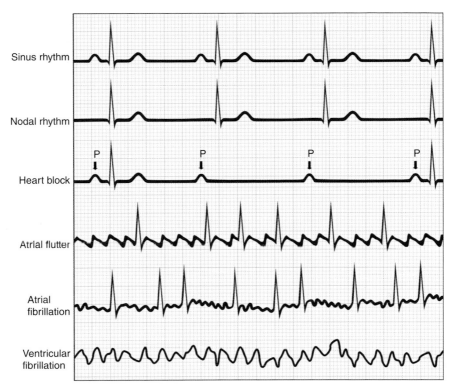

Figure 6.9   Examples of some normal and abnormal ECG tracings. Courtesy of shutterstock/
Alila Sao Mai.

viscosity (thickness) of the blood. Blood pressure generally measures atrial
pressure because of the vessel size and volume of blood. In fact, when taking an
animal's pulse, it is the arteries that are palpated (felt). Blood pressure is measured
using a sphygmomanometer (Figure 6.7).

Circulation

There are two types of circulation in the body: pulmonary circulation and systemic
circulation (Figure 6.10).

Pulmonary circulation is the flow of blood from the right side of the heart, to
the lungs, and back to the left side of the heart. This is where the oxygenation of
blood occurs.

Systemic circulation is the flow of blood from the heart, to the tissues, and then
back to the heart. It is during systemic circulation that the blood becomes deoxygenated due to gas exchange at the tissue level.

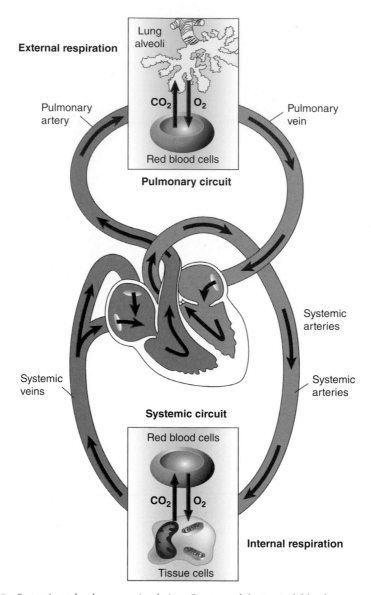

Figure 6.10   Systemic and pulmonary circulation. Courtesy of shutterstock/blamb.

Related Terms

Aorta	Largest artery in the body.
Aortic valve	Valve between the left ventricle and aorta.
Apex	Pointed end of the heart (Figure 6.11).
Artery	Largest vessel in the body; carries blood away from the heart.

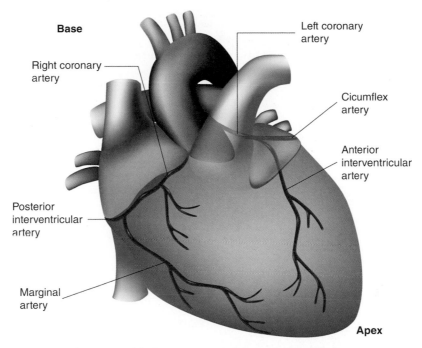

Base

Right coronary artery

Left coronary artery

Cicumflex artery

Anterior interventricular artery

Posterior interventricular artery

Marginal artery

Apex

Figure 6.11   External anatomy of the heart. Courtesy of shutterstock/Alila Sao Mai.

Atrioventricular bundle	Specialized muscle fibers in the interventricular septum; carry electrical impulses to the ventricles. Also called the **bundle of His.**
Atrioventricular node (AV node)	Specialized tissue in the interatrial septum; carries impulses from the SA node to the AV node.
Atrioventricular valves (AV valves)	Valves between the atria and ventricles.
Atrium (plural: atria)	Two upper heart chambers.
Base	Cranial portion of the heart (Figure 6.11).
Bicuspid valve	Valve between the left atrium and left ventricle. Also called the **mitral valve** or left **AV valve.**
Capillaries	Smallest blood vessels.
Carbon dioxide (CO_2)	Gas released by tissue cells and transported to the heart and lungs for exhalation.
Coronary arteries	Supply blood and oxygen to the myocardium (Figure 6.11).
Deoxygenated blood	Oxygen-poor blood.
Diastole	The relaxation phase of the heartbeat.
Endocardium	Inner lining of the heart.

Endothelium	Epithelial cells lining the heart cavities and vessels.
Myocardium	Muscle layer of the heart.
Oxygen (O$_2$)	Gas that enters the blood through the lungs and travels to the heart to be pumped to the rest of the body.
Oxygenated blood	Oxygen-rich blood.
Pericardium	Membrane surrounding the heart (Figure 6.12).

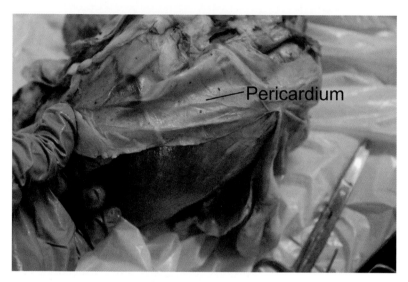

Figure 6.12   Pericardium on a dissected sheep heart.

Pulmonary artery	Artery that carries deoxygenated blood from the heart to the lungs.
Pulmonary circulation	Flow of blood from the heart, to the lung, and back to the heart.
Pulmonary valve	Valve between the right ventricle and pulmonary artery.
Pulmonary veins	Veins that carry oxygenated blood from the lungs to the heart.
Pulse	Heartbeat felt through the walls of the arteries.
Semilunar valves	Valves between the entrances of the aorta and pulmonary artery. Referred to as semilunar because they are shaped like a half moon.
Septum	Partition
Sinoatrial node	Pacemaker of the heart.
Sinus rhythm	Normal heart rhythm.

Systemic circulation	Flow of blood from the body cells to the heart and back out to the body cells.
Systole	Contraction phase of the heart.
Valves	Structures in veins and in the heart that temporarily close an opening so that blood can flow in one direction (Figure 6.13).

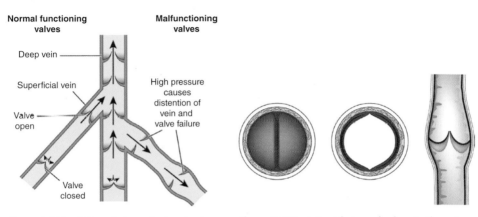

Figure 6.13A   External view of valves in the veins. Courtesy of shutterstock/blamb.

Figure 6.13B   Internal view of valves in the veins. Courtesy of shutterstock/blamb.

Vein	Thin-walled vessel that carries blood towards the heart.
Vena cavae **(Singular: vena cava)**	Largest vein in the body.
Ventricles	Two lower chambers of the heart.

Pathology and Procedures

Aneurysm	Sac (dilation) formed by weakening of a blood vessel.Can lead to hemorrhage and stroke (Figure 6.14).
Arrhythmia	Abnormal heart rhythm. Also called **dysrhythmia**.
Asystole	Without contraction; lack of heart activity.
Atherosclerosis	Hardening of arteries due to plaque buildup (Figure 6.15).
Auscultation	Listening with a stethoscope to sounds within the body. Thoracic auscultation is used to listen to heart and breath sounds. Abdominal auscultation is often used to listen to gut sounds. (Figure 6.16).
Cardiac hypertrophy	Enlargement of the heart due to increased cell size (Figure 6.17).

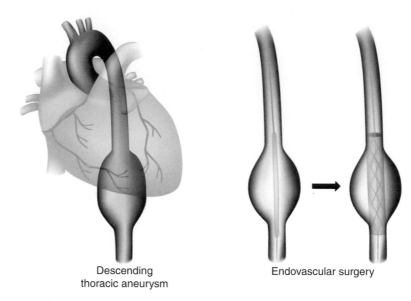

Descending
thoracic aneurysm

Endovascular surgery

Figure 6.14   Thoracic aneurysm. Courtesy of shutterstock/Alila Sao Mai.

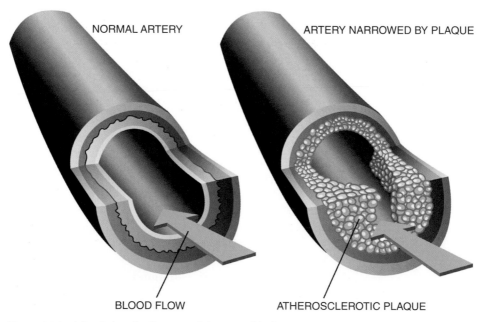

NORMAL ARTERY

ARTERY NARROWED BY PLAQUE

BLOOD FLOW

ATHEROSCLEROTIC PLAQUE

Figure 6.15   Atherosclerosis. Courtesy of shutterstock/Rob3000.

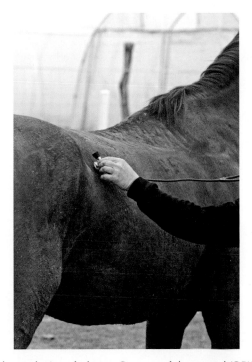

Figure 6.16   Abdominal auscultation of a horse. Courtesy of shutterstock/OPIS.

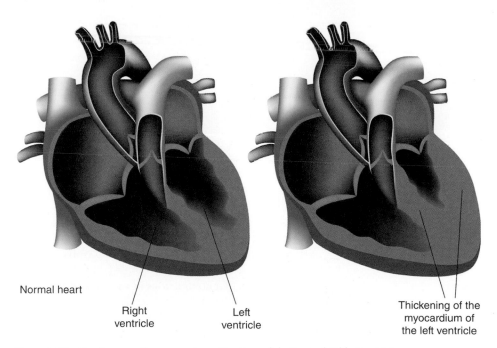

Normal heart

Right
ventricle

Left
ventricle

Thickening of the
myocardium of
the left ventricle

Figure 6.17   Cardiomyopathy comparison. Courtesy of shutterstock/Alila Sao Mai.

Cardiac tamponade	Compression of the heart due to fluid or blood in the pericardial sac.
Congenital heart disease (CHD)	Abnormalities of the heart at birth.
Congestive heart failure (CHF)	Heart is unable to pump its required amount of blood.
Capillary refill time (CRT)	The time it takes for the mucous membranes to return to a normal pink color after applying finger pressure.
Defibrillation	Use of electrical shock to restore normal heart rhythm(Figure 6.18).

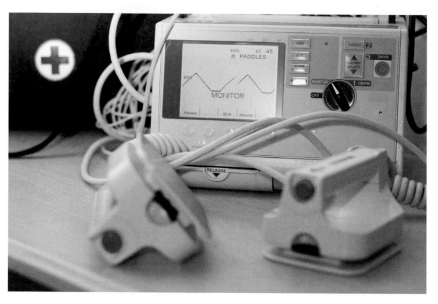

Figure 6.18　A defibrillator. Courtesy of shutterstock/Renewer.

Echocardiogram (ECHO)	High-frequency sound waves and echoes that produce an image of the heart (Figure 6.19).
Embolism	Blockage of a vessel by a clot or foreign material.
Embolus (Plural: emboli)	A detached, moving clot.
Fibrillation	Rapid, random, and irregular contractions of the heart.
Flutter	Rapid but regular contractions of the atria and ventricles. Can be further isolated as an **atrial flutter** or **ventricular flutter** depending on the chambers involved.
Heartworm disease	Infestation of the parasite *Dirofilaria immitis* in the right ventricle and pulmonary arteries. Transmitted after a blood meal from a mosquito (Figure 6.20).

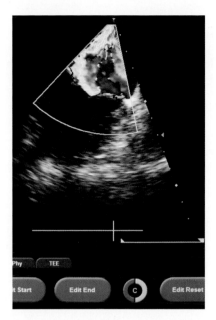

Figure 6.19   Echocardiogram and color Doppler flow. Courtesy of shutterstock/Renewer.

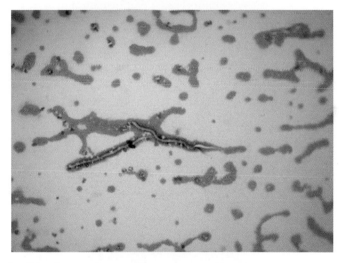

Figure 6.20   Bloodfilm showing the microfilariae (larvae) of heartworm.

Hypertension	Increased blood pressure.
Hypotension	Decreased blood pressure.
Hypoxia	Decreased oxygen to tissues.
Infarction	Area of dead tissue.
Ischemia	Lack of blood flow to tissues.
Mitral valve prolapse (MVP)	Displacement of the bicuspid valve leading to incomplete closure of the valve during ventricular contraction.

> **TECH TIP 6.4 Ischemia vs. Hypoxia**
>
> Be careful with the differences between ischemia and hypoxia. Ischemia is a lack of blood flow to tissues. This can lead to tissue necrosis, and this tissue turns a black color.
>
> Hypoxia is a lack of oxygen to tissues. This can lead to cyanosis, or an abnormal blue color.
>
> Ultimately a lack of blood flow to tissues leads to a lack of oxygen to tissues because red blood cells carry oxygen.

Murmur	An extra heart sound.
Occlusion	Blockage; obstruction or closure of body passage.
Patent	Open; unobstructed. Term can be used to describe vessels and catheters.
Patent ductus arteriosus (PDA)	Condition in which the small duct between the aorta and pulmonary artery, which normally closes after birth, remains open. The duct itself is called the ductus arteriosus. PDA causes continuous murmur, fatigue, and exercise intolerance. It is the most common heart malformation in dogs and is most often seen in Collies, Shelties, Old English Sheepdogs, and Pomeranians (Figure 6.21).
Perfusion (tissue perfusion)	Passage of fluid through the blood vessels of a specific organ; blood flow through the tissue.

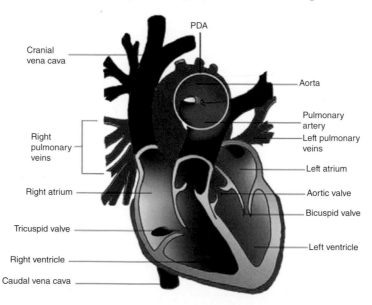

Figure 6.21　Cross section of a heart with a patent ductus arteriosus. This duct should close soon after birth. If it remains open, oxygenated and deoxygenated blood will mix. Courtesy of BrownCow. Public domain, from WikiCommons.

Pericardial effusion

Escape of fluid into the pericardial sac leading to cardiac tamponade. An **effusion** is an escape of fluid and can occur anywhere in the body (Figure 6.22).

Premature ventricular contraction (PVC, VPC)

Ventricles are triggered to contract by the Purkinje fibers rather than the SA node.

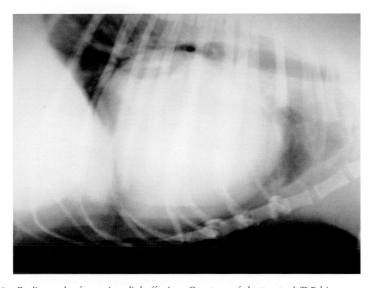

Figure 6.22   Radiograph of a pericardial effusion. Courtesy of shutterstock/P Fabian.

Shock

Inadequate tissue perfusion. Blood pools in the capillarics to increase the blood volume of the patient, which then decreases its flow to vital organs.

Sphygmomanometer

Instrument that measures arterial blood pressure.

Stent

Small expander inserted into tubular structures such as vessels to provide support and prevent collapse (Figure 6.23).

Stethoscope

Instrument used to listen to sounds within the body (Figure 6.24).

Tetralogy of Fallot

Congenital malformation of the heart that combines four structural defects: pulmonary artery stenosis, ventricular septal defect, aortic right shift, and right ventricular hypertrophy (Figure 6.25).

Thrill

Vibration felt on palpation of the chest. Usually caused by turbulence in the heart.

Thrombus (Plural: thrombi)

Stationary clot attached to the wall of a vessel (Figure 6.26).

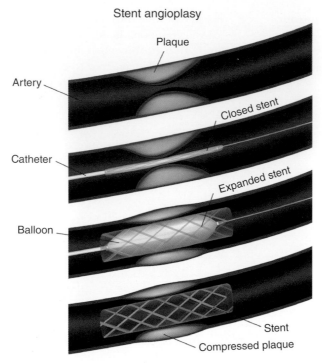

Stent angioplasy

Plaque

Artery

Closed stent

Catheter

Expanded stent

Balloon

Stent

Compressed plaque

Figure 6.23   Stent placement to prevent vessel collapse. Courtesy of shutterstock/Alila Medical Images.

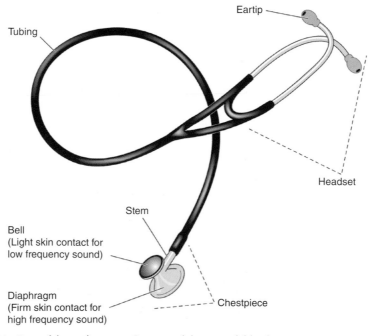

Eartip

Tubing

Headset

Stem

Bell
(Light skin contact for
low frequency sound)

Diaphragm
(Firm skin contact for
high frequency sound)

Chestpiece

Figure 6.24   Parts of the stethoscope. Courtesy of shutterstock/blamb.

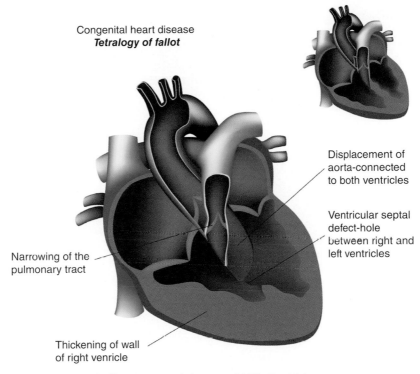

Congenital heart disease
Tetralogy of fallot

Displacement of
aorta-connected
to both ventricles

Ventricular septal
defect-hole
between right and
left ventricles

Narrowing of the
pulmonary tract

Thickening of wall
of right venricle

Figure 6.25   Tetralogy of Fallot. Courtesy of shutterstock/Alila Sao Mai.

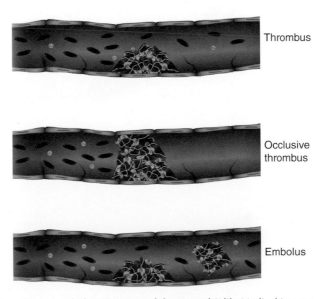

Thrombus

Occlusive
thrombus

Embolus

Figure 6.26   Thrombus vs. embolus. Courtesy of shutterstock/Alila Medical Images.

Ventricular septal defect (VSD)

Small hole(s) in the interventricular septum. Causes shunting of the blood and therefore deoxygenated blood is pumped to the rest of the body (Figure 6.27).

Vasoconstriction

Narrowing of a vessel (Figure 6.28).

Vasodilation

Expansion of a vessel (Figure 6.28).

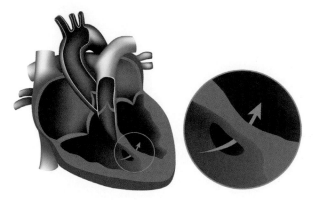

Figure 6.27   Ventricular septal defect. Courtesy of shutterstock/Alila Sao Mai.

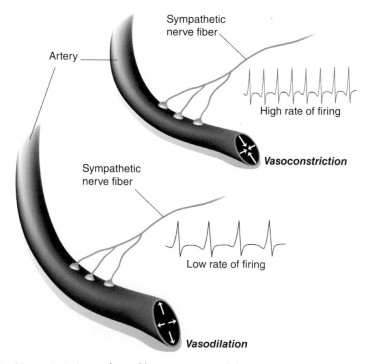

Figure 6.28   Vasoconstriction and vasodilation. Courtesy of shutterstock/Alila Sao Mai.

Building the Terms

Table 6.1   Chapter 6 Combining Forms.

Combining Forms	Definition	Combining Forms	Definition
Angi/o	Vessel	**Necr/o**	Death
Aort/o	Aorta	**Ox/o**	Oxygen (O_2)
Arter/o	Artery	**Pericardi/o**	Pericardium
Arteri/o	Artery	**Phleb/o**	Vein
Ather/o	Plaque (fatty substance)	**Sphygm/o**	Pulse
Atri/o	Atrium	**Steth/o**	Chest
Capn/o	Carbon dioxide (CO_2)	**Thorac/o**	Chest
Cardi/o	Heart	**Thromb/o**	Clot
Cholesterol/o	Cholesterol	**Valv/o**	Valve
Coron/o	Heart	**Valvul/o**	Valve
Cyan/o	Blue	**Vascul/o**	Vessel
Electr/o	Electricity	**Vas/o**	Vessel; vas deferens; duct
Hem/o	Blood	**Ven/i**	Vein
Isch/o	To hold back; back	**Ven/o**	Vein
Man/o	Pressure	**Ventricul/o**	Ventricle
My/o	Muscle		

Table 6.2   Chapter 6 Prefixes.

Prefix	Definition	Prefix	Definition
brady-	slow	**inter-**	between
endo-	in; within	**peri-**	surrounding; around
hyper-	above; excessive; increased	**tachy-**	fast
hypo-	deficient; below; under; less than normal; decreased		

Table 6.3 Chapter 6 Suffixes.

Suffix	Definition	Suffix	Definition
-al, -ar, -ic, -ous	pertaining to	-oma	tumor; mass; collection of fluid
-centesis	surgical puncture to remove fluid	-osis	abnormal condition
-ectomy	removal; excision; resection	-oxia	oxygen
-emia	blood condition	-pathy	disease condition
-gram	record	-plasty	surgical repair
-graph	instrument for recording	-rrhaphy	suture
-graphy	process of recording	-sclerosis	hardening
-ia	condition		
-itis	inflammation	-stenosis	tightening; narrow; stricture
-lysis	breakdown; destruction; separation; loosening	-tension	pressure
-megaly	enlargement	-tomy	incision; process of cutting
-meter	measure	-ule	small; little
-ole	small; little		

Now it's time to put these word parts together. If you memorize the meaning of the combining forms, prefixes, and suffixes, then this will get easier each time. Remember your five basic rules to medical terminology when building and defining these terms. You'll notice some word parts are repeated from the previous chapter.

Parts			Medical Term	Definition
Angi/o	+ -gram		= Angiogram	: _____
Angi/o	+ -pathy		= Angiopathy	: _____
Angi/o	+ -plasty		= Angioplasty	: _____
Angi/o	+ -rrhaphy		= Angiorrhaphy	: _____
Hem/o	+ Angi/o	+ -oma	= Hemangioma	: _____
Aort/o	+ -ic	+ Stenosis	= Aortic stenosis	: _____

*Remember that stenosis
can be a term by itself,
not just a suffix.
The definition is the same.*

endo-	+ Arter/o	+ -ectomy	= Endarterectomy	: _____
Arteri/o	+ -al	+ Anastomosis	= Arterial anastomosis	: _____
Arteri/o	+ -ectomy		= Arteriectomy	: _____
Arteri/o	+ -graphy		= Arteriography	: _____
Arteri/o	+ -sclerosis		= Arteriosclerosis	: _____
Arteri/o	+ -tomy		= Arteriotomy	: _____
Arteri/o	+ -ole		= Arteriole	: _____
Atri/o	+ -al		= Atrial	: _____
Atri/o	+ Ventricul/o	+ -ar	= Atrioventricular	: _____
hyper-	+ Capn/o	+ -ia	= Hypercapnia	: _____
hypo-	+ Capn/o	+ -ia	= Hypocapnia	: _____
brady-	+ Cardi/o	+ -ia	= Bradycardia	: _____
Cardi/o	+ -megaly		= Cardiomegaly	: _____
Cardi/o	+ My/o	+ -pathy	= Cardiomyopathy	: _____
Cardi/o	+ -itis		= Carditis	: _____
endo-	+ Cardi/o	+ -itis	= Endocarditis	: _____

*Remember your rules
for "endo-" when attached
to an organ.*

tachy-	+ Cardi/o	+ -ia	= Tachycardia	: _____
hyper-	+ Cholesterol/o	+ -emia	= Hypercholesterolemia	: _____
Cyan/o	+ -osis		= Cyanosis	: _____
Cyan/o	+ -osis	+ -ic	= Cyanotic	: _____
Electr/o	+ Cardi/o	+ -gram	= Electrocardiogram	: _____
Electr/o	+ Cardi/o	+ -graph	= Electrocardiograph	: _____
hypo-	+ -oxia		= Hypoxia	: _____
hypo-	+ -oxia	+ -ic	= Hypoxic	: _____
mitral	+ Valvul/o	+ -itis	= Mitral valvulitis	: _____
Necr/o	+ -osis		= Necrosis	: _____
Pericardi/o	+ -centesis		= Pericardiocentesis	: _____
Phleb/o	+ -itis		= Phlebitis	: _____
Thorac/o	+ -ic		= Thoracic	: _____
Thorac/o	+ -tomy		= Thoracotomy	: _____
Thromb/o	+ -lysis		= Thrombolysis	: _____
Thromb/o	+ -osis		= Thrombosis	: _____
Valv/o	+ -tomy		= Valvotomy	: _____
Valvul/o	+ -plasty		= Valvuloplasty	: _____
Vascul/o	+ -ar		= Vascular	: _____
Vascul/o	+ -itis		= Vasculitis	: _____
Ven/o	+ -ous		= Venous	: _____
Ven/o	+ -ule		= Venule	: _____

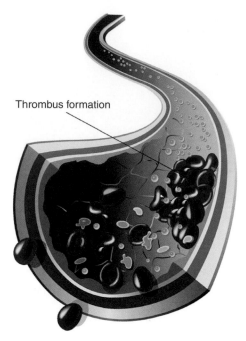

Thrombus formation

Figure 6.29   Thrombosis. Courtesy of shutterstock/Rob3000.

Abbreviations

Table 6.4   Chapter 6 Abbreviations.

Abbreviation	Definition
AF	Atrial fibrillation
AS	Aortic stenosis
BP	Blood pressure
bpm	Beats per minute/breaths per minute
CHF	Congestive heart failure
CO_2	Carbon dioxide
CVS	Cardiovascular system
CVP	Central venous pressure
ECHO	Echocardiogram
EKG	Electrocardiogram; (ECG)
H_2O	Water

Table 6.4   (*Continued*).

Abbreviation	Definition
HR	Heart rate
MI	Myocardial infarction
MVP	Mitral valve prolapse
O₂	Oxygen
PAC	Premature atrial contraction
PDA	Patent ductus arteriosus
PVC	Premature ventricular contraction
V fib	Ventricular fibrillation
VPC	Ventricular premature contraction; ventricular premature complexes
VSD	Ventricular septal defect
VT	Ventricular tachycardia (**V tach**)

Case Study

You'll notice some terms from the previous chapters

A 6-month-old Dalmatian named Bailey is brought to the clinic with lethargy. The owner states that Bailey has been resistant to going for walks and begins panting after walking around the yard. Bailey has tachycardia and a delayed CRT. MM are cyanotic and a Grade IV murmur can be heard on thoracic auscultation. The doctor orders radiographs and blood work.

   The blood work is unremarkable; however, the thoracic radiographs show a slight cardiomegaly. EKG and ECHO are done and PDA is diagnosed.

   Surgery is performed to tie off the PDA and Bailey has a routine recovery. On the 2-week post op exam, the owner is delighted with Bailey's recovery. She states that Bailey's energy has gone up and she's much more frisky at home and at the dog park.

Case Study Questions

1. Why was Bailey lethargic and resistant to walking around?
   a. Blood on the right side of the heart (deoxygenated) was mixing with blood on the left side of the heart (oxygenated) and then getting pumped to the rest of the body.
   b. Fluid was collecting between the heart and membrane surrounding the heart, which impeded the heart from beating.
   c. The bicuspid valve was protruding into the right atrium, disrupting the normal blood flow.

2. What color were Bailey's MM?
   a. Pink
   b. Blue
   c. Black
3. Which of the following describes Bailey's symptoms?
   a. Slow heart rate
   b. Fast heart rate
   c. Increased blood pressure
4. On radiographs, what abnormality was seen?
   a. Enlarged heart
   b. Fluid in the lungs
   c. None of the above
5. True or False: A Grade II murmur implies a loud heart sound.

Exercises

6-A: Fill in the following blanks regarding the flow of blood through the heart.

1. Vena cavae to the _____
2. Left AV valve to the _____
3. Pulmonary valve to the _____
4. Pulmonary artery to the _____
5. Lungs to the _____

6-B: Give the term for the following definitions.

1. _____: Upper chambers of the heart
2. _____: Surgical repair of a vessel
3. _____: Breakdown of a clot
4. _____: Lack of blood flow to tissues
5. _____: Supply blood and O_2 to myocardium
6. _____: Largest vein in the body
7. _____: An extra heart sound
8. _____: Membrane surrounding the heart
9. _____: Listening to sounds within the body
10. _____: Narrowing of a vessel
11. _____: Valve between the left atrium and ventricle
12. _____: Inadequate tissue perfusion
13. _____: A detached, moving clot
14. _____: Contraction phase of the heartbeat

6-C: Define the following terms.

1. Arrhythmia _____
2. Stethoscope _____
3. Thrill _____
4. Hypertension_____
5. Fibrillation _____
6. Sinoatrial node _____
7. Myocardium _____
8. Cardiomegaly _____
9. Hypoxia _____
10. Hypercapnia _____

6-D: Define the following:

1. _____: -oxia
2. _____: -tension
3. _____: Capn/o
4. _____: Phleb/o
5. _____: Coron/o
6. _____: brady-
7. _____: stenosis
8. _____: -lysis
9. _____: Thromb/o
10. _____: Ather/o
11. _____: Vascul/o
12. _____: -ole

6-E: Define the following abbreviations.

1. _____: VSD
2. _____: CHF
3. _____: V fib.
4. _____: PDA
5. _____: ECHO
6. _____: ECG
7. _____: PVC
8. _____: V tach.
9. _____: AS
10. _____: BP
11. _____: BPM
12. _____: CO_2
13. _____: AF
14. _____: MI
15. _____: PAC

6-F: Circle the correct term in parentheses.

1. What procedure would be used for cardiac tamponade? (pericardiocentesis, thoracocentesis)
2. Technique that can evaluate tissue perfusion: (auscultation, CRT)
3. EKG wave used to evaluate ventricular function: (P, QRS)
4. Causes cyanosis: (hypercapnia, hypoxia)
5. Causes tissue necrosis: (ischemia, hypoxia)
6. Given for an embolism: (thrombolytic, vasodilator)
7. Instrument used to listen to murmur: (electrocardiograph, stethoscope)
8. Felt on thoracic palpation: (thrill, Grade I murmur)
9. Heartworm infestation leads to: (venous congestion, arterial congestion)
10. Greyhounds and race horses may have: (cardiac hypertrophy, pericardial effusion)

6-G: Match the following terms with their descriptions.

1.	_____ Inflammation of veins	A.	Carditis
2.	_____ Inflammation of the heart	B.	Endocarditis
3.	_____ Inflammation of the inner lining of the heart	C.	Mitral valvulitis
4.	_____ Inflammation of vessels	D.	Pericarditis
5.	_____ Inflammation of the membrane surrounding the heart	E.	Phlebitis
6.	_____ Inflammation of the valve between the left atrium and left ventricle	F.	Vasculitis

Answers can be found starting on page 571.

Go to www.wiley.com/go/taibo/terminology to find additional learning materials for this chapter:

- A crossword puzzle
- Flashcards
- Audio clips to show how to pronounce terms
- Case studies
- Review questions
- The figures from the chapter in PowerPoint

Chapter 7

The Respiratory Tract

Respiration is the exchange of oxygen and carbon dioxide between the body and the atmosphere (Figure 7.1). It includes the acts of inspiration (inhalation) and expiration (exhalation). When the animal inhales the room air, oxygen diffuses from the lungs into the blood, and carbon dioxide from the blood to the lungs. Simultaneously at the tissue level, oxygen diffuses from the blood into the tissue cells as carbon dioxide leaves the tissue cells and goes into the blood. The gas exchange that occurs within the lungs is referred to as external respiration and the gas exchange that occurs at the tissue level is referred to as internal respiration. The organs necessary for respiration to occur include the nasal sinuses, pharynx, larynx, and bronchi of the upper respiratory tract, and the bronchioles and alveoli of the lower respiratory tract. Muscles necessary for respiration to occur include the diaphragm, shoulder girdle, thoracic muscles, and intercostals.

Anatomy of the Respiratory Tract

When an animal inhales, the oxygen enters the nose through two openings called the nostrils (nares). Once through the nostrils, the air is divided as it moves into the nasal cavity due to a partition in the nose, called a nasal septum. As the air passes through the nasal cavity, it is filtered through cilia which collect any foreign material that was inhaled. Cilia are thin hairs attached to the mucous membrane epithelium lining the respiratory tract.

As introduced in Chapter 3, within the facial bones are air spaces called sinuses which are also lined with mucous membrane epithelium. These sinuses produce mucus which helps to lubricate the respiratory tract and warm the room air that is inhaled. The mucus aids the cilia in trapping foreign debris that has been inhaled. The best example of this function is if you have been working in your yard and mowing the lawn. After completing the task, try blowing your nose. You'll see the debris that the nasal passage has caught as you worked in the yard.

Veterinary Medical Terminology Guide and Workbook, First Edition. Angela Taibo.
© 2014 John Wiley & Sons, Inc. Published 2014 by John Wiley & Sons, Inc.
Companion website: www.wiley.com/go/taibo/terminology

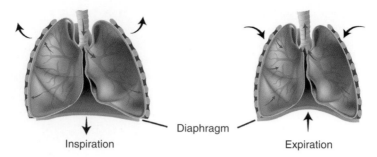

Inspiration   Diaphragm   Expiration

Figure 7.1   Stages of respiration. Courtesy of shutterstock/Alila Medical Images.

After passing through the nasal cavity, air then enters the pharynx (throat). The pharynx is divided into three sections based on their location: the nasopharynx, oropharynx, and laryngopharynx. The nasopharynx is above, or cranial to, the soft palate of the mouth, or behind the nasal cavity. The oropharynx is directly behind the mouth between the soft palate, the tongue, and epiglottis. Finally, the laryngopharynx is the caudal portion of the pharynx that enters the larynx (voice box). If having difficulty remembering the locations, just try memorizing the combining forms: Nas/o for nose, Or/o for mouth, and Laryng/o for voice box. The three sections of the pharynx work together to direct food and air in the appropriate direction.

When swallowing food, the nasopharynx closes to prevent the food from going into the nasal cavity. Simultaneously, the laryngopharynx prepares to direct the food toward the esophagus. In Chapter 4 the epiglottis was introduced as a leaf-like piece of cartilage covering the trachea to prevent aspiration of food. The epiglottis directs the food swallowed or air inhaled into the appropriate tracts. The laryngopharynx is the common passageway where the epiglottis lies and directs the food toward the GI tract and air toward the respiratory tract.

From the epiglottis, air enters the larynx (voice box). Within the larynx are two lip-like structures called vocal folds (vocal cords). The structure containing these folds is called the glottis. It is these two folds that create sound as air passes through. If "debarking" a dog, these two folds are cut to prevent the animal from making sounds, though this procedure isn't widely done in veterinary medicine in today's society. If placing an endotracheal tube in a patient before surgery, the epiglottis and vocal folds are our guide to proper tube placement. Once the epiglottis is pulled down, the vocal folds become visible. If the tube is placed between the vocal folds then it is assured that it is in the respiratory tract and more specifically, in the trachea.

After air passes the larynx, it enters the trachea (windpipe). The trachea is easily recognized by its cartilaginous rings. Unlike the esophagus which is a collapsible tube that merely expands with the presence of food, the trachea is a rigid, stiff tube that's always open in diameter.

Label Figure 7.2 using the terms in Table 7.1 regarding the flow of air through the respiratory tract. Structures are listed in order of occurrence.

Table 7.1   Structure of the Respiratory Tract.

Trachea (1)	Windpipe.
Bronchus (2) (plural: bronchi)	The bifurcation of the trachea that is a passageway into the air spaces of the lungs. The space in which the bronchi lie is called the **mediastinum (7)**.
Bronchioles (3)	Smallest branches of the bronchi.
Alveolus (4) (plural: alveoli)	Air sacs in the lungs located at the ends of the bronchioles.
Capillary (5)	Smallest blood vessel. O_2 and CO_2 diffuse across the walls of this vessel to and from the alveoli.
Erythrocytes (6)	Red blood cells **(RBC)**. Transport oxygen from the lungs to the rest of the body.

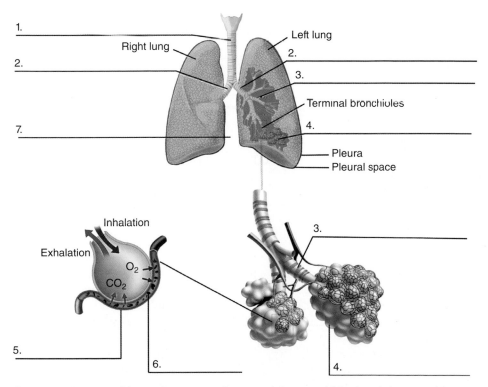

Figure 7.2   Anatomy of the respiratory tract. Courtesy of shutterstock/blamb and shutterstock/ Andrea Danti.

Each lung is surrounded by a double-folded membrane called the pleura. The outer fold of the membrane is called the parietal pleura, which lines the thoracic cavity. The inner fold of the membrane is called the visceral pleura, which lines the lungs. The small space between the pleural membranes and surrounding each lung is termed the pleural space. Within this space is a thin, watery fluid which helps to lubricate the pleural membranes and moisten the pleura during respiration. This pleural fluid also acts as an adhesive for the lungs to move with the thoracic cavity during respirations.

The final structure in the respiratory tract is a thin, muscular partition separating the thoracic and abdominal cavities, the diaphragm. As the diaphragm contracts, it causes the thoracic cavity to expand and the lungs to spread. As the lungs spread, they fill with air (inhalation). When the diaphragm relaxes, the thoracic cavity returns to its normal size which causes the lungs to expel their air (exhalation).

Related Terms

Alveoli	Air sacs in the lungs.
Bifurcation	Splitting into two branches.
Bronchus	Bifurcation of the trachea; passageway into
(plural: bronchi)	the air spaces of the lungs. Also called **Bronchial tubes**.
Bronchioles	Smallest branches of the bronchi; lead to the alveoli.
Capillary	Smallest blood vessel.
Cilia	Thin hairs attached to the mucous membrane epithelium lining the respiratory tract.
Carbon dioxide (CO_2)	Gas released by tissue cells and transported to the heart and lungs for exhalation.
Diaphragm	Thin, muscular partition separating the thoracic and abdominal cavities.
Epiglottis	Leaf-like piece of cartilage over the trachea (windpipe) to prevent aspiration of food.
Expiration	Breathing out; exhalation.
Glottis	Opening to the larynx (voice box).
Inspiration	Breathing in; inhalation.
Internal respiration	Gas exchange occurring at the tissue level.
Larynx	Voice box.
Mediastinum	Space between the lungs.
Mucous membranes	Specialized form of epithelial tissue that secretes mucus.
Mucus	Slimy substance produced by mucous membranes; contains epithelial cells, salts, white blood cells, and glandular secretions.
Nasal cavity	Proximal aspect of the respiratory tract within the nose.

Olfactory	Condition of smelling.
Oxygen (O_2)	Gas that enters the blood through the lungs and travels to the heart to be pumped to the rest of the body.
Pharynx	Throat.
Pleura	Membrane surrounding each lung.
Pleural cavity	Space between the pleural membranes and surrounding each lung. Also called **pleural space**.
Respiration	Exchange of oxygen and carbon dioxide between the body and the atmosphere.
Respiratory system	Group of organs working together to transfer oxygen from the air to the blood and to transfer carbon dioxide from the blood to the air.
Trachea	Windpipe.
Ventilation	Exchange of gas (air) in an enclosed space.
Vocal cords (vocal folds)	Folds of mucous membranes in the larynx that vibrate to create sound.

Pathology and Procedures

Agonal	Respirations near death.
Antitussives	Substances used to control and prevent coughing.
Asphyxia	Blockage of breathing leading to hypoxia; **suffocation**.
Aspiration	Inhalation of a foreign substance into the respiratory tract.
Asthma	Chronic, inflammatory disorder marked by dyspnea (difficulty breathing) and wheezing (Figure 7.3).

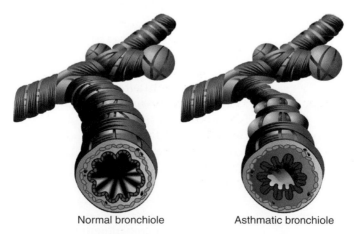

Normal bronchiole   Asthmatic bronchiole

Figure 7.3   Asthma. Courtesy of shutterstock/Rob3000.

Atelectasis	Incomplete dilation of a lung (alveoli).
Auscultation	Listening with a stethoscope to sounds within the body.
Bronchodilators	Drugs that cause dilation or expansion of the bronchus.
Chest tube	Hollow tube placed into the thoracic cavity to remove air or fluid.
Chronic obstructive pulmonary disease (COPD)	Disease in horses consisting of chronic bronchitis, bronchiolitis, and emphysema. Commonly called **heaves** or **broken wind** (Figure 7.4).

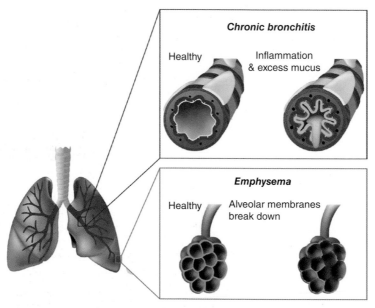

Chronic bronchitis

Healthy

Inflammation & excess mucus

Emphysema

Healthy

Alveolar membranes break down

Figure 7.4   Chronic obstructive pulmonary disease (COPD). Courtesy of shutterstock/Alila Sao Mai.

Cough	Forced expulsion of air from the lungs.
Diaphragmatic hernia	Displacement of abdominal organs through the opening in the diaphragm (Figure 7.5).
Emphysema	Lung disease caused by enlargement of the alveoli. This occurs due to changes, or loss of elasticity, in the alveolar wall.
Endotracheal intubation	Placement of a tube through the mouth and into the windpipe to establish an airway (Figure 7.6).
Epistaxis	Nosebleed.
Hyperpnea	Increased depth of breathing.
Hyperventilation	Abnormal, rapid, deep breathing.
Hypopnea	Slow or shallow breathing.

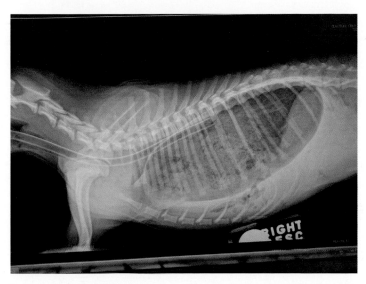

Figure 7.5   Radiograph of a diaphragmatic hernia. Note the abdominal viscera in the thoracic cavity. Courtesy of Beth Romano, AAS, CVT.

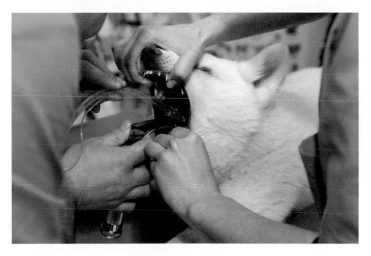

Figure 7.6   Placement of an endotracheal tube. Courtesy of shutterstock/sima.

Metastasis	To spread beyond control; spreading of a tumor to a secondary location (Figure 7.7).
Mucolytics	Substances used to break down or dissolve mucus.
Palliative	Relieving symptoms, but not curing.
Paroxysmal	Sudden occurrence such as a spasm or seizure. An example is a **cough**.

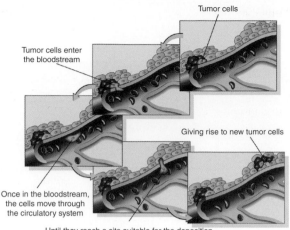

Tumor cells

Tumor cells enter
the bloodstream

Giving rise to new tumor cells

Once in the bloodstream,
the cells move through
the circulatory system

Until they reach a site suitable for the deposition
and reintegramento in tissues

Figure 7.7A Stages of metastasis. Courtesy of shutterstock/Rob3000.

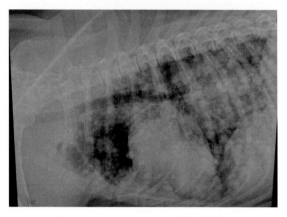

Figure 7.7B Metastasis in the lungs. Normal lungs are clear black on a radiograph. Courtesy of Beth Romano, AAS, CVT.

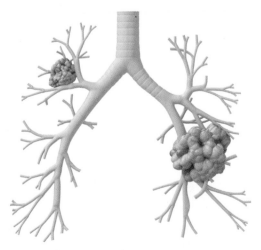

Figure 7.7C Metastasis in the bronchioles. Courtesy of shutterstock/Sebastian Kaulitzki.

TECH TIP 7.1   Can animals get lung cancer?

A curiosity that students often have is if animals can get lung cancer. Lung cancer as a primary disease isn't often seen in veterinary medicine. It is possible, however, for animals to get lung cancer from secondhand smoke. Owners who smoke in their houses put their animals at risk.

In veterinary medicine, we typically take thoracic radiographs to check for metastasis of a cancer that originated elsewhere in the body. If the cancer has metastasized to the lungs, then the prognosis is poor.

Percussion	Tapping a surface to determine the density of the underlying structure. For example, if tapping the surface of a chest or abdomen filled with air, the sound produced is a hollow ping. If filled with fluid, the sound is more of a thunk or thud.
Phlegm	Thick mucus excreted in large quantities.
Pleural effusion	Escape of fluid into the pleural cavity.
Pneumonia	Acute inflammation and infection of the alveoli (Figures 7.8 and 7.9).

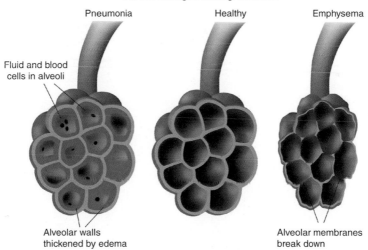

Alveoli changes in lung diseases

Pneumonia   Healthy   Emphysema

Fluid and blood cells in alveoli

Alveolar walls thickened by edema

Alveolar membranes break down

Figure 7.8   Comparison of lung diseases. Courtesy of shutterstock/Alila Sao Mai.

Pulse oximeter	Instrument for measuring oxygen concentration in arterial blood (Figure 7.10).
Purulent	Containing pus (Figure 7.11).
Rales and crackles	Crackling noises heard on inspiration due to fluid in the alveoli. Also called **crepitant.**
Rhonchi	Wheezing. High-pitched whistling sounds heard during inspiration.

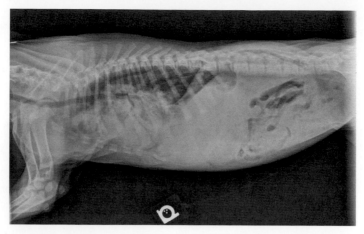

Figure 7.9　Radiograph of a dog with pneumonia. Courtesy of Beth Romano, AAS, CVT.

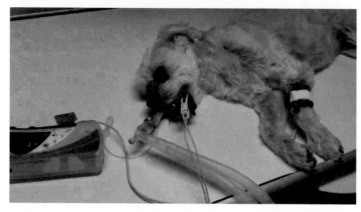

Figure 7.10　Dog attached to pulse oximeter going into surgery. Courtesy of Greg Martinez, DVM; www.youtube.com/drgregdvm.

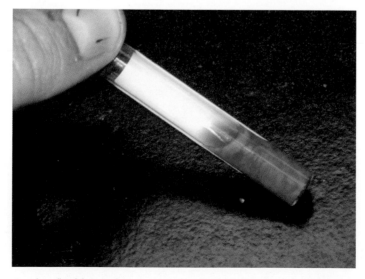

Figure 7.11　Purulent fluid from a thoracentesis. Courtesy of AK Traylor, DVM; Microscopy Learning Systems.

Sputum   Mucous secretion from the lungs, bronchi, and
                                    trachea.
Stridor   Strained shrill heard during inspiration due to an
                                    airway obstruction.
Tidal volume   Amount of gas passing in and out of the lungs
                                    during a respiratory cycle.
Transtracheal wash   Introduction of sterile saline into the trachea
                                    through a catheter and then withdrawl of that
                                    fluid for cytology.
Vesicular sounds   Soft sounds heard on auscultation due to small
                                    bronchioles and alveoli. Also called a **vesicular
                                    murmur.**

Building the Terms

Table 7.2   Chapter 7 Combining Forms.

Combining Forms	Definition	Combining Forms	Definition
Alveol/o	Alveoli; air sacs	**Ox/o**	Oxygen (O_2)
Bronch/o	Bronchial tube	**Pector/o**	Chest
Bronchiol/o	Bronchioles	**Pharyng/o**	Pharynx; throat
Capn/o	Carbon dioxide (CO_2)	**Phragm/o**	Wall
Cyan/o	Blue	**Phren/o**	Diaphragm
Diaphragmat/o	Diaphragm	**Pleur/o**	Pleura
Epiglott/o	Epiglottis	**Pneum/o**	Lung; air; gas
Furc/o	Forking; branching	**Pneumon/o**	Lung; air; gas
Gastr/o	Stomach	**Pulmon/o**	Lung
Glott/o	Glottis	**Py/o**	Pus
Hem/o	Blood	**Rhin/o**	Nose
Laryng/o	Larynx; voice box	**Sinus/o**	Sinus
Lob/o	Lobe	**Spir/o**	To breathe; breathing
Mediastin/o	Mediastinum	**Tel/o**	Complete
Nas/o	Nose	**Thorac/o**	Chest
Olfact/o	Smelling	**Trache/o**	Trachea; windpipe
Onc/o	tumor	**Tuss/i**	Cough

Table 7.3 Chapter 7 Prefixes.

Prefix	Definition	Prefix	Definition
a-, an-	no; not; without	**hyper-**	above; excessive; increased
anti-	against	**hypo-**	deficient; below; under; less than normal; decreased
bi-	two; both	**meta-**	change; beyond
brady-	slow	**para-**	near; beside; abnormal; apart from; along the side of
dia-	through; complete	**tachy-**	fast
dys-	bad; painful; difficult; abnormal	**trans-**	across; through
em-	in		

Table 7.4 Chapter 7 Suffixes.

Suffix	Definition	Suffix	Definition
-al, -ar, -ary, -eal, -ic	pertaining to	**-osis**	abnormal condition
-ation	process; condition	**-plasty**	surgical repair
-centesis	surgical puncture to remove fluid or gas	**-pnea**	breathing
-dynia	pain	**-ptysis**	spitting
-ectasia	stretching; dilation; expansion	**-rrhea**	flow; discharge
-ectasis	stretching; dilation; expansion	**-scopy**	visual examination
-ectomy	removal; excision; resection	**-spasm**	sudden involuntary contraction of muscles
-ema	condition	**-sphyxia**	pulse
-ia	condition	**-stasis**	stopping; controlling
-itis	inflammation	**-stenosis**	tightening; narrowing; stricture
-logy	study of	**-stomy**	new opening to the outside of the body
-lytic	to reduce; destroy; separate; breakdown	**-thorax**	chest; pleural cavity
-meter	measure	**-tomy**	incision; process of cutting into

Now it's time to put these word parts together. If you memorize the meaning of the combining forms, prefixes, and suffixes, then this will get easier each time. Remember your five basic rules to medical terminology when building and defining these terms. You'll notice some word parts are repeated from the previous chapter.

	Parts		Medical Term		Definition
Alveol/o	+ -ar	=	Alveolar	:	_____
Bronchi/o	+ -ectasis	=	Bronchiectasis	:	_____

Sometimes called bronchiectasia.

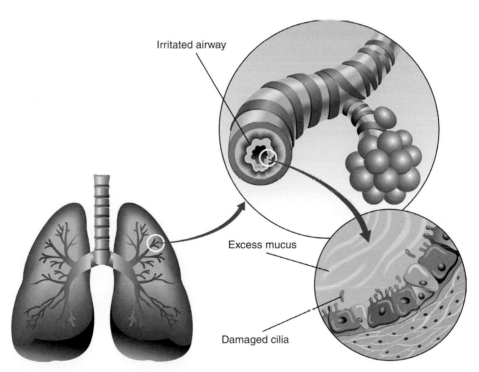

Irritated airway

Excess mucus

Damaged cilia

Figure 7.12   Chronic bronchitis. Courtesy of shutterstock/Rob3000.

	Parts		Medical Term		Definition
Bronch/o	+ -itis	=	Bronchitis	:	_____
Bronch/o	+ -spasm	=	Bronchospasm	:	_____
Bronch/o	+ -scopy	=	Bronchoscopy	:	_____
Bronchiol/o	+ -itis	=	Bronchiolitis	:	_____
hyper-	+ Capn/o + -ia	=	Hypercapnia	:	_____
hypo-	+ Capn/o + -ia	=	Hypocapnia	:	_____

Cyan/o	+ -osis	= Cyanosis	: _____
Diaphragmat/o	+ -ic	= Diaphragmatic	: _____
Epiglott/o	+ -itis	= Epiglottitis	: _____
Hem/o	+ -ptysis	= Hemoptysis	: _____
Hem/o	+ -thorax	= Hemothorax	: _____
Laryng/o	+ -eal	= Laryngeal	: _____
Laryng/o	+ -itis	= Laryngitis	: _____
Laryng/o	+ -scopy	= Laryngoscopy	: _____
Laryng/o	+ -spasm	= Laryngospasm	: _____
Lob/o	+ -ectomy	= Lobectomy	: _____
Mediastin/o	+ -al	= Mediastinal	: _____
Nas/o	+ Gastr/o + -ic	= Nasogastric	: _____
para-	+ Nas/o + -al	= Paranasal	: _____
an-	+ -oxia	= anoxia	: _____
hypo-	+ -oxia	= hypoxia	: _____
Onc/o	+ -logy	= Oncology	: _____
Pector/o	+ -al	= Pectoral	: _____
Pharyng/o	+ -eal	= Pharyngeal	: _____
Pharyng/o	+ -plasty	= Pharyngoplasty	: _____
Pharyng/o	+ -tomy	= Pharyngotomy	: _____
Pharyng/o	+ -stomy	= Pharyngostomy	: _____
Phren/o	+ -ic	= Phrenic	: _____
Pleur/o	+ -al	= Pleural	: _____
Pleur/o	+ -dynia	= Pleurodynia	: _____
a-	+ -pnea	= apnea	: _____
brady-	+ -pnea	= bradypnea	: _____
dys-	+ -pnea	= dyspnea	: _____
tachy-	+ -pnea	= tachypnea	: _____
Pneum/o	+ -thorax	= Pneumothorax	: _____
Pneumon/o	+ -ectomy	= Pneumonectomy	: _____

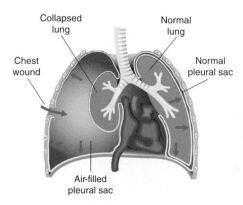

Figure 7.13A   Diagram of a pneumothorax. Courtesy of shutterstock/Rob3000.

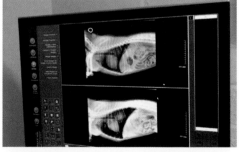

Figure 7.13B   Radiograph of a dog treated for pneumothorax. Top: Radiograph of the dog following a thoracentesis. Bottom: Note the air surrounding the heart from the pneumothorax. Courtesy of Greg Martinez, DVM.; www.youtube.com/drgregdvm.

| Pulmon/o | + -ary | = Pulmonary | :_____ |
| Py/o | + -thorax | = Pyothorax | :_____ |

Also called empyema.

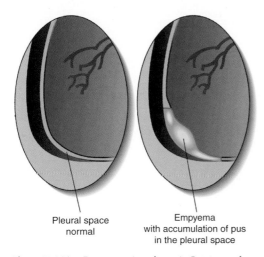

Pleural space
normal

Empyema
with accumulation of pus
in the pleural space

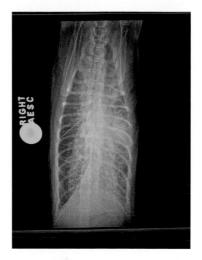

Figure 7.14A   Empyema (pyothorax). Courtesy of shutterstock/Rob3000.

Figure 7.14B   Radiograph of a dog with pyothorax.

Rhin/o	+ itis	= Rhinitis	:_____
Rhin/o	+ -plasty	= Rhinoplasty	:_____
Rhin/o	+ -rrhea	= Rhinorrhea	:_____
Sinus/o	+ -itis	– Sinusitis	:_____
Sinus/o	+ -tomy	= Sinusotomy	:_____
Spir/o	+ -meter	= Spirometer	:_____
dia-	+ -meter	= Diameter	:_____
Thorac/o	+ -centesis	= Thoracocentesis	:_____

Also called a thoracentesis.

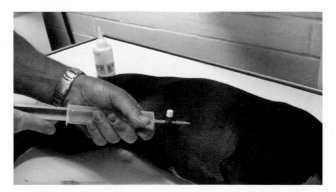

Figure 7.15   Thoracentesis in a dog with pneumothorax from HBC. Ideally it would be best to shave and surgically prep the site. This dog was hit by car and emergency service acted quickly. Courtesy of Greg Martinez, DVM; www.youtube.com/drgregdvm.

Thorac/o + -ic   = Thoracic   : _____
Thorac/o + -tomy   = Thoracotomy   : _____
Thorac/o + -scopy   = Thoracoscopy   : _____

Also called thorascopy.

Trache/o + -al   + stenosis = Tracheal stenosis : _____
Trache/o + -plasty   = Tracheoplasty   : _____
Trache/o + -stomy   = Tracheostomy   : _____
Trache/o + -tomy   = Tracheotomy   : _____
trans-   + Trache/o + -al   = Transtracheal   : _____

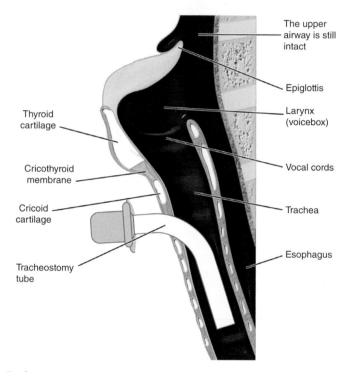

The upper airway is still intact

Epiglottis

Thyroid cartilage

Larynx (voicebox)

Cricothyroid membrane

Vocal cords

Cricoid cartilage

Trachea

Tracheostomy tube

Esophagus

Figure 7.16   Tracheostomy. Courtesy of shutterstock/blamb.

Abbreviations

Table 7.5   Chapter 7 Abbreviations.

Abbreviation	Definition
ABG	Arterial blood gas; measurement of O_2 and CO_2 in arterial blood.
BG	Blood gas; measurement of O_2 and CO_2 in arterial and venous blood.
BRSV	Bovine respiratory syncytial virus: Virus in calves caused by a pneumovirus. Causes dyspnea and eventually death.

Table 7.5   (*Continued*).

Abbreviation	Definition
COPD	Chronic obstructive pulmonary disease.
CPCR	Cardiopulmonary cerebral resuscitation; new name for CPR.
CPR	Cardiopulmonary resuscitation.
ET tube	Endotracheal tube.
IBR	Infectious bovine rhinotracheitis; infectious disease in cattle caused by a herpes virus. Causes rhinorrhea, rhinitis, tracheitis, and fever.
OPP	Ovine progressive pneumonia; virus in sheep caused by lentivirus. Causes chronic pneumonia and eventually goes to the brain, causing death.
pCO_2, P_{CO2}	Partial pressure of carbon dioxide; measures dissolved carbon dioxide in the blood.
pO_2, P_{O2}	Partial pressure of oxygen; measures dissolved oxygen in the blood (plasma).
PE	Pulmonary embolism.
Pulse Ox	Pulse oximeter; pulse oximetry.
RR	Respiratory rate.
URI	Upper respiratory infection.

Case Study

In this case study you'll notice some terms from the previous chapters.

Nelson, a 4-year-old Yorkie, has been rushed into the clinic after being attacked by an Akita. The owner claims that the Akita came out of nowhere and grabbed Nelson. Nelson is dyspneic and has obvious puncture wounds on his face, neck, and chest. He's spitting blood and has swelling below his lower jaw.
1.   Where is Nelson's swelling?
    a. Submandibular
    b. Paranasal
    c. Maxillary
2.   What other clinical signs is Nelson displaying?
    a. Rapid breathing and hemoptysis
    b. Difficulty breathing and hemoptysis
    c. Slow breathing and hemorrhea

Radiographs show that Nelson has a pneumothorax.
3.   Why is Nelson dyspneic?
    a. Pus in the chest cavity
    b. Blood in the chest cavity
    c. Air in the chest cavity

4. What procedure can relieve the condition in number 3?
   a. Abdominocentesis
   b. Thoracentesis
   c. Cystocentesis

After the procedure was performed in number 4, Nelson's respirations improved. Some puncture wounds were deep and had to be repaired surgically. An ET tube was placed and Nelson went to surgery.

5. Where was the tube placed?
   a. Into the lungs
   b. Within the windpipe
   c. Through the chest cavity

Nelson was placed on antibiotics and pain medication and eventually sent home.

Exercises

7-A: Give the term for the following definitions.

1. _____: Membrane surrounding the lungs
2. _____: Space between the lungs
3. _____: Throat
4. _____: Nares
5. _____: Bifurcation of the trachea that acts as a passageway into the lungs.
6. _____: Air sacs in the lungs
7. _____: Voice box
8. _____: Thin hairs lining the respiratory tract
9. _____: Smallest branches of the bronchi
10. _____: Leaf-like piece of cartilage over trachea
11. _____: Space between pleural membranes
12. _____: Windpipe

7-B: Define the following terms.

1. Epistaxis _____
2. Agonal _____
3. Atelectasis _____
4. Inspiration _____
5. Olfactory _____
6. Mucolytics _____
7. Percussion _____
8. Palliative _____
9. Bronchodilators _____
10. Diaphragm _____

7-C: Complete the term.

1. Not breathing: _____pnea
2. Lack of O_2 to tissue: _____oxia
3. Blood in the chest cavity: hemo _____
4. Inflammation of sinuses: _____itis
5. Visual exam of the voice box: _____scopy
6. New opening to the windpipe: _____stomy
7. Pertaining to the throat: _____eal
8. Abnormal condition of blue color: _____osis
9. Removal of a lung: _____ectomy
10. Surgical repair of the nose: rhino _____
11. Pus in the chest cavity: _____thorax
12. Excessive carbon dioxide: Hypercap _____

7-D: Define the following abbreviations.

1. _____: ABG
2. _____: ET tube
3. _____: CPCR
4. _____: OPP
5. _____: BRSV

6. _____: URI
7. _____: PE
8. _____: RR
9. _____: pCO_2
10. _____: Pulse ox

7-E: Circle the correct answer.

1. T or F Aspiration is the same as inspiration.
2. T or F Slimy substance produced in the respiratory tract is spelled mucous.
3. T or F The definition of agonal is respirations near death.
4. T or F A pneumothorax is air in the lungs.
5. T or F Acute is a sudden onset.
6. T or F Antitussives are used to dilate the airways.
7. T or F Alveoli lose their elasticity in emphysema.
8. T or F Pneumonia is defined as acute inflammation and infection of the alveoli.
9. T or F Dyspnea and apnea are the same thing.
10. T or F A purulent wound contains pus.

7-F: Match the following terms with their descriptions.

1. _____ Strained shrill due to obstruction
2. _____ Soft sounds due to small alveoli
3. _____ Caused by fluid in the alveoli
4. _____ Abnormal, rapid, deep breathing
5. _____ Wheeze

A.   Hyperventilation
B.   Rales and crackles
C.   Ronchi
D.   Stridor
E.   Vesicular sounds

Answers can be found starting on page 571.
Answers can be found starting on page 571.

Go to www.wiley.com/go/taibo/terminology to find additional learning materials for this chapter:

- A crossword puzzle
- Flashcards
- Audio clips to show how to pronounce terms
- Case studies
- Review questions
- The figures from the chapter in PowerPoint

Chapter 8

Hematology

Hematology is the study of the blood. Blood has three main components: cellular, fluid, and acellular dissolved substances. Cellular components include erythrocytes (red blood cells), leukocytes (white blood cells), and thrombocytes (platelets). The fluid component of blood is water and acellular dissolved substances is a broad category which includes vitamins, minerals, proteins, gases, wastes, and much more. Each component of blood has a specialized function. Forty-five percent of blood is made up of blood cells. The remaining 55% is fluid and acellular dissolved substances (Figure 8.1).

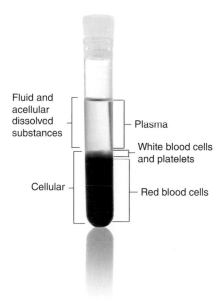

Figure 8.1 Anatomy of blood. Courtesy of shutterstock/Nixx Photography.

Veterinary Medical Terminology Guide and Workbook, First Edition. Angela Taibo.
© 2014 John Wiley & Sons, Inc. Published 2014 by John Wiley & Sons, Inc.
Companion website: www.wiley.com/go/taibo/terminology

Anatomy and Physiology of Blood and Blood-Forming Organs

Within the bone marrow are hematopoietic cells called stem cells. These cells are capable of differentiating into precursors of red blood cells, white blood cells, and platelets.

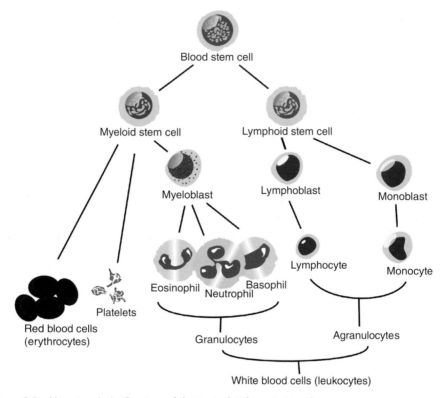

Figure 8.2 Hematopoiesis. Courtesy of shutterstock/Athanasia Nomikou.

Erythrocytes

Erythrocytes are the most abundant of the blood cells. Their function is to transport oxygen from the lungs to the tissues. Within the erythrocytes is an oxygen-carrying pigment called hemoglobin, which allows the red blood cells to transport oxygen. If a red blood cell is lacking hemoglobin, then it is unable to transport oxygen to tissues and the animal will become hypoxic and cyanotic.

Red blood cells, or RBCs, are produced in the bone marrow. The stimulus for red blood cell production is hypoxia. When an animal becomes hypoxic, their kidneys begin secreting a hormone called erythropoietin (EPO). EPO then stimulates the stem cells in the bone marrow to differentiate into red blood cells (RBCs). The stem cells in the bone marrow can become anything that the body needs.

As the red blood cells are being produced, three changes occur in the cell. The cell size decreases, the cell color changes from basophilic (blue) to eosinophilic (red), and the cell loses its nucleus. During its earliest stages, an RBC has a nucleus containing ribosomes which actively produce hemoglobin to put into the RBC. After reaching maturity, the nucleus is no longer needed because the cell has been filled with the proper amount of hemoglobin. Once an RBC is fully mature, the bone marrow releases it into the peripheral blood (circulation) to transport oxygen. Morphologically, the RBC is biconcave in shape. That slight "pinch" in the center of the cell is referred to as central pallor.

An RBC can stay in circulation for three months. When the cell is done fulfilling it role, the body destroys the RBC using a group of cells called macrophages in the liver, spleen, and bone marrow. The breakdown of RBCs is termed hemolysis.

Table 8.1 RBC Morphology Terms.

Morphology	Definition
Agglutination	Clumping of RBCs; technically this is the joining of antibodies and antigens.
Rouleaux	Stacking of RBCs; this is due to a "sticky" surface on the cells from high levels of antibodies.
Anisocytosis	Unequal sizes of RBCs.
Poikilocytosis	Irregular shapes of RBCs.
Normocytic	RBCs are normal in size.
Macrocytic	RBCs are larger in size.
Microcytic	RBCs are smaller in size.
Normochromic	RBCs are normal in color.
Hyperchromic	RBCs are more red than normal; this is an artifactual finding due to hemolysis.
Hypochromic	RBCs have less red color than normal; this is due to a lack of hemoglobin.
Spherocytosis	Presence of spherocytes; RBCs are rounded, lacking central pallor. Seen with hemolytic anemias.

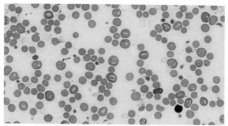

Figure 8.3A Bloodfilm of a dog with hemolytic anemia. Note the spherocytes which are smaller and a more solid pink. There is also anisocytosis.

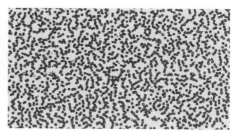

Figure 8.3B Equine bloodfilm showing rouleaux.

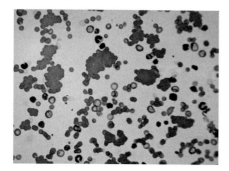

Figure 8.3C Bloodfilm from a dog with hemolytic anemia showing agglutination.

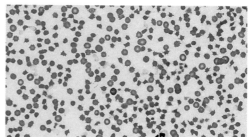

Figure 8.3D Feline bloodfilm with poikilocytosis.

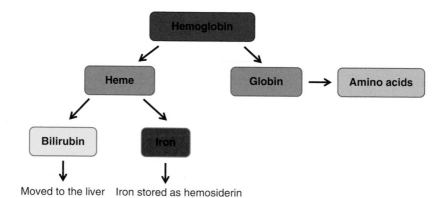

Figure 8.4 The breakdown and recycling of hemoglobin.

After hemolysis occurs, hemoglobin is released. The body has no use for the free hemoglobin so the macrophages breakdown the hemoglobin and recycle its component parts. Hemoglobin is made up of a heme molecule and a globin molecule (Figure 8.4). Globin is a protein which the body breaks down further into amino acids that can be recycled. The heme molecule is made up of iron and a yellow pigment called bilirubin. Iron is stored within cells for future use when the

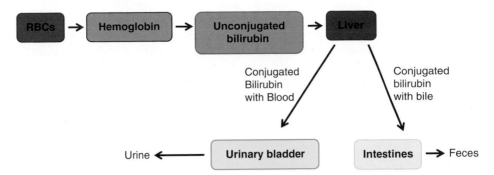

Figure 8.5   The path of bilirubin in the body.

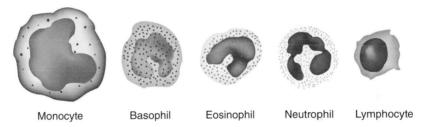

Figure 8.6   The five different types of white blood cells. Courtesy of shutterstock/MiAdS.

body needs to make more hemoglobin. That iron storage within cells is called hemosiderin. The bilirubin is excreted in stool and urine after being conjugated (processed) in the liver (Figure 8.5).

Leukocytes

There are five different kinds of white blood cells (WBCs) (Figures 8.6 and 8.7). Each has a specific function and a specific stimulus for its production. White blood cells are divided into two categories based on their cytoplasmic morphology. Leukocytes with granules in their cytoplasm are termed granulocytes and those without granules in their cytoplasm are termed agranulocytes.

Granulocytes include neutrophils, eosinophils, and basophils. The granules within each cell are packages that contain various substances including enzymes which are released during an immune response. When the substances within the granules are released, it is termed degranulation. Each granulocyte responds to a specific stimulus or chemical mediator. All three granulocytes have a segmented (pinched) nucleus.

Neutrophils are the most numerous of the granulocytes and contain neutral-staining granules in their nucleus. Neutrophils are bacterial phagocytes (eating cells) so the stimulus for their production is a bacterial infection. Eosinophils have pink- or red-staining granules. Eosin/o means red, rosy, or pink.

The granules within the eosinophil contain substances that respond to allergies or parasites. Therefore, the stimulus for eosinophil production is the presence of allergies or parasites. Basophils are the rarest of all the white blood cells and they contain blue-staining granules. Basophils increase in severe or exaggerated hypersensitivities. Their function therefore is anaphylaxis.

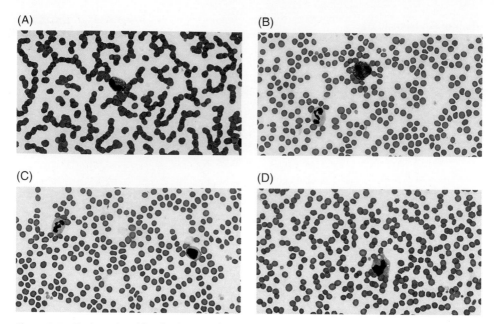

Figure 8.7 Equine white blood cells. (A) Basophil. (B) Neutrophil and eosinophil. (C) Neutrophil and lymphocyte. (D) Monocyte.

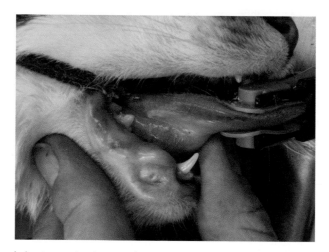

Figure 8.8 Anaphylactic reaction in a cat during anesthesia. The tongue and throat began to swell during surgery due to a reaction to the anesthetic drugs that were used. A tracheostomy had to be performed. Courtesy of AK Traylor, DVM; Microscopy Learning Systems.

TECH TIP 8.1 Allergies vs. Anaphylaxis

Allergies are abnormal hypersensitivities that are not life threatening. An example is an animal that's allergic to chicken and breaks out in a skin rash. Anaphylaxis is an exaggerated hypersensitivity that is generally life threatening. An example is an animal that's allergic to chicken and its throat swells shut when it eats chicken.

Table 8.2   Leukocytes.

Leukocytes	Stimulus	Function
Neutrophil	Inflammation, infection, bacterial products	Primary bacterial phagocyte
Eosinophils	Allergies, parasites	Anti-allergy (antihistamine) Anti-parasite (acid)
Basophils	Exaggerated hypersensitivity	Anaphylaxis
Lymphocytes	Antigens	Produce antibodies
Monocytes	Inflammation, infection, bacterial products	Macrophage

Agranulocytes include lymphocytes and monocytes. These cells are mononuclear, which means there's no pinching in their nucleus. Lymphocytes are the most numerous of agranulocytes and their function is to produce antibodies, which are proteins that are produced in response to antigens (foreign proteins). They neutralize the antigens by hooking onto them. Examples of antigens include viruses and parasites. The diagnostic feature of lymphocytes is their high nucleus to cytoplasm ratio(N:C ratio). Monocytes are literally the garbage can of the blood vessels because these cells are macrophages (large eating cells). They eat everything from bacteria to older cells that are no longer needed. The diagnostic feature of monocytes is their ameboid-looking nucleus. The stimulus for monocyte production is the same as that for the neutrophil because its main priority is to eat what neutrophils left behind.

With the exception of lymphocytes, the four remaining white blood cells are produced in the bone marrow and originate from stem cells. The lymphocytes are produced in lymphoid tissue such as the spleen, lymph nodes, and thymus gland. Imagine when you get sick with the flu—your lymph nodes swell because they're producing lymphocytes to battle the virus.

Thrombocytes

Platelets are produced by stem cells in the bone marrow and their function is to aid in the clotting process (Figure 8.9). When platelets are needed, the stem cells in the bone marrow differentiate into a cell called a megakaryocyte. Platelets are cytoplasmic fragments of the megakaryocyte.

Serum or Plasma?

After removing the cellular components of blood, fluid and acellular substances are left. The fluid portion of blood is simply water. Dissolved in the water are the acellular-dissolved substances such as proteins, gases, and wastes. This mixture of fluid and acellular matter is normally clear or straw in color in most animals.

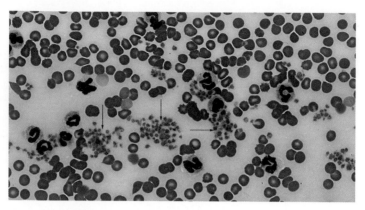

Figure 8.9 Clumps of platelets on a canine bloodfilm.

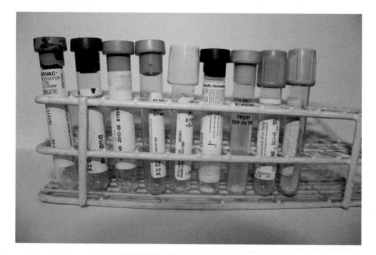

Figure 8.10 Various types of vacutainer tubes used in blood collection.

Table 8.3 Blood Tubes.

Tube	Contents	Use	Fluid Portion
Red top tube (RTT)	Nothing	Blood chemistry (Biochemistry)	Serum
Green top tube (GTT)	Heparin	Blood gas analysis	Plasma
Blue top tube (BTT)	Sodium citrate	Coagulation studies	Plasma
Grey top tube (GTT)	Oxylate	Blood glucose test	Plasma
Lavender top tube (LTT)	EDTA	Complete blood count	Plasma

Serum is the fluid portion of coagulated (clotted) blood. Plasma is the fluid portion of anticoagulated or circulating blood. The difference between them is in the blood tubes in which the fluids were collected. Some blood tubes contain an anticoagulant so when blood is mixed with that anticoagulant and then spun down in a centrifuge, the fluid that results is called plasma. If blood is placed in a blood tube that's lacking an anticoagulant, then the blood will clot. After centrifuging the clotted blood, the fluid that results is termed serum. The difference is that plasma still contains all the clotting proteins in the blood, whereas serum has used up all of its clotting proteins.

Coagulation, or blood clotting, is far too complicated to thoroughly discuss in this book. The following is a very condensed version of the clotting process (Figure 8.11).

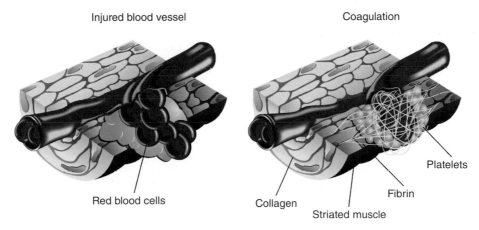

Figure 8.11A   Clotting after damage to a vessel. Courtesy of shutterstock/Rob3000.

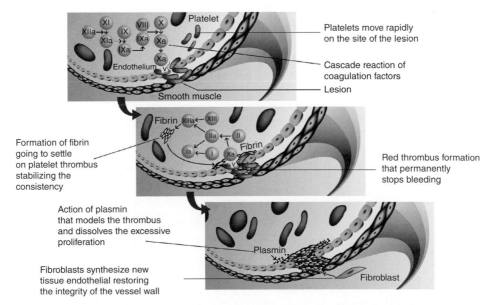

Figure 8.11B   Steps of coagulation. Note the multiple, intricate steps involved as well as the number of clotting proteins involved. Courtesy of shutterstock/Rob3000.

When an animal is injured, the first on the scene are the platelets, which are the body's first line of defense to stop the bleeding. As the platelets clump together and plug the bleed, clotting proteins in the plasma are activated to form a clot, the reinforcement. Multiple clotting proteins are required to form a stable clot. Some of these clotting proteins include prothrombin, thrombin, and fibrinogen. After these proteins are activated, they work together in a series of steps to produce a stable fibrin clot. Fibrin is the protein strands that make up the clot. Animals with a bleeding disorder are typically lacking one or more of these clotting proteins. To detect a bleeding disorder in animals, we draw blood to measure the levels of the various clotting proteins.

Two proteins that dominate a protein measurement are albumin and globulins. Albumin maintains oncotic pressure, or water concentration, in the blood. If albumin is decreased, then water no longer stays in the blood and the animal begins to feel dehydrated. Globulins are proteins that aid in immunity. There are three kinds of globulins: alpha, beta, and gamma. The gamma globulins, or immunoglobulins, are actually antibodies produced in response to antigens.

Blood Banking

A common question is whether animals have blood types. Each species has its own typing system. Cats use the feline AB blood group system; The blood types for cats include A, B, and AB. Dogs use the DEA blood type system, or dog erythrocyte antigen system. Dogs are typed based on the antigens on the surface of their red blood cells. Examples of DEAs include 1.1, 1.2, and 7.

There are a variety of tests available to determine blood types in cats; however, canine testing is still difficult. Most of the canine blood type tests available are only able to detect the presence of DEA 1.1. The best test for compatibility between a donor and recipient is considered to be the crossmatch. Without going into detail, this test involves combining blood components from the recipient and donor in a test tube. If the animals are not compatible, the red blood cells from each animal will attack each other and it is possible to visualize clumping of the red blood cells (Figure 8.12).

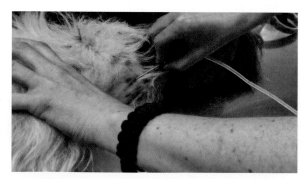

Figure 8.12A Jugular venipuncture to obtain blood from a canine donor. Courtesy of Greg Martinez, DVM.; www.youtube.com/drgregdvm.

(A)   (B)

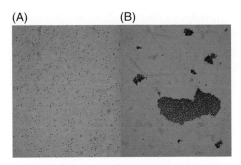

Figure 8.12   Microscopic view of a crossmatch to determine compatibility. Note in (A) the red blood cells are spread out, indicating compatibility. In (B), the red blood cells are clumped, indicating that the two animals are not compatible. The red blood cells are attacking each other.

Other than blood typing, blood banking isn't much different from human medicine. Blood components are often used rather than whole blood for transfusions. Examples of blood components used include plasma and packed red blood cells.

Anemia

Anemia is a decrease in red blood cells and/or hemoglobin. There are three general causes of anemia: decreased production, destruction, and loss. Below is a summary of the types of anemia and their causes.

Aplastic anemia	Decrease in red blood cells and/or hemoglobin due to no production. Examples of no production include bone marrow problems and renal failure (no EPO).
Hemolytic anemia	Decrease in red blood cells and/or hemoglobin due to destruction. The body is destroying its own red blood cells.
Hemorrhagic anemia	Decrease in red blood cells and/or hemoglobin due to loss. The animal is bleeding out and losing red blood cells.

Related Terms

Agranulocytes	White blood cells lacking granules in their cytoplasm;lymphocytes and monocytes.
Albumin	Plasma protein that maintains blood volume.
Anemia	Decrease in red blood cells and/or hemoglobin.
Antibody (Ab)	Proteins produced by white blood cells in response to antigens.
Antigens (Ag)	Foreign substance (protein) that stimulates the production of antibodies.
Basophils	Granulocytic white blood cell seen in anaphylaxis.
Bilirubin	Metabolite of hemoglobin breakdown; conjugated in the liver.
Coagulation	Blood clotting.

Eosinophil	Granulocytic white blood cell seen with allergies and parasites.
Erythrocyte	Red blood cell (RBC).
Erythropoietin (EPO)	Hormone secreted by the kidneys to stimulate RBC production.
Exsanguination	Extensive blood loss due to internal or external hemorrhage.
Fibrin	Protein threads that form the basis of a clot.
Fibrinogen	Plasma protein that is converted to fibrin in the clotting process.
Globulins	Plasma proteins such as alpha, beta, and gamma globulins.
Granulocytes	White blood cells containing granules in their cytoplasm; neutrophils, eosinophils, and basophils.
Heme	Iron-containing portion of hemoglobin.
Hemoglobin (Hb)	Oxygen-carrying pigment of red blood cells.
Homeostasis	State of equilibrium of the body's internal environment.
Leukocyte	White blood cell (WBC).
Lymphocyte	Agranulocyte that produces antibodies.
Macrophages	Monocytes that migrate from the blood to the tissue; large phagocytes. Exist in liver, spleen, and bone marrow.
Megakaryocyte	Precursor to a platelet formed in the bone marrow.
Neutrophil	Granulocytic WBC that is the body's primary bacterial phagocyte.
Plasma	Fluid portion of anticoagulated or circulating blood.
Prothrombin	Plasma protein that is converted to thrombin in the clotting process.
Reticulocyte	Immature stage of a red blood cell seen when blood is stained in new methylene blue stain. Ribosomes appear dark blue inside the cell.
Serum	Fluid portion of coagulated blood.
Stem cell	Bone marrow cell that can become any cell type.
Thrombin	An enzyme that results from the activation of prothrombin. It converts fibrinogen to fibrin in the clotting process.
Thrombocyte	Platelet; clotting cell.

Pathology and Procedures

Anticoagulant	Agent that prevents coagulation of blood.
Biochemistries	Test to measure enzymes and electrolytes in the body. Also called **blood chemistries**.
Bleeding time	Coagulation test used to measure the time required for a small wound to stop bleeding. In animals, the incision is generally made in the buccal mucosa.

Bone marrow biopsy	Procedure to obtain a bone marrow sample for cytology.
Complete blood count	Blood panel that includes WBC count, RBC count, and platelet count.
Disseminated intravascular coagulation (DIC)	Formation of clots throughout microcirculation which leads to hemorrhage due to consumption of clotting factors.
Dyscrasia	Any abnormal or pathological condition of blood.
Hematocrit	The percentage of red blood cells in a volume of blood. Also called **packed cell volume (PCV)**.

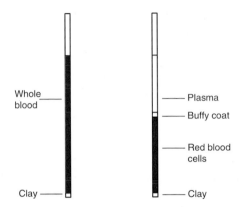

Figure 8.13A   Anatomy of a hematocrit tube used for a packed cell volume. The left shows a hematocrit tube with whole blood. The right shows the same tube after being spun in a centrifuge.

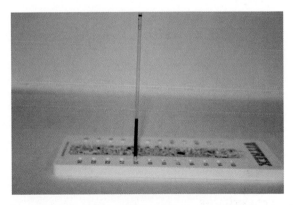

Figure 8.13B   Actual spun hematocrit that will be used to measure PCV.

| Hemophilia | Bleeding disorder in which the animal is lacking one or more clotting proteins. The disorder can be further classified based on which proteins are missing. Examples include hemophilia A, hemophilia B, and hemophilia C. |

Hemorrhage	Escape of blood through ruptured blood vessels.
Icterus	Yellowish coloration of the plasma (Figure 8.14). Caused by increased bilirubin.

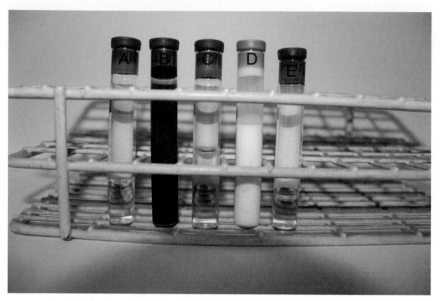

Figure 8.14 Plasma colors. Please note that the samples in each tube are strictly plasma, not whole blood. The colors are as follows: (A) clear, (B) hemolytic, (C) icteric, (D) lipemic, (E) straw.

Leukemia	Increase in the number of cancerous white blood cells.
Lipemia	Fat in the blood. This term is most often used to describe a white plasma color (Figure 8.14).
Phlebotomy	Venipuncture; the act of drawing blood.
Transfusion	Transfer of blood and blood components from one animal to another.
Von Willebrand's disease	Congenital bleeding disorder in which the animal is lacking Von Willebrand's clotting factor. Breeds commonly seen include Doberman Pinscher, Collie, Shetland Sheepdog, Scottish Terrier, and Irish Wolfhound. It is the most common inherited bleeding disorder in dogs.
Warfarin toxicity	Coumarin compound found in rodenticides. Once ingested, it binds to the Vitamin K in the animal's body, which is needed for proper function of certain clotting factors.
White blood cell differential	Test to count the different types of white blood cells on a slide.

Building the Terms

Table 8.4   Chapter 8 Combining Forms.

Combining Forms	Definition	Combining Forms	Definition
Albumin/o	Albumin	**Leuk/o**	White
Bas/o	Base	**Lip/o**	Fat
Bilirubin/o	Bilirubin	**Lymph/o**	Lymph
Chrom/o	Color	**Mon/o**	One; single
Coagul/o	Clotting; coagulation	**Morph/o**	Shape; form
Cyt/o	Cell	**Myel/o**	Bone marrow; spinal cord
Eosin/o	Red; rosy; dawn	**Neutr/o**	Neutrophil; neutral; neither
Erythr/o	Red	**Nucle/o**	Nucleus
Granul/o	Granules	**Phag/o**	Eat; swallow
Hem/o	Blood	**Phleb/o**	Vein
Hemat/o	Blood	**Poikil/o**	Irregular; varied
Hemoglobin/o	Hemoglobin	**Sider/o**	Iron
Home/o	Sameness; unchanging; constant	**Spher/o**	Round; globe-shaped
Is/o	Same; equal	**Thromb/o**	Clot
Kary/o	Nucleus		

Table 8.5   Chapter 8 Prefixes.

Prefix	Definition	Prefix	Definition
a-, an-	no; not; without	**mega-**	large
anti-	against	**micro-**	small
dys-	bad; abnormal; difficult; abnormal	**mono-**	single; one
hyper-	excessive; increased; above	**pan-**	all
hypo-	deficient; below; under; less than normal; decreased	**poly-**	many; much
macro-	large		

Table 8.6 Chapter 8 Suffixes.

Suffix	Definition	Suffix	Definition
-ar, -ic	pertaining to	**-oid**	resembling
-blast	immature; embryonic	**-osis**	abnormal condition
-cyte	cell	**-pathy**	disease condition
-cytosis	increase in the number of cells	**-penia**	deficiency
-emia	blood condition	**-phage**	eat; swallow
-emic	pertaining to a blood condition	**-phil**	attraction for
-genous	producing	**-philia**	increase in the number of cells; attraction for
-globin	protein	**-plasia**	development; formation; growth
-globulin	protein	**-poiesis**	formation
-logy	study of	**-rrhage**	bursting forth
-lysis	breakdown; destruction; separation; loosening	**-stasis**	stopping; controlling; place
-lytic	to reduce; destroy; separate; breakdown	**-tomy**	incision; process of cutting into

---

TECH TIP 8.2 Increases and Decreases "-cytosis" vs. "-philia"

The suffixes "cytosis" and "philia" are defined as an increase in cell numbers. The rule that works best for white blood cells is as follows: If the cell that is increased is a granulocyte, then the suffix "-philia" is used. If the cell that is increased is an agranulocyte, then the suffix "-cytosis" is used.

Neutrophilia	Increase in neutrophils
Eosinophilia	Increase in eosinophils
Basophilia	Increase in basophils
Lymphocytosis	Increase in lymphocytes
Monocytosis	Increase in monocytes

When the white blood cells are decreased, the suffix stays the same regardless of cell type.

Neutropenia	Decrease in neutrophils
Eosinopenia	Decrease in eosinophils
Monocytopenia	Decrease in monocytes; also called **monopenia**
Lymphocytopenia	Decrease in lymphocytes; also called **lymphopenia**

Because basophils are rare in the healthy patient, there is no such thing as a basopenia.

Now it's time to put these word parts together. If you memorize the meaning of the combining forms, prefixes, and suffixes, then this will get easier each time. Remember your five basic rules to medical terminology when building and defining these terms. You'll notice some word parts are repeated from the previous chapter.

Parts			Medical Term	Definition
hypo-	+ Albumin/o + -emia		= Hypoalbuminemia	: _____
hyper-	+ Bilirubin/o + -emia		= Hyperbilirubinemia	: _____
Coagul/o	+ -pathy		= Coagulopathy	: _____
Cyt/o	+ -logy		= Cytology	: _____
pan-	+ Cyt/o	+ -penia	= Pancytopenia	: _____
Erythr/o	+ -blast		= Erythroblast	: _____
Erythr/o	+ -cytosis		= Erythrocytosis	: _____

*Pay attention to when "-osis" is attached to cyt/o to produce the new suffix "-cytosis." Erythrocytosis is also referred to as **polycythemia**.*

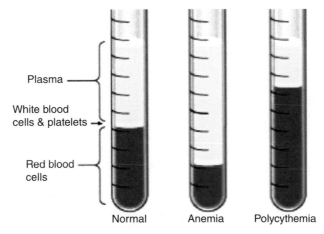

Plasma

White blood cells & platelets →

Red blood cells

Normal   Anemia   Polycythemia

Figure 8.15   Comparison of three spun blood tubes. Courtesy of Greg Martinez, DVM; www.youtube.com/drgregdvm.

Erythr/o	+ Cyt/o	+ -penia	= Erythrocytopenia	: _____
Erythr/o	+ -poiesis		= Erythropoiesis	: _____
Granul/o	+ Cyt/o	+ -penia	= Granulocytopenia	: _____
Hemat/o	+ -logy		= Hematology	: _____
Hemat/o	+ -poiesis		= Hematopoiesis	: _____
Hem/o	+ -lytic		= Hemolytic	: _____

Hem/o   + -lysis   = Hemolysis   : _____
                                                            This term is usually
                                                            used to describe
                                                            red blood cells.

Hem/o   + -stasis   = Hemostasis   : _____
Hemoglobin/o + -pathy   = Hemoglobinopathy : _____
Leuk/o   + Cyt/o   + -penia   = Leukocytopenia   : _____
                                                            Also called leukopenia.

Leuk/o   + -cytosis   = Leukocytosis   : _____
Lymph/o   + -blast   = Lymphoblast   : _____
Mon/o   + Nucle/o   + -ar   = Mononuclear   : _____

Role of an antigen-presenting cell

① Phagocytosis of enemy cell (antigen)

② Fusion of lysosome and phagosome

③ Enzymes start to degrade enemy cell

④ Enemy cell broken into small fragments

⑤ Fragments of antigen presented on APC surface

⑥ Leftover fragments released by exocytosis

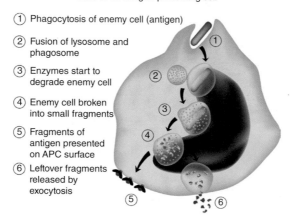

Figure 8.16A   Steps of phagocytosis with a monocyte. A monocyte is also a phagocyte. Courtesy of shutterstock/Alila Sao Mai.

Mon/o   + -blast   = Monoblast   : _____
Morph/o   + -logy   = Morphology   : _____
poly-   + Morph/o + Nucle/o + -ar   = Polymorphonuclear : _____
Myel/o   + -blast   = Myeloblast   : _____
Myel/o   + -genous   = Myelogenous   : _____
Myel/o   + -oid   = Myeloid   : _____
Myel/o   + -poiesis   = Myelopoiesis   : _____
Myel/o   + dys-   + -plasia   = Myelodysplasia   : _____
                                                            This term is most often
                                                            used to describe white
                                                            blood cells instead of
                                                            bone marrow. It is an
                                                            ineffective maturation
                                                            of white blood cells
                                                            in the bone marrow.

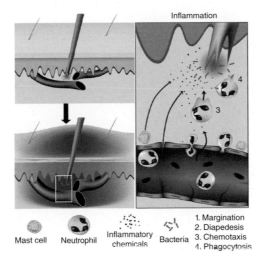

Figure 8.16B   Inflammatory response of neutrophils. Courtesy of shutterstock/Alila Sao Mai.

Phag/o	+ -cyte		= Phagocyte	: _____
Thromb/o	+ -cytosis		= Thrombocytosis	: _____
Thromb/o	+ -osis		= Thrombosis	: _____
Thromb/o	+ Cyt/o	+ -penia	= Thrombocytopenia	: _____

This is the most common acquired bleeding disorder in dogs.

Abbreviations

Table 8.7   Chapter 8 Abbreviations.

Abbreviation	Definition
AIHA	Autoimmune hemolytic anemia; disease in which the body destroys its own good RBCs.
IMHA	Immune-mediated hemolytic anemia
CBC	Complete blood count
Diff	White blood cell differential
HCT	Hematocrit
PCV	Packed cell volume
EPO	Erythropoietin
BMBT	Buccal mucosal bleeding time

(Continued)

Table 8.7   (*Continued*).

Abbreviation	Definition
RBC	Red blood cell
WBC	White blood cell
Plt	Platelet
TP	Total protein; test to measure dissolved substances in the plasma.
Hb	Hemoglobin; also abbreviated **Hgb**
hpf	High power field; used when counting cells in a microscope
lpf	Low power field; used when counting cells in a microscope
qns	Quantity not sufficient
VWD	Von Willebrand's Disease
Baso	Basophils
Eos	Eosinophils
Lymph	Lymphocytes
Mono	Monocytes
Seg	Neutrophils
ESR	Erythrocyte sedimentation rate; rate at which red blood cells settle in a blood tube. In dogs, the rate increases in cases of inflammation. Also called **sed rate**.
MCH	Mean corpuscular hemoglobin; test to measure the average hemoglobin per cell.
MCHC	Mean corpuscular hemoglobin concentration; test to measure hemoglobin concentration.
MCV	Mean corpuscular volume; test to measure the average size of red blood cells.
PT	Prothrombin time; coagulation test that measures the activity of certain clotting proteins.
PTT	Partial thromboplastin time; coagulation test that measures the activity of certain clotting proteins.
DIC	Disseminated intravascular coagulation
g/dl	Grams/deciliter; unit of measurement used on total protein.
µl	Microliters; unit of measurement for blood cell counts

Case Study

You'll notice some terms from the previous chapters.

A 4-month-old Irish Wolfhound named Gandolf is brought to the clinic after the owner notices prolonged bleeding at the site of recent tooth loss. On P/E Gandolf has blood on his gingiva where his deciduous teeth recently fell out. Doctor orders a CBC. The results are as follows:

Patient	Normal Range
RBC ct	6.77×10^6 RBC/µl $(5.00-10.00 \times 10^6$ RBC/µl)
WBC ct	8,422 WBC/µl (6,000–17,000 WBC/µl)
Plt ct	101,000 plt/µl (200,000–500,000 Plt/µl)

1. What does Gandolf have?
   a. Anemia
   b. Leukemia
   c. Thrombocytopenia
2. True or False: Gandolf's condition is the most common inherited bleeding disorder of dogs.

Exercises

8-A: Give the term for the following definitions.

1. _____: Red blood cell
2. _____: Granulocyte seen with allergies
3. _____: Agranulocyte that produces antibodies
4. _____: Oxygen carrying pigment of RBCs
5. _____: Hormone secreted by kidneys to stimulate erythropoiesis.
6. _____: Stopping or controlling of blood
7. _____: Immature monocyte
8. _____: Blood clotting
9. _____: Venipuncture
10. _____: Increase in cancerous WBCs
11. _____: Fat in the plasma
12. _____: Escape of blood from ruptured blood vessels.

8-B: Define the following terms.

1. Hemostasis _____
2. Neutropenia _____
3. Eosinophilia _____
4. Morphology _____
5. Thrombosis _____

6. Bilirubin _____
7. Antigen _____
8. Megakaryocyte _____
9. Packed cell volume _____
10. Dyscrasia _____

8-C: Answer the following questions.

1. What is the stimulus for lymphopoiesis?_____
2. What clotting factor is missing in Von Willebrand's disease?

   _____
3. What causes aplastic anemia?_____
4. What is the function of a neutrophil?_____
5. Which organ conjugates bilirubin?_____
6. List three locations of macrophages. _____
7. If blood is placed in a green TT then the fluid that results is called

   _____.
8. What is the difference between leukemia and
   leukocytosis?_____
9. Another name for erythrocytosis is _____.
10. The synonymous abbreviation for HCT is _____.
11. True or False: Thrombosis is the same as thrombocytosis.
12. What color is the plasma with hyperbilirubinemia?_____

8-D: Define the following abbreviations.

1. _____: CBC	6. _____: Hgb
2. _____: DIC	7. _____: AIHA
3. _____: hpf	8. _____: TP
4. _____: qns	9. _____: IMHA
5. _____: Diff	10. _____: lpf

8-E: Give the term for the following definitions.

1. Resembling bone marrow: myel_____
2. Pertaining to one nucleus: mono_____
3. Destruction of RBCs: _____lysis
4. Deficiency in all cells: _____penia
5. Disease condition of clotting: coagulo_____
6. Increase in WBCs: leuko_____
7. Blood condition of decreased albumin: hypo_____
8. RBCs are unequal in size: _____osis
9. State of equilibrium of the body's internal environment:
   _____stasis
10. Decrease in RBCs and/or Hb due to loss: _____anemia

8-F: Match the following terms with their descriptions.

1. _____ Protein threads forming   A. Agranulocytes
   the basis of a clot
2. _____ Segs, eos, basos   B. Albumin
3. _____ Enzyme that converts   C. Fibrin
   fibrinogen to fibrin
4. _____ Lymphs, monos   D. Granulocytes
5. _____ Maintains blood volume   E. Thrombin

Answers can be found starting on page 571.

Go to www.wiley.com/go/taibo/terminology to find additional learning materials for this chapter:

- A crossword puzzle
- Flashcards
- Audio clips to show how to pronounce terms
- Case studies
- Review questions
- The figures from the chapter in PowerPoint

Chapter 9

Immunology

Immunology is the study of the body's immune system. Three different systems work together to defend the body against foreign organisms such as bacteria, viruses, parasites, and fungi. The systems include the blood system, the lymphatic system, and the immune system itself.

The Lymphatic System

The lymphatic system is made up of lymph vessels, lymph nodes, lymph fluid, and lymphoid organs. The lymphatic system has several functions besides immunity. It acts as a drainage system to collect any materials such as proteins that have leaked out of the circulatory system and transport them back to the blood. A second function is to transport substances. Examples include transporting fat that was absorbed by the intestinal villi to the bloodstream or transporting metabolic waste products from tissue to the bloodstream. Finally, it stores lymphocytes which produce antibodies in response to antigens.

   Lymphoid organs include the spleen and thymus gland. The spleen has three functions: it destroys old erythrocytes, filters the blood of foreign materials and organisms, and stores erythrocytes and platelets. In veterinary medicine, splenomegaly (enlargement of the spleen) is frequently seen (Figure 9.1). The organ becomes enlarged due to neoplasias, inflammation, or excessive hemolysis. When enlarged, the risk of splenic rupture increases so a splenectomy is performed. Once removed, the macrophages in the liver and bone marrow take over the functions of the spleen.

   The thymus gland is located in the cranial mediastinum (Figure 9.2). The sole function of the thymus is to aid in immunity through the modification and storage of lymphocytes. The thymus gland is most active in younger animals and tends to decrease in function as the animal gets older.

Veterinary Medical Terminology Guide and Workbook, First Edition. Angela Taibo.
© 2014 John Wiley & Sons, Inc. Published 2014 by John Wiley & Sons, Inc.
Companion website: www.wiley.com/go/taibo/terminology

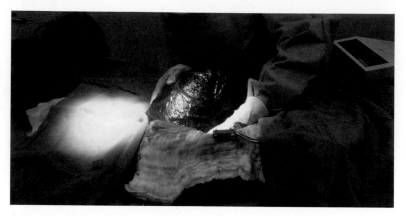

Figure 9.1 Splenomegaly in a dog. Courtesy of Deanna Roberts, BA, AAS, CVT.

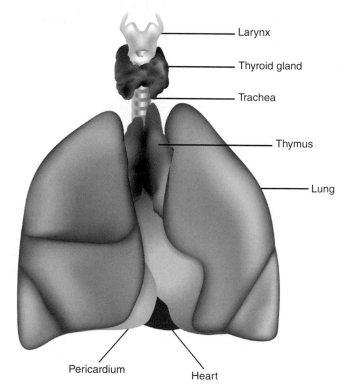

Figure 9.2 Diagram showing the location of the thymus gland. Courtesy of shutterstock/GRei.

Lymph fluid, or lymph, is a combination of water, lymphocytes, wastes, and a small amount of plasma proteins. As blood circulates, a small amount of fluid filters out of the capillaries and into the tissue spaces between cells (Figure 9.3). This fluid within the tissues is called interstitial fluid. As the fluid shifts through the interstitial space, it passes through tiny vessels called lymph capillaries. Once

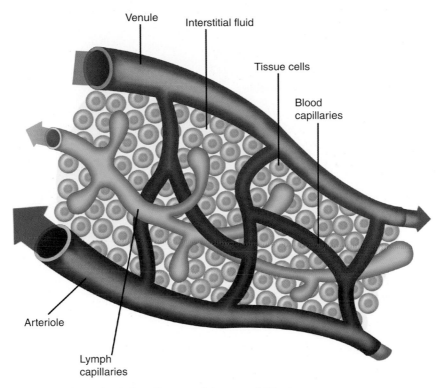

Venule   Interstitial fluid

Tissue cells

Blood
capillaries

Arteriole

Lymph
capillaries

Figure 9.3 Lymphatic circulation. Courtesy of shutterstock/Alex Luengo.

TECH TIP 9.1 Do Animals Have Tonsils?

Tonsils are small masses of lymphoid tissue. Tonsils can be found in several areas of an animal's body, but are most commonly associated with the throat.

---

in the lymph capillaries, the fluid is referred to as lymph. The function of lymph is to transport waste products of metabolism from the tissues to blood and to transport nutrients from the blood into the tissues. Lymph moves through the capillaries and into larger lymph vessels which are similar to veins in that the vessels only allow movement in one direction. The flow of lymph is always toward the thoracic cavity.

Along the lymphatic vessels are areas of stationary lymph tissue, called lymph nodes, which filter the lymph as it circulates around the body (Figure 9.4). Lymphocytes are stored within the lymph nodes (Figure 9.5). If an animal becomes sick, its lymph nodes will swell due to the proliferation (multiplication) of lymphocytes and the excessive amount of cells being destroyed during the filtration of lymph fluid. Lymph nodes can also become swollen due to neoplasias such as lymphoma. If the lymph vessels become obstructed, then the lymphatic fluid can't

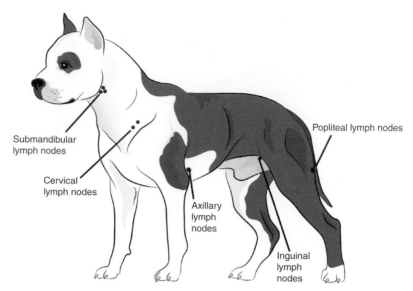

Figure 9.4 Lateral view of a dog showing the location of main lymph nodes. Courtesy of shutterstock/tiggra.

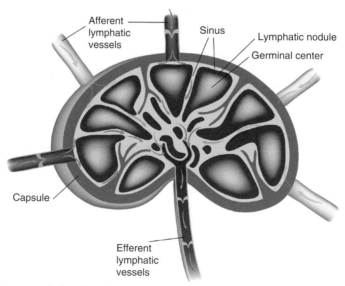

Figure 9.5 Anatomy of a lymph node. Courtesy of shutterstock/Alila Sao Mai.

drain. The fluid begins to accumulate in the tissue spaces, causing a condition called edema (Figure 9.6).

All lymph vessels merge into two large ducts in the chest, called lymphatic ducts. The right lymphatic duct empties into the venous system and drains lymph from the cranial right side of the body. The left lymphatic duct, also

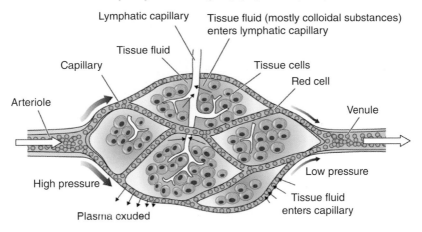

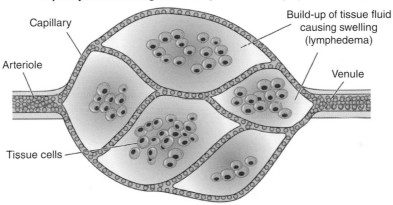

Figure 9.6   Illustration of lymphedema. Courtesy of shutterstock/blamb.

called the thoracic duct, enters the circulatory system and drains the left cranial side of the body.

The Blood System

As introduced in Chapter 8, neutrophils are granulocytes that act as bacterial phagocytes. Monocytes are agranulocytes that are phagocytic cells used to back up the neutrophils. Their responsibility is to remove any remnants that neutrophils left behind. This is one aspect of the body's natural defense mechanisms and is termed natural immunity. Every animal is born with this defense mechanism.

When bacteria are introduced to the body through a wound, neutrophils are the first to respond. They are the inflammatory mediators. The neutrophils that are circulating in the blood begin to move across the vessel walls and into the tissues to engulf the bacteria. The process by which the neutrophils migrate from the vasculature to the tissue is termed diapedesis. Once at the site of infection, the neutrophils engulf the bacteria.

Monocytes soon follow to remove any remaining bacteria and cells. Once monocytes leave the vessels, they become tissue macrophages capable of engulfing any foreign organisms including bacteria. If the animal has an infestation of worms and the worms have recently been killed, then the tissue macrophages will remove the dead worms.

The Immune System

Acquired immunity is the third type of immunity. Based on the name, the animal acquires immunity from an outside source. There are two types of acquired immunity: acquired active immunity and acquired passive immunity.

Passive immunity is the transfer of antibodies from a donor to a recipient. Mammals obtain passive immunity with the ingestion of colostrum soon after birth. Colostrum has a high concentration of antibodies from the mother. Animals may also receive maternal antibodies while in utero through the placenta. In birds, maternal antibodies are transferred to the yolk of the egg where the developing chick can absorb them. Examples of passive immunity aren't just isolated to maternal antibodies. Other examples include the administration of antitoxins after snake bites or injections of immunoglobulins (antibodies) in patients with poorly developed immune systems.

Active immunity is immunity that the animal acquires after being exposed to an antigen. The most obvious example is the administration of a vaccine. A vaccine is a suspension containing a killed or modified live virus that is given via injection. After receiving the vaccination, the animal undergoes an immune response which creates a memory to prevent future infections. Another example which isn't as common in animals as in humans is simply getting sick and creating antibodies toward the virus. Those newly created antibodies remain in the body to prevent future sickness from the same virus.

Once an animal undergoes an immune response, two specialized cell types are activated: B-lymphocytes and T-lymphocytes.

B-lymphocytes develop from stem cells in the bone marrow and are activated by binding to the antigens. Once activated, the B-lymphocytes differentiate (transform) into plasma cells, which produce immunoglobulins (antibodies) that neutralize the antigens by attaching to them. There are five different immunoglobulins with specialized functions: IgA, IgD, IgE, IgG, and IgM. This immune response is termed humoral immunity.

T-lymphocytes are produced in the bone marrow and then stored in the thymus gland (Figure 9.7). T-lymphocytes don't produce antibodies; instead, they attack the antigens directly. T-lymphocytes proliferate in the presence of antigens, and then the resultant cells, T-cells, destroy the antigens. There are four subsets of

TECH TIP 9.2 **What Does Each Immunoglobulin Do?**

IgA   Exists in secretions of the body including saliva, bile, synovial fluid,
         intestinal secretions, and respiratory secretions, including mucus.
         IgA acts as the body's first line of defense in the mucous membranes.
IgD   Exists on the surface of B-lymphocytes and in serum. Its function is
         unknown.
IgE   Exists in skin, lungs, and mucous membranes. IgE is increased in animals
         with allergies and therefore plays a role in allergic reactions. It is also
         increased in animals with parasites.
IgG   The most abundant of the immunoglobulins. Produced in response to
         antigens. It is the only immunoglobulin that can cross the placenta and it
         plays a major role in passive transfer of maternal antibodies.
IgM   First immunoglobulin produced in an immune response. Produced in
         response to antigens.

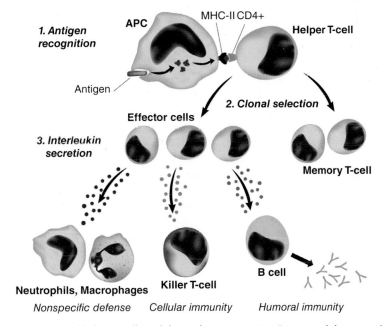

Figure 9.7   Illustration of helper T-cells and their roles in immunity. Courtesy of shutterstock/Alila
Medical Images.

T-cells with more specialized functions. This immune response is known as
cell-mediated immunity.

Helper T-cells   Stimulate antibody production from B-lymphocytes and
                     stimulate cytotoxic T-cells.
Cytotoxic T-cells   Directly attack and destroy the antigen.

| Suppressor T-cells | Deactivate, or suppress, the B-lymphs and T-lymphs when they're no longer needed. |
| Memory T-cells | Initiate a quicker immune response in the future due to a previous encounter with the same antigen. These cell populations are dedicated to one specific antigen. |

Related Terms

Acquired immunity	Formation of antibodies after exposure to an antigen.
Antibody (Ab)	Proteins produced by white blood cells in response to antigens.
Antigen (Ag)	Foreign substance (protein) that stimulates the production of antibodies.
Histiocyte	A macrophage. Histiocytes are named based on their tissue locations.
Immunity	The body's ability to resist organisms and toxins; also called immune response.
Immunoglobulins	Antibodies (gamma globulins) produced by plasma cells (Figure 9.8).

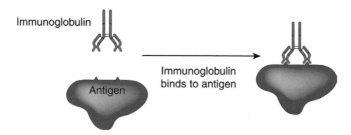

Figure 9.8   Immunoglobulins attacking antigens. Courtesy of shutterstock/blamb.

Interstitial fluid	Fluid in the spaces between cells; extracellular fluid in tissues.
Lymph	Watery fluid found in lymphatic vessels.
Lymph capillaries	Tiniest lymphatic vessels.
Lymph node	Stationary, bean-shaped structure along lymphatic vessels.
Lymph vessels	Vessels that carry lymph throughout the body.
Macrophages	Monocytes that migrate from the blood to the tissue; large phagocytes. Exist in liver, spleen, and bone marrow.
Spleen	Organ in the cranial abdomen that stores, produces, and destroys blood cells.
Thymus gland	Organ in the cranial mediastinum that produces and stores lymphocytes.

Pathology and Procedures

Allergen	Substance that causes a specific hypersensitivity.
Allergy	Abnormal hypersensitivity to an antigen.
Anaphylaxis	Exaggerated hypersensitivity to a foreign substance.
Autoimmune disease	Disease in which the body makes antibodies against its own good cells and tissues.
Carrier	An animal that harbors a disease without displaying signs of infection. The animal can still transmit the disease to others.
Edema	Excess fluid (interstitial fluid) in tissues.
ELISA	**Enzyme-linked immunosorbent assay.** Test to detect the presence of antibodies or antigens in a patient sample (Figure 9.9). Commonly used in-house ELISA tests include heartworm, parvo, feline leukemia, and feline immuno deficiency virus. Also called a **Snap® Test** (Figure 9.9).

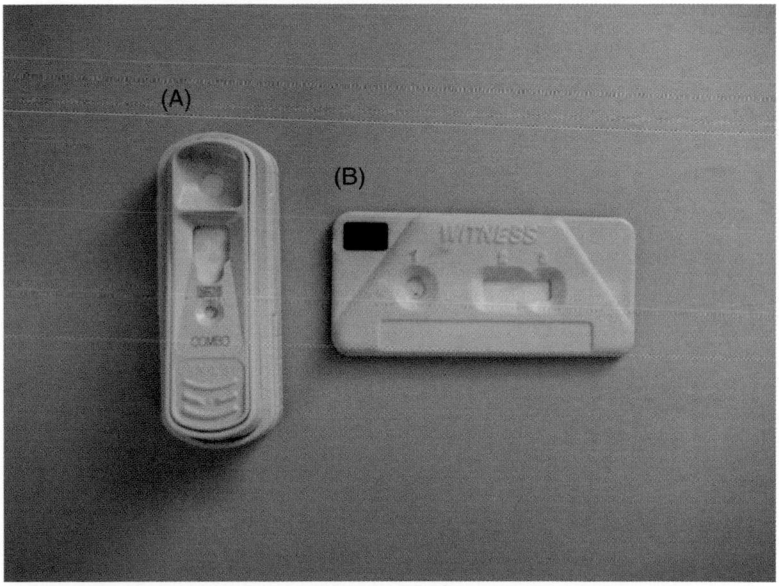

Figure 9.9   Examples of ELISA tests used in-house. (A) FeLV/FIV combo test. (B) K-9 heartworm test.

Feline infectious peritonitis (FIP)	Disease caused by a coronavirus in cats (Figure 9.10)

(A)

(B)

(C)

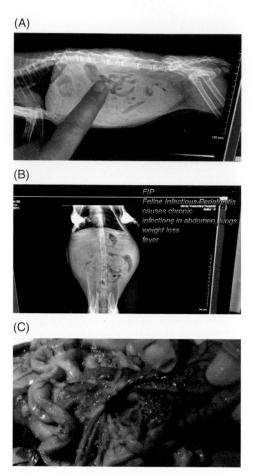

Figure 9.10 FIP case. Courtesy of Greg Martinez, DVM; www.youtube.com/drgregdvm.
(A) Lateral radiograph of fluid in the abdomen. (B) Ventral radiograph showing the inflammation
in the abdomen. (C) Small masses on the abdominal viscera.

Feline immunodeficiency virus (FIV)	Retrovirus causing immunosuppression. Also known as **feline AIDS**.
Feline leukemia virus (FeLV)	Retrovirus that causes leukocytosis, immunosuppression, and lymphoma. The virus is passed through saliva and excretions.
Hypersplenism	Condition marked by splenomegaly and excessive cell destruction causing anemia, leukopenia, and thrombocytopenia. Bone marrow biopsy shows increased cell numbers in response to the pancytopenia.
Immunofluorescent antibody test (IFA)	Test used to detect antigens or antibodies using fluorescent dye. Widely used in veterinary medicine in reference laboratories.

Immunosuppression	Impaired immune response; also known as **immunocompromised.**
Lymphoma	Malignant tumor of lymphoid tissue; also called **lymphosarcoma.** This is the most common neoplasm of lymph nodes.
Opportunistic	Organism which is normally nonpathogenic that becomes pathogenic in certain conditions.
Remission	Symptoms lessen and the patient feels better.
Relapse	Symptoms return after an apparent recovery.
Resistant	Does not easily affect; not susceptible. This term is often used to describe the relationship between a microorganism and antibiotics.
Retrovirus	RNA virus that multiplies by using the host's DNA. An example would be FIV (Figure 9.11).

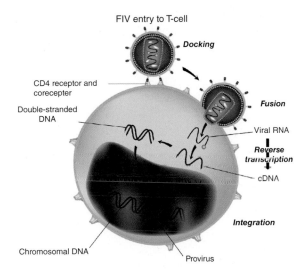

FIV entry to T-cell

Docking

CD4 receptor and corecepter

Double-stranded DNA

Fusion

Viral RNA

Reverse transcription

cDNA

Integration

Chromosomal DNA

Provirus

Figure 9.11 Mode of entry and replication of a retrovirus, in this case FIV. Courtesy of shutterstock/ Alila Sao Mai.

Susceptible	Easily affected; lacking resistance. This term is often used to describe the relationship between a microorganism and antibiotics.
Toxin	A poison.
Vaccine	Suspension containing a killed or weakened microorganism given via injection to induce immunity.
Vaccination	Administration of a suspension containing a killed or weakened microorganism to induce immunity. Also called **immunization.**
Zoonotic	Disease capable of being transmitted from animals to humans.

Building the Terms

Table 9.1 Chapter 9 Combining Forms.

Combining Forms	Definition	Combining Forms	Definition
Aden/o	Gland	**Lymphangi/o**	Lymph vessel
Axill/o	Armpit	**Splen/o**	Spleen
Chem/o	Drug; chemical	**Staphyl/o**	Clusters; uvula
Cyt/o	Cell	**Strept/o**	Twisted chains
Immun/o	Immune; protection; safe	**Thym/o**	Thymus gland
Lymph/o	Lymph	**Tonsill/o**	Tonsils
Lymphaden/o	Lymph node (gland)	**Tox/o**	Poison

Table 9.2 Chapter 9 Prefixes.

Prefix	Definition
ana-	up; apart; backward; again; anew
auto-	self; own
inter-	between

Table 9.3 Chapter 9 Suffixes.

Suffix	Definition	Suffix	Definition
-ary	pertaining to	**-itis**	inflammation
-coccus; -cocci	berry-shaped bacterium	**-logy**	study of
-cyte	cell	**-oid**	resembling
-cytosis	increase in the number of cells	**-oma**	tumor; mass; collection of fluid
-ectomy	removal; excision; resection	**-pathy**	disease condition
-globulin	protein	**-penia**	deficiency
-ic	pertaining to	**-poiesis**	formation
-ism	process; condition	**-therapy**	treatment

Now it's time to put these word parts together. If you memorize the meaning of the combining forms, prefixes, and suffixes, then this will get easier each time. Remember your five basic rules to medical terminology when building and defining these terms. You'll notice some word parts are repeated from the previous chapters.

Parts	Medical Term	Definition
Lymph/o + -oid	= Lymphoid	:_____
Lymph/o + -poiesis	= Lymphopoiesis	:_____

Term can be used to describe lymphocytes or lymph fluid.

Parts	Medical Term	Definition
Lymph/o + Cyt/o + -osis	= Lymphocytosis	:_____
Lymph/o + Cyt/o + -penia	= Lymphocytopenia	:_____

Also called lymphopenia.

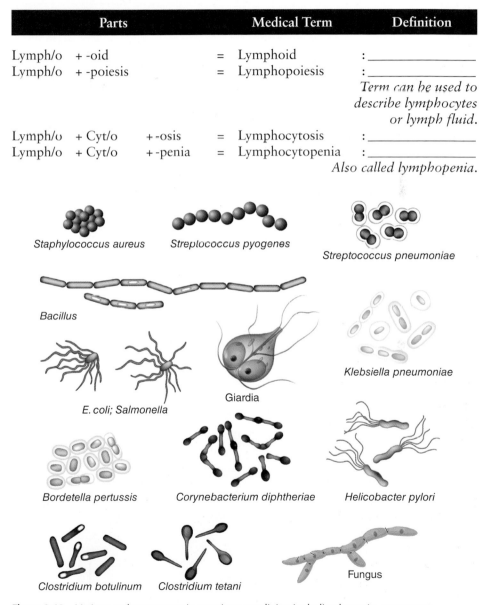

Staphylococcus aureus   Streptococcus pyogenes

Streptococcus pneumoniae

Bacillus

Klebsiella pneumoniae

E. coli; Salmonella

Giardia

Bordetella pertussis   Corynebacterium diphtheriae   Helicobacter pylori

Clostridium botulinum   Clostridium tetani

Fungus

Figure 9.12 Various pathogens seen in veterinary medicine including bacteria, protozoans, and fungus. Courtesy of shutterstock/Sebastian Kaulitzki, shutterstock/Alila Sao Mai, and shutterstock/blamb.

Lymphaden/o	+ -itis	= Lymphadenitis	: _____
Lymphaden/o	+ -pathy	= Lymphadenopathy	: _____
Lymphangi/o	+ -oma	= Lymphangioma	: _____
Splen/o	+ -ectomy	= Splenectomy	: _____
Splen/o	+ -megaly	= Splenomegaly	: _____
Staphyl/o	+ -cocci	= Staphylococci	: _____
Strept/o	+ -coccus	= Streptococcus	: _____
Thymo	+ -ectomy	= Thymectomy	: _____

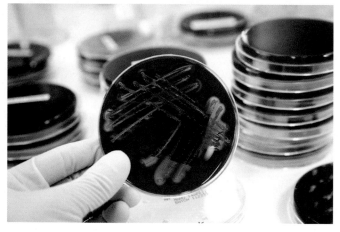

Figure 9.13 Streptococcus on a blood agar plate showing beta hemolysis. Courtesy of shutterstock/attem.

Thym/o	+ -oma	= Thymoma	: _____
Tonsill/o	+ -ectomy	= Tonsillectomy	: _____
Tonsill/o	+ -itis	= Tonsillitis	: _____
Tox/o	+ -ic	= Toxic	: _____
Chem/o	+ -therapy	= Chemotherapy	: _____

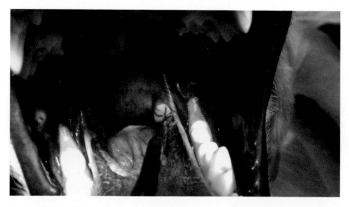

Figure 9.14 Dog with tonsillitis. Courtesy of Greg Martinez, DVM; www.youtube.com/drgregdvm.

Abbreviations

Table 9.4   Chapter 9 Abbreviations.

Abbreviation	Definition
CA	Cancer
ELISA	Enzyme-linked immunosorbent assay
FeLV	Feline leukemia virus
FIV	Feline immunodeficiency virus
IFA	Immunofluorescent antibody test
IgA, IgD, IgE, IgG, IgM	Immunoglobulins
LN	Lymph node
mets	Metastasis
sol.; soln	Solution
tab	Tablet
bx	Biopsy
dx	Diagnosis
DDx	Differential diagnosis
fx	Fracture
hx	History
Rx	Prescription/medication
sx	Surgery
Tx	Treatment
TR	Treatment
LRS	Lactated Ringer's Solution
PSS	Physiological Saline Solution

Case Study

You'll notice some terms from the previous chapters.

Ms. Petersen has just brought in her new kitten, Tofino. She found Tofino in the parking garage at her office. Based on Tofino's pearly white teeth, it's estimated that he's around 8 months old. Tofino is frisky during the exam, chasing the stethoscope and playing with the veterinarian's pen. Before giving his vaccinations, venipuncture is performed so an FeLV/FIV snap test can be done. Tofino turns up positive for FeLV Ag and negative FIV Ab.

Because Tofino shows no signs of the disease, additional blood is drawn and sent to a reference lab for an IFA. The IFA can detect intracellular Ags, whereas the snap test can only detect the Ags circulating freely in the blood. The IFA comes out negative for FeLV Ag.

When seen 8–12 weeks later, another snap test is done and still comes out positive for FeLV Ag. Tofino is still acting fine.

1. What is Tofino?
   a. A carrier
   b. Susceptible
   c. Autoimmune
2. What is another name for the snap test?
   a. Retrovirus
   b. ELISA
   c. Allergen
3. Where can the IFA detect the antigens?
   a. In tissues
   b. Inside cells
   c. Outside cells

Exercises

9-A: Give the term for the following definitions.

1. _____: Disease capable of being transmitted from animals to humans
2. _____: Another name for a macrophage
3. _____: Stationary lymph tissue along lymph vessels
4. _____: Substance that causes a hypersensitivity
5. _____: Excess fluid in tissue
6. _____: Lymphs that differentiate to plasma cells
7. _____: Lymphoid organ that produces, filters, and stores blood.
8. _____: Disease in which the body makes antibodies against its own cells and tissues
9. _____: Removal of the spleen
10. _____: A poison

9-B: Define the following terms.

1. Lymphangioma _____
2. Lymphadenitis _____
3. Toxic _____
4. Resistant _____
5. Tonsillitis _____
6. Lymphocytosis _____
7. Thymoma _____
8. Lymphoid _____
9. Immunosuppression _____
10. Interstitial Fluid _____

9-C: Answer the following questions.

1. Give an example of a retrovirus: _____
2. Where are inguinal lymph nodes found? _____
3. Which T-cells inhibit the B-lymphs? _____
4. Define an immune response in which a recipient receives antibodies from a donor. _____
5. Where are axillary lymph nodes found? _____

9-D: Define the following abbreviations.

1. _____: ELISA   6. _____: Rx
2. _____: IFA   7. _____: mets
3. _____: LN   8. _____: bx
4. _____: FeLV   9. _____: Tx
5. _____: FIV   10. _____: Sx

9-E: Match the following terms with their descriptions.

1. _____ Fluid found in lymphatic vessels   A. Acquired immunity
2. _____ Formation of Abs after exposure to an Ag   B. Immunoglobulins
3. _____ Malignant tumor of lymphoid tissue   C. Lymph
4. _____ Normally nonpathogenic disease that becomes pathogenic   D. Lymphoma
5. _____ Antibodies   E. Opportunistic

Answers can be found starting on page 571.

Go to www.wiley.com/go/taibo/terminology to find additional learning materials for this chapter:

- A crossword puzzle
- Flashcards
- Audio clips to show how to pronounce terms
- Case studies
- Review questions
- The figures from the chapter in PowerPoint

The Endocrine System

The endocrine system can be the most overwhelming system to learn (Figure 10.1). By comparison, systems such as the cardiovascular system and gastrointestinal systems aren't as intimidating because we have a basic understanding of the purpose of the heart and stomach.

The endocrine system is made up of glands that secrete hormones into the bloodstream. Hormones are chemical messengers that have a lock-and-key effect in which

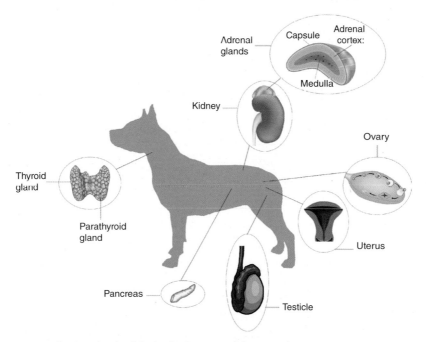

Figure 10.1 Endocrine glands of the body. Courtesy of shutterstock/serg741.

Veterinary Medical Terminology Guide and Workbook, First Edition. Angela Taibo.
© 2014 John Wiley & Sons, Inc. Published 2014 by John Wiley & Sons, Inc.
Companion website: www.wiley.com/go/taibo/terminology

Table 10.1   Endocrine Glands.

Adrenal glands	Pair of suprarenal endocrine glands. These glands are made up of a **cortex** (outer section) and a **medulla** (inner section).
Ovaries	Pair of female organs on either side of the pelvis that produce estrogen and progesterone.
Pancreas	Organ under the stomach that produces insulin, glucagon, and digestive enzymes.
Parathyroid glands	Four small endocrine glands on the posterior aspect of the thyroid gland that regulate calcium.
Pineal gland	Endocrine gland in the brain which synthesizes melatonin. It is believed that the pineal gland influences sexual development and sleep-wake cycles.
Pituitary gland	Endocrine gland at the base of the brain made of an anterior and posterior portion. Commonly known as the "master gland."
Testicles	Male gonads that produce spermatozoa and the hormone testosterone.
Thymus gland	Gland in the cranial mediastinum that produces and stores lymphocytes.
Thyroid gland	Endocrine gland in the neck that produces thyroid hormones which help regulate metabolism. It is the largest of the endocrine glands and is responsible for the storage of iodine.

they bind to sites on other organs and tissues to trigger an action. These hormones only bind to specific sites called target tissues. The goal of the endocrine system is to maintain homeostasis, which is the state of equilibrium of the body's internal environment. For example, the pancreas produces the hormone insulin, which decreases blood sugar, as well as the hormone glucagon, which increases blood sugar.

Endocrine Glands

The Pituitary Gland

The pituitary gland, or hypophysis, is commonly known as the "master gland" of the body because it secretes hormones that control all other endocrine glands. The pituitary is divided into two lobes, the adenohypophysis (anterior portion) and the neurohypophysis (posterior portion).

The adenohypophysis produces hormones which stimulate other organs to produce more specialized hormones. The neurohypophysis produces hormones that directly stimulate a target organ. Figures 10.2 (A and B) are diagrams of the pituitary and its functions. Note the differences between the anterior and posterior lobes.

The pituitary gland is attached by a stalk, the infundibulum, to the hypothalamus of the brain. The hypothalamus is the portion of the brain that secretes releasing and inhibiting factors that affect the pituitary gland.

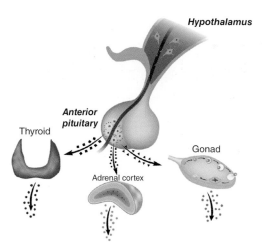

Figure 10.2A   Secretions from the anterior pituitary. Courtesy of shutterstock/Alila Sao Mai.

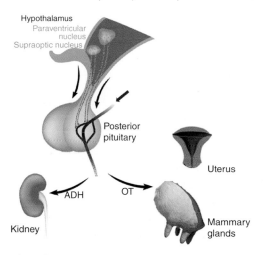

Figure 10.2B   Secretions from the posterior pituitary. Courtesy of shutterstock/Alila Sao Mai.

Together, the hypothalamus and pituitary work on the principle of negative feedback. When the concentration of a certain hormone reaches a normal range, the hypothalamus and pituitary are inhibited. If the hormone levels drop below normal levels, the hypothalamus begins secreting its releasing factors to stimulate the pituitary to secrete more hormones.

Figure 10.3 lists the hormones that are released from the pituitary.

Thyroid Gland

The thyroid gland is a butterfly-shaped gland found in the neck on either side of the larynx (Figure 10.4). This gland regulates metabolism, stores iodine, and regulates calcium levels. The thyroid produces and secretes the hormones thyroxine (T_4), triiodothyronine (T_3), and calcitonin.

Table 10.2   Pituitary Hormones.

ADH	Antidiuretic hormone; secreted from the posterior pituitary and controls the reabsorption of water by the kidneys. Also called **vasopressin**.
Oxytocin	Secreted by the posterior pituitary; causes the uterus to contract and stimulates milk secretion.
ACTH	Adrenocorticotropic hormone; released by the anterior pituitary and stimulates the adrenal cortex to secrete steroids.
FSH	Follicle-stimulating hormone; released by the anterior pituitary and stimulates the maturation of the ovum.
GH	Growth hormone; released by the anterior pituitary and stimulates the growth of bones and tissues. Also known as **somatotropin**.
LH	Luteinizing hormone; released by the anterior pituitary to promote ovulation.
MSH	Melanocyte -stimulating hormone; released by the anterior pituitary and stimulates the production of melanin, which gives the skin its pigment.
PRL	Prolactin; released by the anterior pituitary and stimulates milk secretion.
TSH	Thyroid-stimulating hormone; released by the anterior pituitary and stimulates the thyroid to produce thyroid hormones.

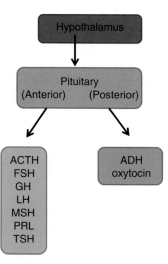

Figure 10.3   Summary of pituitary secretions.

T_3 is made up of three iodine atoms, which is where its chemical name comes from. T_4 is made up of four iodine atoms which is where its lesser known chemical name comes from, tetraiodothyronine. Together, these two hormones regulate the body's metabolism.

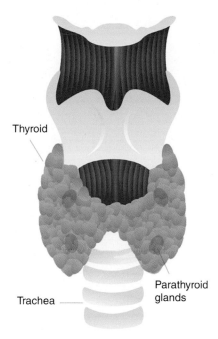

Thyroid

Parathyroid
glands

Trachea

Figure 10.4   Anatomical location of the thyroid and parathyroid glands. Courtesy of shutterstock/
Zuzanae.

Calcitonin controls the absorption of calcium from the blood into the bones.
When a patient becomes hypercalcemic, calcitonin is secreted to stimulate the
calcium to move from the blood to the bones to be stored.

Parathyroid Glands

The parathyroid glands are four endocrine glands on the posterior aspect of
the thyroid gland. They secrete a hormone called parathormone (PTH) which
regulates calcium and phosphorus levels in the blood. When secreted from the
parathyroid glands, PTH acts on the kidneys, controlling calcium reabsorption
and phosphorus excretion. Calcium gets reabsorbed back into the bloodstream and phosphorus is excreted in the urine. PTH also causes the release of
calcium from the bones back into the bloodstream when the patient becomes
hypocalcemic.

Adrenal Glands

The adrenal glands are located on the cranial aspect of each kidney. Each adrenal
gland is divided into two parts, the adrenal cortex and the adrenal medulla
(Figure 10.5).

The adrenal cortex is the outer section of the adrenal gland that secretes
steroid hormones called corticosteroids. Steroids, or corticosteroids, are derived

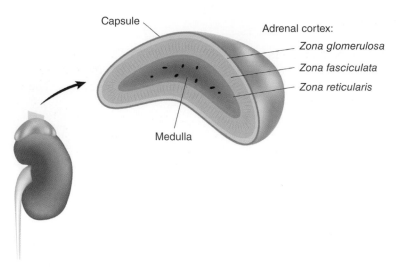

Capsule

Adrenal cortex:

Zona glomerulosa

Zona fasciculata

Zona reticularis

Medulla

Figure 10.5   Anatomy of the adrenal gland. Courtesy of shutterstock/Alila Sao Mai.

from fats and are used in the production of hormones. There are three types of corticosteroids produced in the adrenal cortex: mineralocorticoids, glucocorticoids, and androgens.

Mineralocorticoids are corticosteroids that regulate electrolytes and water balance. The principle mineralocorticoid is aldosterone. Aldosterone acts on the kidneys to control the reabsorption of sodium back into the bloodstream and the excretion of potassium in the urine. If an animal has hyponatremia (decreased sodium), aldosterone is released by the adrenal gland to stimulate the kidneys to reabsorb sodium back into the bloodstream. Where sodium goes, water follows. When sodium is reabsorbed, water is also reabsorbed.

Glucocorticoids are corticosteroids that regulate the metabolism of carbohydrates, fats, and proteins, and they have an anti-inflammatory effect. The principle glucocorticoid is cortisol, which regulates the metabolism of carbohydrates, fats, and proteins. When carbohydrate levels are low, cortisol is released to promote the body's cells to produce glucose using fats and proteins. This process is known as gluconeogenesis and occurs in the liver.

Cortisone is a glucocorticoid that is released in cases of stress and has anti-inflammatory effects. Cortisone inhibits the immune system, which can decrease inflammation.

Androgens are corticosteroids responsible for male sex characteristics.

The adrenal medulla is the inner section of the adrenal gland. It secretes catecholamines, which are hormones derived from amino acids. There are two types of catecholamines, epinephrine and norepinephrine. Epinephrine, also known as adrenaline, is a catecholamine that acts on the sympathetic nervous system to increase heart rate, blood pressure, and glucose levels. Norepinephrine, also known as noradrenaline, is a catecholamine that promotes vasoconstriction (vessel contraction), increases blood pressure, and increases heart rate.

The Pancreas

The pancreas is both an endocrine and exocrine organ. The exocrine functions were discussed in Chapter 4. To review, the exocrine functions of the pancreas include the production of the digestive enzymes amylase, lipase, and trypsin. The endocrine functions of the pancreas include the production of insulin and glucagon to maintain normal blood glucose levels. While the majority of pancreatic cells have exocrine function, a small section of specialized cells in the pancreas produce hormones to regulate blood glucose. These cells are known as the islets of Langerhans.

Insulin is a hormone produced by the beta cells of the islets of Langerhans to decrease blood glucose (Figure 10.6). Insulin promotes the glucose in blood to move into tissue cells when an animal is hyperglycemic or when cells require energy to function. If glucose is not needed in the body's cells, it is stored in the liver in the form of glycogen.

Glucagon is a hormone produced by the alpha cells of the islets of Langerhans to increase blood glucose. When an animal is hypoglycemic, glucagon breaks down the glycogen back into glucose.

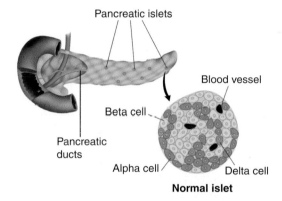

Figure 10.6A   Islet cells of the pancreas. Courtesy of shutterstock/Alila Medical Images.

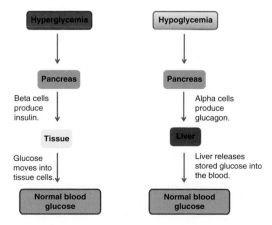

Figure 10.6B   Functions of the islet cells when blood glucose is out of range.

The Thymus Gland

As introduced in Chapter 9, the thymus gland produces and stores lymphocytes. The endocrine function of the thymus is to secrete the hormone thymosin, which promotes the maturation of T-lymphocytes. This gland is more prominent in the young as their immune systems are developing.

The Pineal Gland

The pineal gland is an endocrine gland found in the brain and whose functions are uncertain. It is believed that it secretes the hormone melatonin during hours of darkness. Melatonin plays a role in the body's "biological clock," meaning it regulates the release of gonadotropins.

Gonadotropins are hormones that stimulate the gonads. Examples include growth hormone and follicle-stimulating hormone.

The Gonads

Gonads are sex organs such as the ovaries and testes. Gonads produce gametes, or sex cells, such as sperm and ova.

The ovaries are a pair of female organs on either side of the pelvis that produce estrogen and progesterone. Estrogen is responsible for the female sex characteristics and it regulates ovulation. Female sex characteristics include mammary gland development and sexual receptivity. Progesterone is produced during pregnancy to protect the embryo and stimulate lactation.

The testes are the male gonads that produce spermatozoa and testosterone. Testosterone is responsible for the male sex characteristics, including the development of horns and tusks in certain species. Testosterone is an androgen that is secreted from both the testes and the adrenal cortex. In females, it is secreted in very small amounts from the adrenal cortex.

Related Terms

Adrenal glands	Pair of suprarenal glands that are made up of a cortex and medulla.
Adrenal cortex	Outer section of the adrenal gland that secretes corticosteroids.
Adrenal medulla	Inner section of the adrenal gland that secretes catecholamines.
Adrenocorticotropic hormone (ACTH)	Hormone produced by the anterior pituitary; stimulates the adrenal cortex.
Aldosterone	Produced by the adrenal cortex; controls sodium reabsorption and potassium excretion.

Antidiuretic hormone (ADH)	Hormone produced by the posterior pituitary that controls reabsorption of water by the kidneys. Also known as **vasopressin.**
Calcitonin	Hormone produced by the thyroid gland to regulate calcium levels.
Catecholamines	Hormones derived from amino acids secreted from the adrenal medulla. Examples include epinephrine and norepinephrine.
Corticosteroids	Hormones derived from fats and secreted by the adrenal cortex. Examples include glucocorticoids and mineralocorticoids. Also called **steroids.**
Cortisol	Glucocorticoid produced by the adrenal cortex to regulate metabolism of carbohydrates, fats, and lipids. Also increases blood glucose.
Electrolytes	Chemical substances necessary for proper functioning of cells.Examples include sodium, potassium, chloride, phosphorus,magnesium, and calcium.
Endocrinologist	Specialist in the study of the endocrine system.
Endocrinology	Study of the endocrine system.
Epinephrine	Catecholamine produced by the adrenal medulla to increase blood pressure, heart rate, and blood glucose. Also known as **adrenaline.**
Estrogen	Hormone produced by the ovaries; responsible for the female secondary sex characteristics.
Follicle-stimulating hormone (FSH)	Hormone produced by the pituitary to stimulate the maturation of ovum.
Glucagon	Hormone produced by the pancreas to increase blood sugar.
Glucocorticoids	Corticosteroids that regulate the metabolism of carbohydrates, fats, and proteins; they have an anti-inflammatory effect. Cortisol is an example.
Glycogen	Stored starch form of glucose in the liver.
Gonadotropins	Hormones that stimulate the gonads. Examples include FSH and GH.
Growth hormone (GH)	Produced by the anterior pituitary to stimulate growth of bones and tissues. Also known as **somatotropin.**
Homeostasis	State of equilibrium of the body's internal environment.
Hormone	Chemical messengers that have a lock-and-key effect in which they bind to sites on other organs and tissues to trigger an action.

Insulin	Hormone produced by the pancreas to decrease blood sugar.
Ketones	Acid by-products of fat metabolism.
Luteinizing hormone (LH)	Produced by the anterior pituitary to promote ovulation
Mineralocorticoid	Corticosteroids produced by the adrenal cortex to regulate electrolytes and water balance.
Norepinephrine	Catecholamine produced by the adrenal medulla to promote vasoconstriction (vessel contraction), increase blood pressure, and increase heart rate. It is a major neurotransmitter of the autonomic nervous system.
Ovaries	Pair of female organs on either side of the pelvis that produce estrogen and progesterone.
Oxytocin	Hormone produced by the posterior pituitary to stimulate the uterus to contract and secrete milk.
Pancreas	Endocrine gland that secretes insulin and glucagon to regulate blood glucose.
Parathormone (PTH)	Hormone produced by the parathyroid glands to regulate calcium and phosphorus.
Parathyroid glands	Four small endocrine glands on the posterior aspect of the thyroid gland that regulate calcium.
Pituitary gland	Endocrine gland at the base of the brain made of an anterior and posterior portion. Commonly known as the "master gland."
Progesterone	Hormone produced by the ovaries during pregnancy to protect the embryo and stimulate lactation.
Prolactin (PRL)	Produced by the anterior pituitary; stimulates milk secretion.
Testes (Singular: testis)	Male gonads that produce spermatozoa and the hormone testosterone.
Testosterone	Hormone produced by the testes; responsible for male sex characteristics.
Thyroid gland	Endocrine gland in the neck that produces thyroid hormones which help regulate metabolism. It is the largest of the endocrine glands and is responsible for the storage of iodine.
Thyroid-stimulating hormone (TSH)	Produced by the anterior pituitary; stimulates the thyroid to produce thyroid hormones.
Thyroxine (T_4)	Produced by the thyroid gland to regulate metabolism. Also known as **tetraiodothyronine**.
Triiodothyronine (T_3)	Produced by the thyroid gland to regulate metabolism.

Pathology and Procedures

Dexamethasone suppression test	Test that measures the body's response to a dexamethasone injection to diagnose Cushing's disease and its cause.

> **TECH TIP 10.1** Dexamethasone is a potent glucocorticoid that mimics the presence of cortisol in the blood.
>
> When used in a low-dose dexamethasone suppression test (LDDS), cortisol levels are measured after its administration to diagnose Cushing's disease.
>
> When used in a high-dose dexamethasone suppression test (HDDS), cortisol levels are measured after its administration to determine the cause of Cushing's disease. Cushing's is most often caused by either a tumor on the adrenal glands or on the pituitary gland. This test isolates the location of the tumor.

Diabetes insipidus (DI)	Metabolic disorder causing a lack of antidiuretic hormone (ADH) secretion.
Diabetes mellitus (DM)	Disorder characterized by a lack of insulin secretion or a resistance to insulin.
Diabetic ketoacidosis (DKA)	Low blood pH due to a build-up of ketones in diabetics.
Glucose curve	Test used to diagnose DM. Blood is drawn every couple of hours to monitor glucose changes in a 24-hour period.

> **TECH TIP 10.2 A Helpful Hint**
>
> When the prefix "hyper-" is attached to a gland, it generally means that the gland is overactive. If the prefix "hypo-" is attached to a gland, it generally means that the gland is underactive.

Hyperadrenocorticism	Disease in which excessive cortisol is produced by the adrenal cortex; commonly called **Cushing's Disease**. Symptoms include excessive thirst, excessive urination, weight gain, poor hair coat, skin changes, muscle weakness, increased appetite, and abdominal distention. Most commonly affects dogs.

Hypoadrenocorticism	Disease causing a lack of cortisol secretion by the adrenal cortex. Commonly called **Addison's Disease**. Symptoms are vague, including vomiting and lethargy. Most commonly affects dogs.

TECH TIP 10.3 Common Names of Diseases

Some of the medical terms that we are familiar with are actually eponyms. An eponym is a medical term or phrase formed from or including a person's name, for example, Addison's disease and Cushing's disease.

Hypercrinism	Condition of excessive secretion from a gland.
Hypocrinism	Condition of deficient secretion from a gland.
Hypergonadism	Excessive hormone secretion from the gonads.
Hypogonadism	Deficient hormone secretion from the gonads.
Hyperinsulinism	Excessive insulin secretion from the pancreas.
Hypoinsulinism	Deficient insulin secretion from the pancreas.
Hyperparathyroidism	Excessive secretion of parathormone from the parathyroid glands.
Hypoparathyroidism	Deficient secretion of parathormone from the parathyroid glands.
Hyperpituitarism	Excessive secretion from the pituitary gland.
Hypopituitarism	Deficient secretion from the pituitary gland.
Hyperthyroidism	Excessive hormone secretion from the thyroid gland. Symptoms include hyperactivity, weight loss, and increased appetite. Most commonly seen in cats.
Hypothyroidism	Deficient hormone secretion from the thyroid gland. Symptoms include lethargy, weight gain, and hair coat changes. Most commonly seen in dogs (Figure 10.7).
Insulinoma	Tumor on the pancreas causing excessive secretion of insulin. Most commonly seen in ferrets.
Panhypopituitarism	Hypopituitarism due to an absence of the pituitary gland. Notice that "pan-" means all. In this term, all of the pituitary gland is absent.

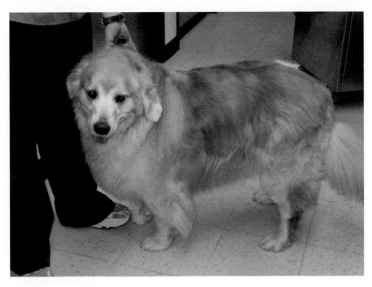

Figure 10.7   Golden retriever with hypothyroidism. Hypothyroid dogs are typically overweight and have a poor hair coat due to the lack of thyroid hormones. Courtesy of AK Traylor, DVM; Microscopy Learning Systems.

TECH TIP 10.4 Tumors

Tumors are a lot like teenagers—they don't listen. In the case of tumors, they cause excessive secretion of one certain substance regardless of whether the body needs it. In the case of an insulinoma, the animal has a tumor that constantly releases insulin. Though the body's cells may send signals to the pancreas to stop releasing insulin, the tumor doesn't listen.

   If the animal had a thyroid tumor, then the tumor secretes excessive amounts of T_3 and T_4. Even if the body sends the proper signals to turn off the thyroid gland, the tumor won't listen and will continually secrete the hormones.

Pheochromocytoma	Tumor in the adrenal medulla causing excessive secretion of catecholamines. Most commonly seen in dogs and cattle.
Pituitarism	Any disorder of the pituitary gland.
T_3 suppression test	Administration of T_3 to diagnose borderline hyperthyroidism.
Thyrotoxicosis	Excessive, life-threatening amounts of thyroid hormones.

Building the Terms

Table 10.3   Chapter 10 Combining Forms.

Combining Forms	Definition	Combining Forms	Definition
Acr/o	Extremities	**Keton/o**	Ketone bodies (ketones)
Aden/o	Gland	**Lact/o**	Milk
Adren/o	Adrenal gland	**Natr/o**	Sodium
Adrenal/o	Adrenal gland	**Pancreat/o**	Pancreas
Andr/o	Male	**Parathyroid/o**	Parathyroid glands
Calc/o	Calcium	**Phys/o**	Growth; growing
Cortic/o	Cortex (outer region)	**Pineal/o**	Pineal gland
Crin/o	To secrete	**Pituitar/o**	Pituitary
Dips/o	Thirst	**Somat/o**	Body
Estr/o	Female	**Ster/o**	Solid structure
Gluc/o	Sugar	**Thym/o**	Thymus gland
Glyc/o; Glycos/o	Sugar	**Thyr/o**	Thyroid gland
Gonad/o	Sex glands	**Thyroid/o**	Thyroid gland
Home/o	Sameness	**Toc/o**	Childbirth
Hormon/o	Hormones	**Toxic/o**	Poison
Insulin/o	Insulin	**Ur/o**	Urine; urinary tract
Kal/i	Potassium		

Table 10.4   Chapter 10 Prefixes.

Prefix	Definition	Prefix	Definition
endo-	in; within	**pan-**	all
eu-	good; normal; true	**poly-**	many; much
hyper-	above; excessive; increased	**tetra-**	four
hypo-	below; deficient; decreased	**tri-**	three
oxy-	rapid; sharp; acid		

Table 10.5   Chapter 10 Suffixes.

Suffix	Definition	Suffix	Definition
-agon	to assemble; gather	**-megaly**	enlargement
-al	pertaining to	**-oid**	resembling
-ectomy	removal; excision; resection	**-oma**	tumor; mass; collection of fluid
-emia	blood condition	**-one**	hormone
-emic	pertaining to a blood condition	**-osis**	abnormal condition
-gen	producing; forming	**-pathy**	disease condition
-in, -ine	a substance	**-stasis**	stopping; controlling
-ism	process; condition	**-tomy**	incision; process of cutting into
-ist	specialist	**-tropic**	turning
-itis	inflammation	**-tropin**	stimulate; act on
-logy	study of	**-uria**	urination; condition of urine

Now it's time to put these word parts together. If you memorize the meaning of the combining forms, prefixes, and suffixes, then this will get easier each time. Remember your five basic rules to medical terminology when building and defining these terms. You'll notice some word parts are repeated from the previous chapters.

Parts			Medical Term	Definition
Acr/o	+ -megaly		= Acromegaly	: _____ *This is caused by excessive secretion of growth hormone by the pituitary gland.*
Adrenal/o	+ -ectomy		= Adrenalectomy	: _____
Adren/o	+ -ectomy		= Adrenectomy	: _____
Adren/o	+ -pathy		= Adrenopathy	: _____
Adren/o	+ -al		= Adrenal	: _____
hyper-	+ Calc/o	+ -emia	= Hypercalcemia	: _____
hypo-	+ Calc/o	+ -emia	= Hypocalcemia	: _____

Gluc/o	+ -uria		=	Glucosuria	: _____
Glyc/o	+ -emic		=	Glycemic	: _____
Glycos/o	+ -uria		=	Glycosuria	: _____
hyper-	+ Glyc/o	+ -emia	=	Hyperglycemia	: _____
hypo-	+ Glyc/o	+ -emia	=	Hypoglycemia	: _____
Hormon/o	+ -al		=	Hormonal	: _____
hyper-	+ Kal/i	+ -emia	=	Hyperkalemia	: _____
hypo-	+ Kal/i	+ -emia	=	Hypokalemia	: _____
hyper-	+ Natr/o	+ -emia	=	Hypernatremia	: _____
hypo-	+ Natr/o	+ -emia	=	Hyponatremia	: _____
Pancreat/o	+ -ectomy		=	Pancreatectomy	: _____
Pancreat/o	+ -ic		=	Pancreatic	: _____
Pancreat/o	+ -itis		=	Pancreatitis	: _____
Pancreat/o	+ -tomy		=	Pancreatotomy	: _____
Parathyroid/o	+ -ectomy		=	Parathyroidectomy	: _____
Pineal/o	+ -pathy		=	Pinealopathy	: _____

TECH TIP 10.5 Rules for Using the Prefix "poly-"

When "poly-" is attached to an action, the meaning of the prefix changes to excessive. For example, the term polyphagia is defined as excessive eating or excessive appetite.

---

poly-	+ -dipsia	=	polydipsia	: _____
poly-	+ -uria	=	polyuria	: _____
Thym/o	+ -ectomy	=	Thymectomy	: _____
Thym/o	+ -oma	=	Thymoma	: _____
Eu-	+ thyroid	=	Euthyroid	: _____
Thyroid/o	+ -itis	=	Thyroiditis	: _____
Thyr/o	+ -megaly	=	Thyromegaly	: _____

Abbreviations

Table 10.6 Chapter 10 Abbreviations.

Abbreviation	Definition
ACTH	Adrenocorticotropic hormone
ADH	Antidiuretic hormone
BG	Blood glucose
Ca	Calcium
Cl	Chloride

Table 10.6   (*Continued*).

Abbreviation	Definition
DI	Diabetes insipidus
DKA	Diabetic ketoacidosis
DM	Diabetes mellitus
FBS	Fasting blood sugar
FSH	Follicle-stimulating hormone
GH	Growth hormone
GTT	Glucose tolerance test; used to diagnose borderline DM
HDDS	High-dose dexamethasone suppression test
K	Potassium
LDDS	Low-dose dexamethasone suppression test
LH	Luteinizing hormone
Mg	Magnesium
Na	Sodium
OT	Oxytocin
PRL	Prolactin
PTH	Parathormone
PU/PD	Polyuria/polydipsia
RAI	Radioactive iodine; treatment for hyperthyroidism
T_3	Triiodothyronine
T_4	Thyroxine; tetraiodothyronine
TSH	Thyroid-stimulating hormone

Case Study

You'll notice some terms from the previous chapters.

A Sheltie named Tubby has come to the clinic for a routine exam with vaccines. Tubby is 10 years and the owners have noticed that Tubby isn't energetic anymore. On P/E, Tubby is overweight by about 15 pounds and has a rough, coarse hair coat. There's hair loss at the base of his tail, creating a "rat tail" appearance. The owners have noticed that Tubby has been eating more than usual. Dr. SkinnyMinny decides to order lab work to measure T$_4$ levels. When the lab results return the following day, the T$_4$ levels are decreased in the blood.

1. What does Tubby have?
   a. Addison's disease
   b. Cushing's disease
   c. Hyperthyroidism
   d. Hypothyroidism
2. Which of the following symptoms describes Tubby?
   a. Polydipsia
   b. Polyphagia
   c. Polyuria
3. Which hormone level was measured?
   a. Thyroxine
   b. Triiodothyronine
   c. Cortisol

Exercises

10-A: Give the other term for the following.

1. _____: Addison's disease
2. _____: Vasopressin
3. _____: Cushing's disease
4. _____: Adrenaline
5. _____: Somatotropin
6. _____: Master gland
7. _____: Steroids
8. _____: Norepinephrine
9. _____: Thyroxine
10. _____: Hypophysis

10-B: Define the following terms.

1. Adrenopathy _____
2. Pancreatitis _____
3. Thymoma _____
4. Hyperglycemia _____
5. Glucosuria _____
6. Acromegaly _____
7. Hyponatremia _____
8. Hyperkalemia _____
9. Hormonal _____
10. Thyromegaly _____

10-C: Fill in the following chart regarding the source and action of hormones.

Hormone	Source	Action
1. GH	_____	_____
2. Insulin	_____	_____
3. PTH	_____	_____
4. ACTH	_____	_____
5. ADH	_____	_____
6. T_4	_____	_____
7. LH	_____	_____
8. Oxytocin	_____	_____
9. FSH	_____	_____
10. Aldosterone	_____	_____

10-D: Define the following abbreviations.

1. _____: PU/PD
2. _____: TSH
3. _____: PTH
4. _____: DM
5. _____: DI
6. _____: DKA
7. _____: ACTH
8. _____: BG
9. _____: PRL
10. _____: LDDS

10-E: Match the following terms with their descriptions.

1. _____	Cortisol	A.	Androgen
2. _____	Aldosterone	B.	Catecholamine
3. _____	Epinephrine	C.	Glucocorticoid
4. _____	FSH	D.	Gonadotropin
5. _____	Testosterone	E.	Mineralocorticoid

Answers can be found starting on page 571.

Go to www.wiley.com/go/taibo/terminology to find additional learning materials for this chapter:

- A crossword puzzle
- Flashcards
- Audio clips to show how to pronounce terms
- Case studies
- Review questions
- The figures from the chapter in PowerPoint

Chapter 11

The Integumentary System

The integumentary system consists of skin, hair, nails, and glands. Because we're dealing with animals, the categories are expanded to include feathers, fur, scales, hooves, horns, and beaks. The functions of the integumentary system are to protect the body, maintain body temperature, lubricate, and provide nerve sensation.

The skin is the largest organ of the body. It protects the body by acting as a barrier against infection from outside organisms and protects the tissues underneath it. The skin produces a pigment to shield the body from ultraviolet exposure and synthesizes vitamin D. Nerve receptors within the different layers of skin allow the animal to feel sensations such as heat, pain, and pressure.

There are two types of glands in the skin layers: sebaceous glands and sweat glands. Sebaceous glands secrete an oily substance called sebum, which lubricates the skin. Sweat glands secrete sweat, which helps to regulate the body's temperature. Sweat is made up of water, lactic acid, and other waste products. The degree of sweating differs in each species. For example, horses sweat excessive amounts, whereas dogs lose a very insignificant amount of sweat. The hair, feathers, or fur on animals help to regulate body temperature.

Skin

There are three layers of the skin. Label the three layers in Figure 11.1 using Table 11.1.

Epidermis

The epidermis, which is composed of several layers of squamous epithelium, is completely cellular—there are no blood vessels in this layer. Epithelium was defined in previous chapters as layers of cells that cover the internal and external surfaces of the

Veterinary Medical Terminology Guide and Workbook, First Edition. Angela Taibo.
© 2014 John Wiley & Sons, Inc. Published 2014 by John Wiley & Sons, Inc.
Companion website: www.wiley.com/go/taibo/terminology

Table 11.1   Skin Layers.

Epidermis (1)	Outermost layer of skin.
Dermis (2)	True layer of skin.
Subcutaneous tissue (3)	Innermost layer of skin.

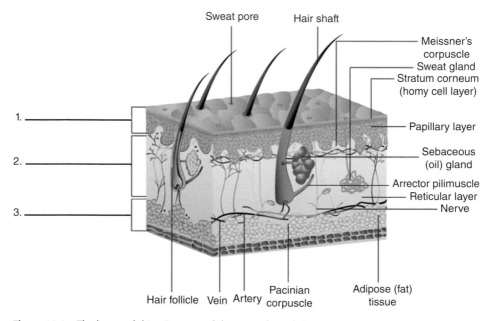

Figure 11.1   The layers of skin. Courtesy of shutterstock/stockshoppe.

body, and there are different types of epithelium depending on the location of the body and the function that is required. The surface of the skin requires protection; therefore, it consists of several layers of squamous (scale-like) cells. Due to the layers of squamous epithelial cells, the epidermis is sometimes referred to as stratified squamous epithelium because of the cells' layered arrangement. Because the epidermis lacks blood vessels, it relies on the layer below, the dermis, to nourish it.

The epidermis is made up of five layers, and literally develops from the inside out (Figure 11.2). The deepest layer of the epidermis is called the basal layer and it is here that new cells are formed. Once a cell is formed, it begins to migrate superficially until it reaches the outer layer, the stratum corneum. Eventually the cells on the surface of the skin slough (flake) off. As skin cells die and slough off, new cells are constantly being formed in the basal layer. During the cell's migration from the basal layer to the surface, it becomes filled with a tough protein called keratin. Keratin is referred to as horny tissue because it is commonly found in the horns of animals. It is the keratin that gives the skin the property of being waterproof.

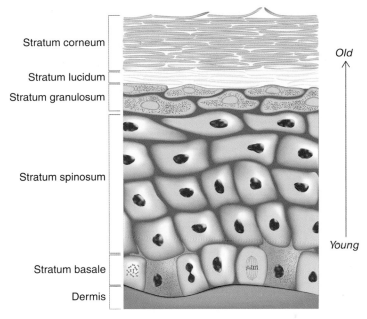

Figure 11.2A   The layers of the epidermis. Courtesy of shutterstock/Alila Medical Images.

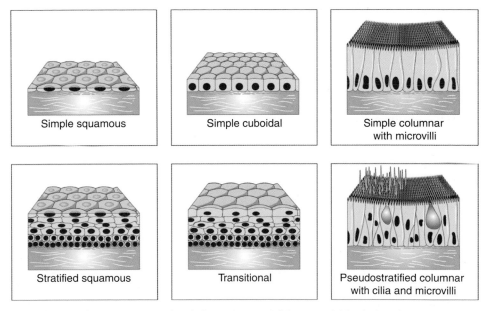

Figure 11.2B   The various types of epithelium. Courtesy of shutterstock/blamb. Simple squamous epithelium can be found in the capillaries, alveoli, glomerulus, and other tissues where diffusion takes place. Simple cuboidal epithelium can be found on the ovaries and nephrons of the kidney. Simple columnar epithelium can found in the intestines. Stratified squamous epithelium is found in the epidermis of the skin. Transitional epithelium is found in parts of the urinary tract. Pseudostratified columnar epithelium can be found in the respiratory tract.

The basal layer of the epidermis also contains a group of cells called melanocytes which produce melanin, the pigment that gives skin its color. Melanin protects the skin from the sun's ultraviolet rays. All animals have melanocytes. Melanocytes that are incapable of producing melanin result in a condition called albinism. These animals have white skin and white hair. Their eyes are a bright red because of the lack of pigment in their retinas, which makes the blood vessels within their eyes visible. Animals that develop melanoma have melanocytes that produce excessive amounts of melanin.

Dermis

The dermis, also called the corium, is considered the true layer of skin because it contains blood vessels, lymph vessels, sweat glands, hair follicles, and nerves. This layer contains connective tissue called collagen which gives the layer the effects of elasticity and longevity. Collagen can be found in bone, tendons, ligaments, and cartilage as well.

Subcutaneous Tissue

The subcutaneous layer is the innermost, fatty layer of the skin. The primary function of this layer is to produce fat to insulate the body. The predominate cell type is the lipocyte, or fat cell.

Hair

Hair is a long structure that contains keratin and grows from a sac called a hair follicle in the dermis. The hair follicle is held in place by a tiny muscle fiber called the arrector pili. When an animal becomes stressed, the arrector pili pulls the hair

Table 11.2   Types of Hair.

Cilia	Thin, tiny hairs; most often associated with the lining of the respiratory tract. The eyelashes can also be classified as cilia.
Fur	Short, very fine, soft hair that functions to protect animals in cold-temperature climates.
Primary hairs	Long, straight hairs that form the outer coat of an animal. Also known as the top coat, overcoat, or guard hairs.
Secondary hairs	Finer, softer hairs that form the inner coat of an animal. Also known as the undercoat. Not all animals have an undercoat. For those that do, it serves as an insulation.
Tactile hairs	Long, brittle hairs on the face that are very sensitive; for example, whiskers.

follicle, causing the hair on the animal to stand up. In humans, this can be caused from cold temperatures.

Animals have different types of hair with different functions. Table 11.2 lists the different types of hair.

When the temperatures in the environment change or the physiology of the animal changes, the hair begins to fall off. This is referred to as shedding. Shedding can be caused due to hormonal changes and dietary changes. If animals aren't groomed on a regular basis, the hair begins to clump (mat) and can cause more serious skin problems.

TECH TIP 11.1   Raising Their Hackles?

When dogs become upset, the hair on the dorsal aspect of their neck and along their spine begins to stand up. This is referred to as raising their hackles. The medical term for the hair standing straight up is piloerection.

Glands

Sebaceous Glands

Sebaceous glands can be found in the dermis along the hair follicles. They produce an oily substance called sebum, which lubricates the skin. Once produced, the sebum moves from the sebaceous gland to the hair follicle and then travels to the surface of the skin. Sebaceous glands are types of exocrine glands.

Sweat Glands

Sweat glands are also found in the dermis and produce a slightly acidic, watery fluid called sweat. The function of sweat is to cool the body and protect it from microorganisms such as bacteria. The acid effect of the sweat helps to destroy the bacteria on the skin's surface. There are two types of sweat glands: eccrine glands and apocrine glands. Eccrine glands secrete sweat directly to the surface of the body, which immediately evaporates to help cool the body. Apocrine glands secrete sweat into the hair follicle, and the sweat then travels to the surface of the skin. Both types of sweat glands are tightly coiled in the dermis.

TECH TIP 11.2   Other Types of Glands

Anal sacs are a combination of sebaceous glands and apocrine glands. Mammary glands are a type of apocrine gland.

Nails

Depending on the species, the nails category can include claws, hooves, antlers, and horns. In this chapter, we'll try to keep things basic with regard to anatomy of these structures. Anatomy will be emphasized in later chapters.

Carnivores have claws which they use for holding and tearing their prey. Most animals are able to retract their claws when they're no longer needed. Claws, like nails, are made up of two keratin plates. The difference between the two is in their shape. The ventral aspect of the claw is called the sole and the dorsal aspect is called the wall. The claw has a white portion on the distal aspect called the cuticle. The proximal aspect of the claw is very vascular dermis called the quick. To the naked eye this is the pink portion of the claw or nail. When performing a nail trim, the cuticle is cut and caution is taken to try and avoid the sensitive quick. Quicking an animal means you trimmed the nail too short, resulting in pain and bleeding.

Claws in birds are referred to as talons. Depending on the species of bird, talons can be used to hunt for prey or for protection against predators. Talon anatomy resembles that of nails.

If nails are long and strong enough to bear weight, they are called hooves. Hooved animals are termed ungulates.

TECH TIP 11.3 Where Are the Pads?

Pads are found on the plantar and palmar surfaces of the feet. They have an extra thick layer of keratin in the epidermis, a vascular dermis, and a subcutaneous layer. Most animals have sweat glands in their pads.

Digitigrade animals walk on their phalanges. Examples include the dog and cat. Plantigrade animals walk on their metacarpals and metatarsals. Primates, like humans, are plantigrade.

Related Terms

Basal layer	Deepest layer of the epidermis, where new cells are produced.
Collagen	Structural protein found in the dermis of the skin.
Dermis	True layer of skin containing blood supply and nerves.
Epidermis	Outermost layer of skin.
Epithelium	Layer of cells that covers the outer and inner body surfaces. Also called **epithelial tissue**.
Hair follicle	Sac in the dermis in which hair grows.
Integumentary system	The skin, hair, nails, and glands, collectively.
Keratin	Hard protein found in the hair, claws, horns, antlers, and epidermis.
Melanin	Pigment that gives skin its color.

Melanocytes	Cells in the epidermis that produce melanin.
Pore	Small opening on the surface of the skin.
Sebaceous glands	Oil-secreting gland of the dermis that's associated with the hair follicles.
Sebum	Oily substance secreted by sebaceous glands.

TECH TIP 11.4

Did you know that lanolin, the substance found in lotions and creams, is actually sebum from sheep? It is a processed and purified form of sheep's sebum.

Squamous epithelium	Flat, scale-like cells of the epidermis.
Subcutaneous tissue	Deep, fatty layer of the skin.
Ungulates	Hooved animals.

Pathology and Procedures

Abrasion	Wound caused by scraping of the skin or mucous membranes.
Abscess	Localized collection of pus.
Acne	Collection of comedones, or blackheads, caused by plugged sebaceous glands (Figure 11.3). Canine and feline acne commonly affects the chin and lips.
Albino/albinism	Congenital absence of pigmentation in the skin, hair, and eyes (Figure 11.4).
Alopecia	Absence of hair in areas where it normally grows (Figure 11.5A).
Atopy	Hypersensitivity reaction characterized by pruritus (itching) and dermatitis. Commonly called **allergic dermatitis.**
Biopsy	Removal of tissue for microscopic examination.
Bulla (Plural: bullae)	Fluid-filled skin elevation; commonly called a **blister or vesicle** (Figure 11.5B).
Burn	Injury to tissue caused by contact with heat, electricity, chemicals, or radiation (Figure 11.6).
Carcinoma	Malignant tumor arising from epithelial tissue.

TECH TIP 11.5

Remember the rule for carcinoma. When another combining form or structure is attached to the term, then you define it as: A malignant tumor of _____ arising from epithelial tissue. For example, carcinoma of the skin is defined as a malignant tumor of the skin arising from epithelial tissue.

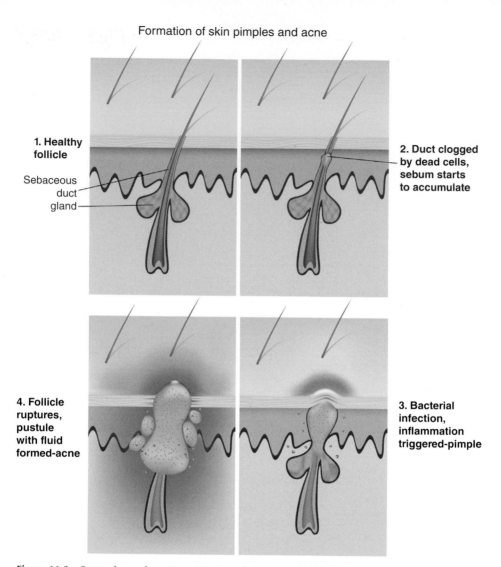

Figure 11.3 Steps of acne formation. Courtesy of shutterstock/Alila Sao Mai.

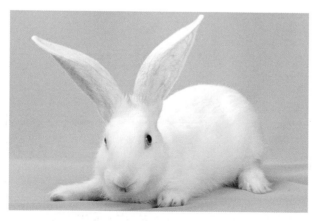

Figure 11.4 Rabbit with albinism. Courtesy of shutterstock/iava777.

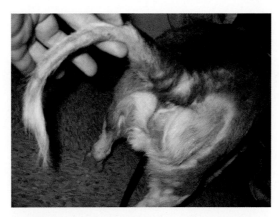

Figure 11.5A   Alopecia in a beagle. Courtesy of AK Traylor, DVM; Microscopy Learning Systems.

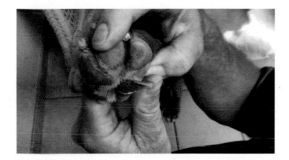

Figure 11.5B   Blister of a dog's paw. Courtesy of Greg Martinez, DVM; www.youtube.com/drgregdvm.

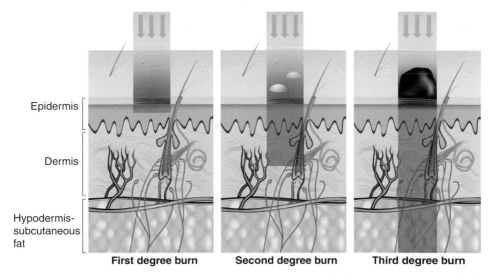

Epidermis

Dermis

Hypodermis-
subcutaneous
fat

First degree burn   Second degree burn   Third degree burn

Figure 11.6   Different degrees of burns. Courtesy of shutterstock/Alila Sao Mai.

| Cauterization | Destruction of tissue using heat, chemicals, or electrical current (Figure 11.7). |

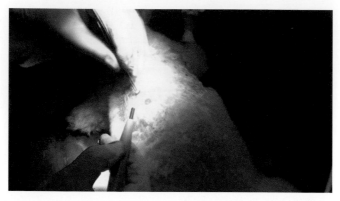

Figure 11.7 Cautery can be used to stop small bleeders and can be used to remove small masses. In this image, cautery is being used to remove small papillomas. Courtesy of Greg Martinez, DVM; www.youtube.com/drgregdvm.

Comedo (Plural:comedones)	Blackheads; plug of keratin and sebum within the opening of a hair follicle.
Contusion	A bruise; injury to tissue without breaking the skin. Characterized by pain, swelling, and tenderness due to broken blood vessels.
Crust	Collection of dried exudate, usually sebum, on the surface of the skin.
Cryosurgery	Use of cold temperatures to destroy tissue (Figure 11.8).

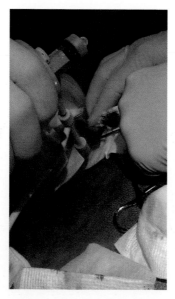

Figure 11.8 Cryosurgery performed to remove a mass on the skin. Courtesy of Beth Romano, AAS, CVT.

Culture	Procedure used to grow microbes in certain types of media.
Cyst	Thick-walled sac containing fluid or semisolid material.
Debridement	Removal of contaminated tissue or foreign material to expose healthy tissue. This in turn aids in healing.
Decubitus ulcers	Bedsores; pressure sores caused by lying in one position over an extended period of time.
Degloving	Injury in which the skin is separated from its underlying structures. Typically seen with traumas such as HBC (hit by car).

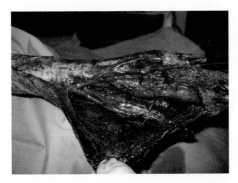 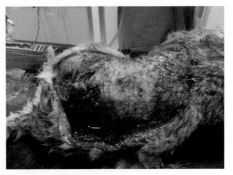

Figure 11.9A Degloving injury in a dog from HBC. Courtesy of Deanna Roberts, BA, AAS, CVT.

Figure 11.9B Degloving injury in a dog from HBC. Courtesy of Beth Romano, AAS, CVT.

| Ecchymosis (Plural: ecchymoses) | Bluish-black mark on the skin (Figure 11.10). |

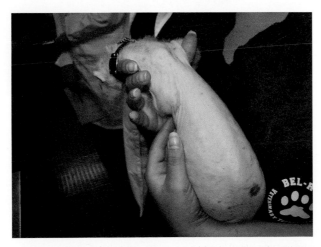

Figure 11.10 Ferret with ecchymosis and petechiae. Courtesy of Amy Johnson, BS, CVT, RLATG.

TECH TIP 11.6 Contusion vs. Ecchymosis

A contusion, or bruise, is typically caused by trauma and involves swelling or a raised area of the skin. Within that raised area is blood from ruptured vessels and bacteria from the trauma. The swelling is also caused by the body's response to the bacterial presence. Contusions cause pain when touched.

Ecchymosis, also called a bruise, is a superficial bluish-black mark on the skin most often caused by internal bleeding. Trauma to the skin is not involved so there is no skin elevation or swelling. The bleeding is typically spontaneous and associated with a bleeding disorder. Generally there is no pain when touched.

Erythema   Widespread redness on the skin. Caused by congestion of the capillary bed due to skin injury or infection (Figure 11.11).

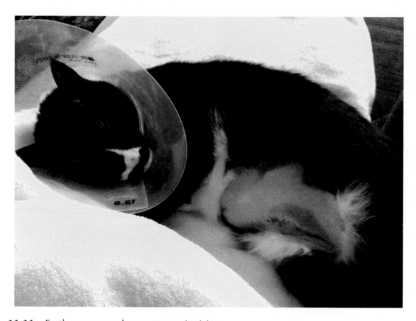

Figure 11.11   Erythema around a cystotomy incision.

Eczema   Generalized term for any superficial inflammation characterized by erythema (redness), pruritus (itching), and oozing blisters which form scabs (Figure 11.12).
Epidermolysis   Loosening of the epidermis leading to the formation of large blisters.

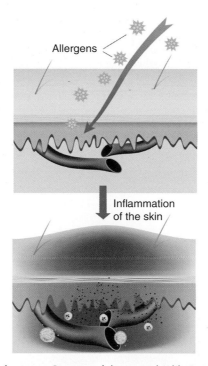

Figure 11.12A Formation of eczema. Courtesy of shutterstock/Alila Sao Mai.

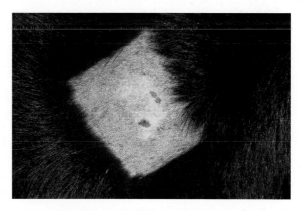

Figure 11.12B Eczema on a dog. Courtesy of shutterstock/richsouthwales.

Fine needle aspirate (FNA)	Collection of fluid or cells for laboratory exam. Most often used on masses for diagnosis (Figure 11.13).
Fissure	Deep crack in the skin.

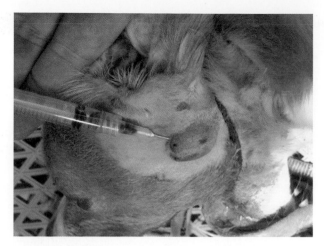

Figure 11.13   A fine needle aspirate on a corgi with a mass below the ear. Courtesy of AK Traylor, DVM; Microscopy Learning Systems.

Fistula	Abnormal tube-like passageway that can occur anywhere on the body. Most often caused by parasites or foreign bodies such as grass-ons (Figure 11.14).

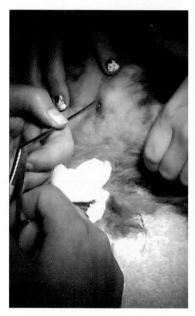
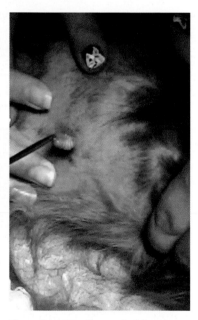

Figure 11.14A   Canine abdomen with a fistula created from an infestation of the bot fly maggot, Cuterebra. Courtesy Beth Romano, AAS, CVT.

Figure 11.14B   Removal of the Cuterebra from the fistula. Courtesy Beth Romano, AAS, CVT.

Flea allergy dermatitis (FAD)	Inflammation of the skin due to hypersensitivity to flea saliva.
Fly strike	In dogs, small bites on the ear tips from adult flies. Commonly seen in older, non-ambulatory dogs. In ruminants, an infestation of maggots on an area of skin covered in urine or feces.

Frostbite	Tissue damage due to exposure to extreme cold.
Gangrene	Death of body tissue (necrosis) associated with loss of blood supply.
Granuloma	Mass of granulation tissue due to a chronic inflammatory process. Typically seen with either an infectious disease or foreign body (Figure 11.15).
Hidrosis	Sweating.

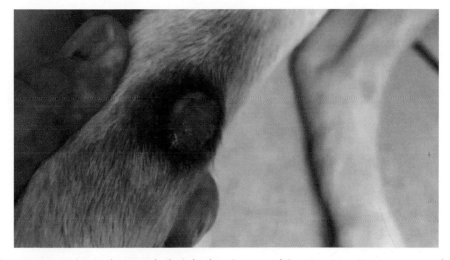

Figure 11.15   Lick granuloma on the leg of a dog. Courtesy of Greg Martinez, DVM; www.youtube.com/drgregdvm.

TECH TIP 11.7 Be Careful!

"Hidr/o" and "Hydr/o" look very similar on paper. "Hidr/o" means sweat; "hydr/o" means fluid or water.

Hyperkeratosis	Excessive growth of the horny layer (stratum corneum) of the dermis.
Infestation	Establishment of a parasite in or on a host.

TECH TIP 11.8 Infestation vs. Infection

The term infection is typically used when an animal has a virus or bacteria. Infestation is used when animals have parasites on or within their bodies.

| Laceration | Wound caused by tearing. Examples include a stab wound or a surgical incision. |
| Lance | To cut or incise with a sharp instrument. |

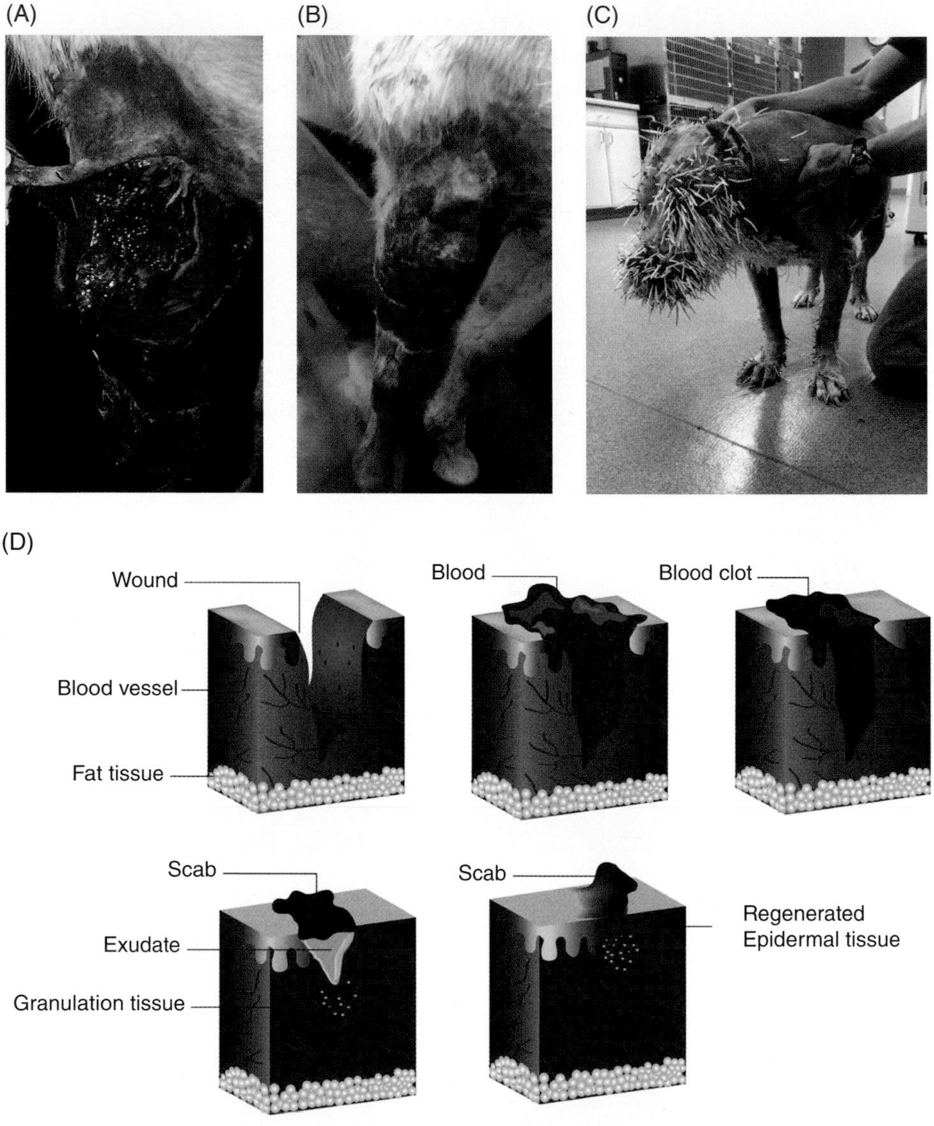

(A)   (B)   (C)

(D)

Wound — Blood vessel — Fat tissue

Blood — Blood clot

Scab — Exudate — Granulation tissue

Scab — Regenerated Epidermal tissue

Figure 11.16 Wounds. (A) Laceration on a horse. Courtesy of Beth Romano, AAS, CVT. (B) Surgically repaired laceration on the horse. Courtesy of Beth Romano, AAS, CVT. (C) Pit bull attacked by a porcupine. Courtesy of Beth Romano, AAS, CVT. (D) Illustration of wound healing. Courtesy of shutterstock/GRei.

Lesion	Abnormal change in tissue. The changes can be pathological or due to trauma. Examples include sores, wounds, and tumors.
Lupus erythematosus (LE)	Generalized term for a disease in which the body makes antibodies against its own good cells and tissues. The disease causes redness on the surface of the skin. A type of autoimmune disease. In dogs there are two types of LE: **discoid lupus erythematosus (DLE)** and **systemic lupus erythematosus (SLE)**. **DLE:** Commonly called "Collie nose," this disease causes redness (erythema), scaling, erosion, crusting, and depigmentation on the nose. Symptoms are often exaggerated with exposure to sunlight. Breeds such as Collies, Shelties, and German Shepherds are most susceptible. **SLE:** Autoimmune disease involving multiple body systems.
Macule	Flat, discolored lesion on the skin; also called **macula**. Freckles are an example.
Mange	An infestation of mites. Commonly seen mites include Demodex and Sarcoptes, which causes scabies (Figure 11.17).

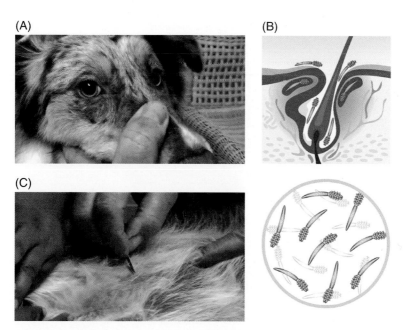

Figure 11.17   Infestation of the mite Demodex. (A) Demodectic mange on an Australian shepherd. Courtesy of Greg Martinez, DVM; www.youtube.com/drgregdvm. (B) Illustration of the site of infestation of Demodex in the skin. Courtesy of shutterstock/spline09. (C) Skin scrape being performed to retrieve mites. Courtesy of Greg Martinez, DVM; www.youtube.com/drgregdvm. (D) Microscopic view of the Demodex mites. (E) Microscopic view of the Sarcoptes mite that causes scabies.

(D)

(E)

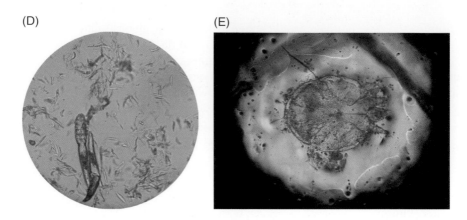

Figure 11.17 *(Continued)*.

Melanoma	Malignant tumor of the skin; malignant tumor of melanocytes (Figure 11.18).

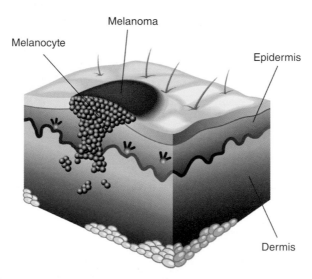

Figure 11.18 Illustration of melanoma. Courtesy of shutterstock/rob3000.

Metastasis	To spread beyond control; spread of a tumor to a secondary location.
Nodule	A small, rounded mass.
Onycholysis	Separation of the nail or claw from the nail bed.
Pallor	Paleness of skin or mucous membranes.
Papilloma	Benign epithelial growth found on the skin or mucous membranes. Commonly called a **skin tag** (Figure 11.19).
Papule	Small, solid, elevated skin lesion less than a centimeter in diameter.

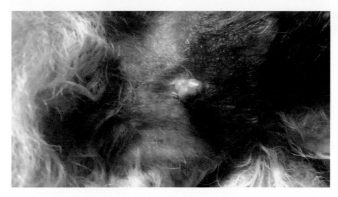

Figure 11.19 Papilloma on the lateral aspect of a poodle. Courtesy of Greg Martinez, DVM; www.youtube.com/drgregdvm.

Paronychia	Inflammation of the tissue surrounding the nails or claws.
Petechia (Plural: petechiae)	Small, pinpoint hemorrhages (Figure 11.11).

TECH TIP 11.9 Petechiae vs. Ecchymosis

Both petechia and ecchymosis are due to bleeding under the skin. The difference between the two is in their size. Petechiae are pinpoint sized marks on the skin. The bluish marks of ecchymosis are much larger, or roughly greater than a couple of centimeters.

Piloerection	Condition in which the hair stands straight up.
Polyp	Mushroom-like growth protruding from the mucous membranes. When attached to the mucous membranes by a stalk, it is termed a pedunculated polyp.
Prutitus	Itching.
Purpura	Condition of hemorrhaging into the skin creating a bruise. Examples include petechiae and ecchymosis.
Purulent	Containing pus (Figure 11.20).

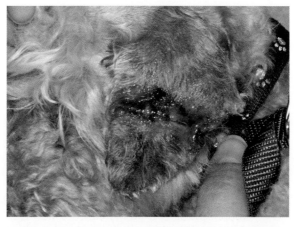

Figure 11.20 Purulent wound on the ear of the poodle after children wrapped a rubber band around it for days. Courtesy of AK Traylor, DVM; Microscopy Learning Systems.

Pus	Collection of white blood cells, usually neutrophils, and debris with fluid.
Pustule	Pus-filled lesion on the skin.
Scar	Mark left on the skin after healing.
Sebaceous cyst	Benign cyst containing sebum. Also called a **steatoma**.
Seborrhea	Excessive production of sebum.
Shedding	Condition of hair coat falling out.
Skin scrape	Scraping of the skin for laboratory exam. Most often used in the diagnosis of parasites or fungal infections (Figure 11.17).
Trichobezoar	Hairball.
Ulcer	Erosion of the skin or mucous membranes.
Urticaria	Red, raised patches on the skin commonly called **hives**. Most often associated with an allergic reaction.
Verruca (Plural: verrucae)	Wart; skin growth caused by a virus.
Wheal	Localized area of swelling that itches.

Coat Types and Color

Dogs

Various terms are used to describe the color and type of coats on dog. Many of the colors and coat patterns are seen in select breeds.

Belton	White coat with colored spots.
Bi-color	Coat with two colors.
Blenheim	Red and white. Typically used with spaniels.
Blue	Solid silver color.
Brindle	Brown coat with black stripes.
Dappled	Splotchy colors with multiple markings.
Harlequin	White coat and large areas of black and blue.
Hound	The typically black, tan, and white patters seen on Hound breeds such as a Beagle.
Long haired	Used to describe dogs with longer, fine hair.
Mantle	Black body with white markings on the head, neck, legs, and tail.
Merle	Marbled appearance. May be seen in reds or blues.
Party	Multi colored.
Phantom	Black and tan coloring patterns. Usually a black body with tan markings on the face, legs, and paws.
Roan	Blended mixture of colors with white.

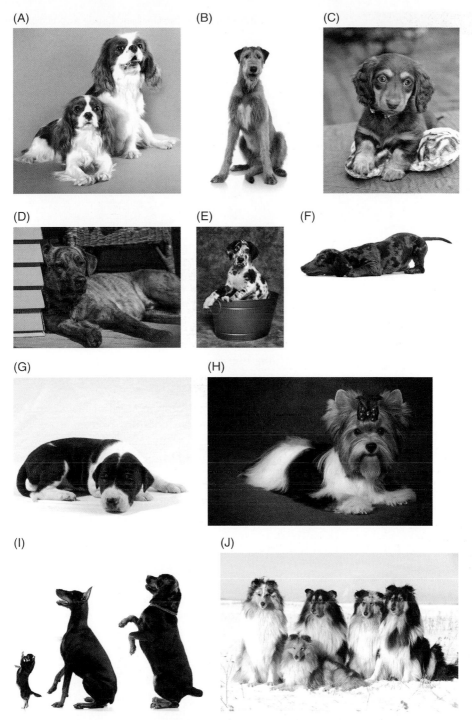

Figure 11.21 Canine coat colors. (A) Blenheim coats on Cavalier King Charles Spaniels. Courtesy of shutterstock/Liliya Kulianionak. (B) Salt and pepper colored Irish Wolfhound. Courtesy of shutterstock/Jagodka. (C) Bi-colored Dachshund. Courtesy of shutterstock/Annmarie Young. (D) Brindle Mastiff. Courtesy of shutterstock/Will Hughes. (E) Harlequin Great Dane puppy. Courtesy of shutterstock/Dee Hunter. (F) Dappled Dachshund. Courtesy of shutterstock/Erik Lam. (G) Mantle colored bull terrier. Courtesy of shutterstock/Mike Neale. (H) Party-colored Yorkshire Terrier. Courtesy of shutterstock/Utekhina Anna. (I) Phantom colored dogs. Courtesy of shutterstock/Alexia Khruscheva. (J) Sable and white, tri-color, and blue merle Collies. Courtesy of shutterstock/Zuzule.

(A)   (B)

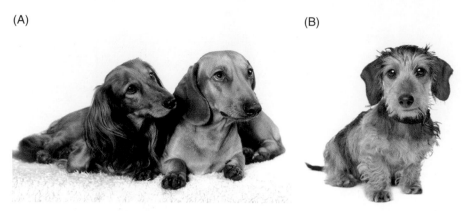

Figure 11.22 Types of canine coats. (A) Long-haired and short-haired dachshunds. Courtesy of shutterstock/Liliya Kulianionak. (B) Wire-haired dachshund. Courtesy of shutterstock/Erik Lam.

Sable and white	Tan and white dogs. Often used to describe herding breeds.
Salt and pepper	Mixture of black and white, giving the appearance of pepper sprinkles.
Tri-color	Three colors in a distinct pattern of black, tan, and white. Often used with herding breeds.
Tuxedo	Black and white patterns resembling a tuxedo.
Wire-haired	Long, wiry, rough coat.

Cats

Feline coat patterns are a bit different than those of dogs; however, some terms used on the canine terms cross over.

Calico	Sometimes called tri-color, these cats have a white base coat with black and tan patterns. In most cases, calicos are females.
Colorpoint	White or cream base coat with colored patterns on the face, paws, and tail.
Ruddy	Red based coat with ticked patterns.
Tabby	Bi-colored coat with striped or spotted patterns.
Tortoise shell	Tri-color coat with the colors blended together. The difference between the torties and calicos is in the white base. Torties have very little white in their coat patterns. Like the calicos, most torties are female.

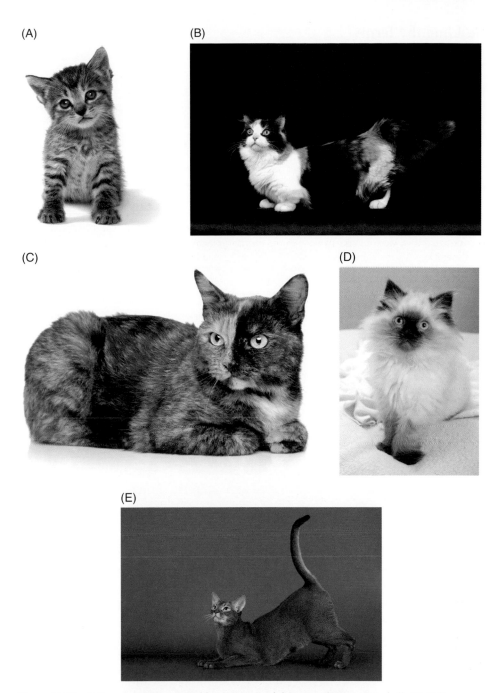

Figure 11.23   Feline coat colors. (A) Tabby. Courtesy of shutterstock/Tony Campbell. (B) Calico munchkin. Courtesy of shutterstock/Linn Currie. (C) Tortoise shell. Courtesy of shutterstock/ Jagodka. (D) Seal-point Ragdoll. Courtesy of shutterstock/cath5. (D) Ruddy Abyssinian. Courtesy of shutterstock/dien.

Building the Terms

Table 11.3   Chapter 11 Combining Forms.

Combining Forms	Definition	Combining Forms	Definition
Adip/o	Fat	**Melan/o**	Black
Albin/o	White	**Myc/o**	Fungus
Bi/o	Life	**Onych/o**	Nail
Carcin/o	Cancer; cancerous	**Pil/o**	Hair
Cutane/o	Skin	**Py/o**	Pus
Derm/o	Skin	**Seb/o**	Sebum
Dermat/o	Skin	**Sebace/o**	Sebum
Erythem/o	Redness; flushed	**Squam/o**	Scale
Erythemat/o	Redness; flushed	**Steat/o**	Fat; sebum
Hidr/o	Sweat	**Therm/o**	Heat
Ichthy/o	Dry; scaly	**Trich/o**	Hair
Kerat/o	Horny; hard; cornea	**Ungu/o**	Nail; Hoof
Lip/o	Fat	**Xer/o**	Dry

Table 11.4   Chapter 11 Prefixes.

Prefix	Definition	Prefix	Definition
epi-	above; upon; on	**meta-**	change; beyond
hyper-	increased; excessive; above	**par-**	other than; abnormal
hypo-	deficient; below; under; less than normal	**per-**	through
intra-	within; into	**sub-**	under; below

Table 11.5 Chapter 11 Suffixes.

Suffix	Definition	Suffix	Definition
-al, -ous	pertaining to	**-lysis**	destruction; breakdown; separation
-cyte	cell	**-oma**	tumor; mass; collection of fluid
-derma	skin	**-opsy**	to view; view of
-ectomy	removal; excision; resection	**-ose**	pertaining to; full of; sugar
-ema	condition	**-osis**	abnormal condition
-ia	condition	**-plasty**	surgical repair
-ism	process; condition	**-rrhea**	flow; discharge
-ist	specialist		
-itis	inflammation		
-logy	study of		

Now it's time to put these word parts together. If you memorize the meaning of the combining forms, prefixes, and suffixes, then this will get easier each time. Remember your five basic rules to medical terminology when building and defining these terms. You'll notice some word parts are repeated from the previous chapters.

Parts				Medical Term		Definition
Adip/o	+	-ose	=	Adipose	:	_____
Dermat/o	+	-itis	=	Dermatitis	:	_____
Dermat/o	+	-logy	+ -ist =	Dermatologist	:	_____
Dermat/o	+	Myc/o	+ -osis =	Dermatomycosis	:	_____
Dermat/o	+	-plasty	=	Dermatoplasty	:	_____
Lip/o	+	-oma	=	Lipoma	:	_____
Onych/o	+	-ectomy	=	Onychectomy	:	_____
Onych/o	+	Myc/o	+ -osis =	Onychomycosis	:	_____
Pil/o	+	Sebace/o	+ -ous =	Pilosebaceous	:	_____
Py/o	+	-derma	=	Pyoderma	:	_____
sub-	+	Cutane/o	+ -ous =	Subcutaneous	:	_____
Trich/o	+	Myc/o	+ -osis =	Trichomycosis	:	_____
sub-	+	Ungu/o	+ -al =	Subungual	:	_____
Xer/o	+	-derma	=	Xeroderma	:	_____

Also called ichthyosis.

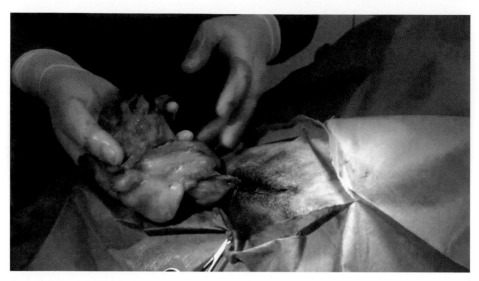

Figure 11.24   Surgery to remove a lipoma from a dog. Courtesy of Greg Martinez, DVM; www.youtube.com/drgregdvm.

Abbreviations

Table 11.6   Chapter 11 Abbreviations.

Abbreviation	Defintion
CA	Cancer
Derm	Skin
DLE	Discoid lupus erythematosus
FAD	Flea allergy dermatitis
FNA	Fine needle aspirate
ID	Intradermal
LE	Lupus erythematosus
SC, SQ, Sub Q	Subcutaneous
SLE	Systemic lupus erythematosus

Case Study

You'll notice some terms from the previous chapters

Bum, a 6-year-old West Highland White Terrier, has just been adopted by Mr. and Mrs. Phillips. They bring him to your clinic to have his skin checked. They noticed areas of bald spots under his eyes and around his legs. On P/E, the areas are isolated to suborbital (below the eye) and on the carpi. The doctor asks you to perform a scotch tape prep, but it turns up nothing so he orders a skin scrape. The figure displays the results.

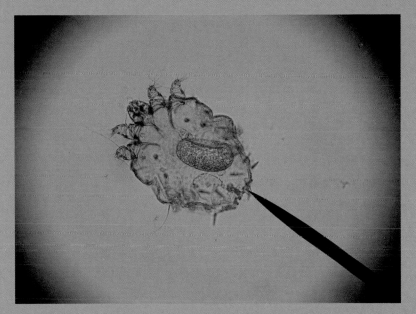

Figure 11.25   Can you identify the parasite?

1. What parasite does Bum have?
   a. Demodex
   b. Sarcoptes
   c. Streptococcus
   d. Staphylococcus
2. Which of the following clinical signs describes Bum?
   a. Pruritus
   b. Alopecia
   c. Acne
3. True or False: Since the parasite was seen on skin scrape and not a scotch tape prep, it was a superficial parasite.

Exercises

11-A: Give the term for the following definitions of the integumentary system.

1. _____: Layer of the epidermis containing melanocytes.
2. _____: True layer of skin.
3. _____: Found along the hair follicle and produces sebum.
4. _____: Structural protein found in the dermis of the skin.
5. _____: Pigment that gives skin its color.
6. _____: Oily substance secreted by sebaceous glands.
7. _____: Small opening on the surface of the skin.
8. _____: Deep, fatty layer of skin.
9. _____: Sac in the dermis in which hair grows.
10. _____: Outermost layer of skin.

11-B: Define the following terms.

1. Percutaneous_____
2. Adipose _____
3. Pyoderma _____
4. Trichomyosis _____
5. Subungual _____
6. Lipoma _____
7. Dermatoplasty _____
8. Onychectomy _____
9. Xeroderma _____
10. Pilosebaceous _____

11-C: Give the medical term for the following:

1. _____: Hairball.
2. _____: Erosion of the skin and mucous membranes.
3. _____: Containing pus.
4. _____: Small, pinpoint hemorrhages.
5. _____: Bluish-black mark on the skin.
6. _____: Sweating
7. _____: Malignant tumor of the skin.
8. _____: Benign cyst containing sebum.
9. _____: Bedsores.
10. _____: Commonly called a skin tag.
11. _____: Spread of a tumor to a secondary location.
12. _____: A bruise.
13. _____: Itching
14. _____: Absence of hair in areas where it normally grows.

15. _____: Commonly called allergic dermatitis.
16. _____: Removal of tissue for microscopic exam.
17. _____: Localized collection of pus.
18. _____: Congenital absence of pigmentation.
19. _____: Plug of keratin and sebum at the hair follicle; blackhead.
20. _____: Abnormal tube-like passageway that can occur anywhere on the body.

11-D: Define the following abbreviations.

1. _____: CA   6. _____: ID
2. _____: LE   7. _____: FAD
3. _____: FNA   8. _____: DLE
4. _____: SQ   9. _____: SC
5. _____: Derm   10. _____: SLE

11-E: Match the following terms with their descriptions.

1. _____ Tough protein found in horny tissue.   A. Abrasion

2. _____ Hooved animals.   B. Keratin

3. _____ Wound caused by scraping.   C. Laceration

4. _____ Wound caused by tearing.   D. Pallor

5. _____ Skin paleness.   E. Ungulates

Answers can be found starting on page 571.

Go to www.wiley.com/go/taibo/terminology to find additional learning materials for this chapter:

- A crossword puzzle
- Flashcards
- Audio clips to show how to pronounce terms
- Case studies
- Review questions
- The figures from the chapter in PowerPoint

Chapter 12

The Nervous System

The nervous system is the most complex of the body systems, controlling all of the body's activities. Some animals have millions of nerve cells in their bodies, while others have up to 1 billion nerve cells which are constantly detecting stimuli, sending messages to the brain to coordinate a response, and then sending messages from the brain to different parts of the body to carry out that response.

Nerves

The neuron, or nerve cell, is the basic structure of the nervous system. This microscopic structure transmits impulses after receiving a stimulus. Label the neuron in Figure 12.1 using Table 12.1.

The Path of the Nervous Impulse

Once there's a change in environment (a stimulus), an impulse is received by the dendrites of the nerve cell. The nervous impulse then passes through the cell body and along the axon. After leaving the axon, the nervous impulse passes through the terminal end fibers and into the synapse to be picked up by the dendrites of another nerve cell. In order to help other neurons recognize the impulse, chemical substances called neurotransmitters are released to excite or inhibit the target cell (Figure 12.2). There are different types of neurotransmitters which create different responses such as acetylcholine, epinephrine, dopamine, endorphins, and serotonin. Table 12.2 lists the neurotransmitters and their effects on the body.

Veterinary Medical Terminology Guide and Workbook, First Edition. Angela Taibo.
© 2014 John Wiley & Sons, Inc. Published 2014 by John Wiley & Sons, Inc.
Companion website: www.wiley.com/go/taibo/terminology

Table 12.1 The Nerve Cell.

Axon (4)	Fiber than carries a nervous impulse along a nerve cell away from the cell body.
Cell body (2)	Part of the nerve cell containing the **nucleus (3)**. A collection of nerve cell bodies is called a **ganglion**.
Dendrites (1)	Branching structures that receive the nervous impulse.
Myelin sheath (5)	Fatty tissue around the axon of a nerve cell. Helps to protect and insulate the axon. The sheath is lobed, creating gaps between layers of myelin along the axon. These gaps are called **nodes of Ranvier**.
Synapse (7)	Space between neurons in which the nervous impulse passes.
Terminal end fibers (6)	Distal portion of the neuron where the impulse leaves the cell.

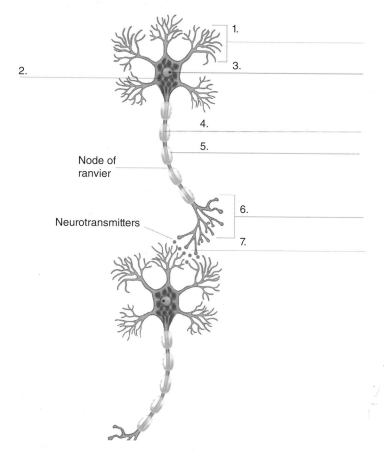

Figure 12.1 Anatomy of a neuron. Courtesy of shutterstock/Alila Sao Mai.

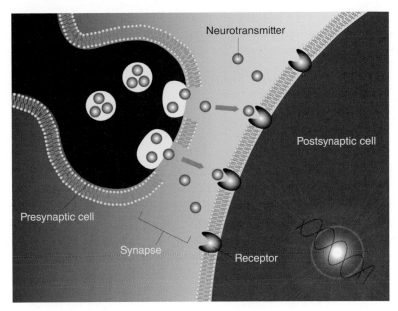

Figure 12.2   The synapse and the effect of neurotransmitters. Courtesy of shutterstock/Meletios.

Table 12.2   Neurotransmitters.

Acetylcholine	Neurotransmitter that causes muscles to contract and aids in "dream" sleep.
Dopamine	Neurotransmitter that inhibits the firing of nerve cells which in turn relaxes the animal.
Endorphins	Neurotransmitters responsible for reducing pain and for pleasure. Endorphins are the body's natural morphine.
Epinephrine	Hormone that acts as a neurotransmitter to increase heart rate and blood pressure.
Norepinephrine	Neurotransmitter that causes vasoconstriction, increased heart rate, and increased blood pressure. Also called **noradrenaline**.
Serotonin	Neurotransmitter responsible for relaxation. When levels are decreased, it leads to stress and behavioral disorders.

Nerves

When dendrites and axons are bundled together, they become visible to the naked eye, forming a structure called a nerve. There are two different kinds of nerves: sensory nerves and motor nerves. Sensory nerves, also called afferent nerves, carry impulses toward the brain. Motor nerves, also called efferent nerves, carry impulses away from the brain. For example, if you were to touch a hot stove, the sensory nerves would carry an impulse to your brain telling you that it's hot. The motor nerves would then send an impulse from your brain to your hand to tell it to move.

Neuroglial Cells

Neuroglial cells, or glial cells, play a supportive role in the nervous system (Figure 12.3). The cells resemble neurons morphologically, but their function is to protect the nerves by attacking foreign material and protect them from infection. Glial cells are far more numerous than neurons and can reproduce and phagocytize foreign microorganisms. There are five different types of glial cells:

Astroglial cells   Commonly called astrocytes, these cells transport electrolytes and water between the capillaries and neurons of the brain, helping to form the blood brain barriers (BBB). They prevent the passage of harmful substances from the blood into the nerve cells of the brain. These cells are shaped like a star, which is where their name comes from.

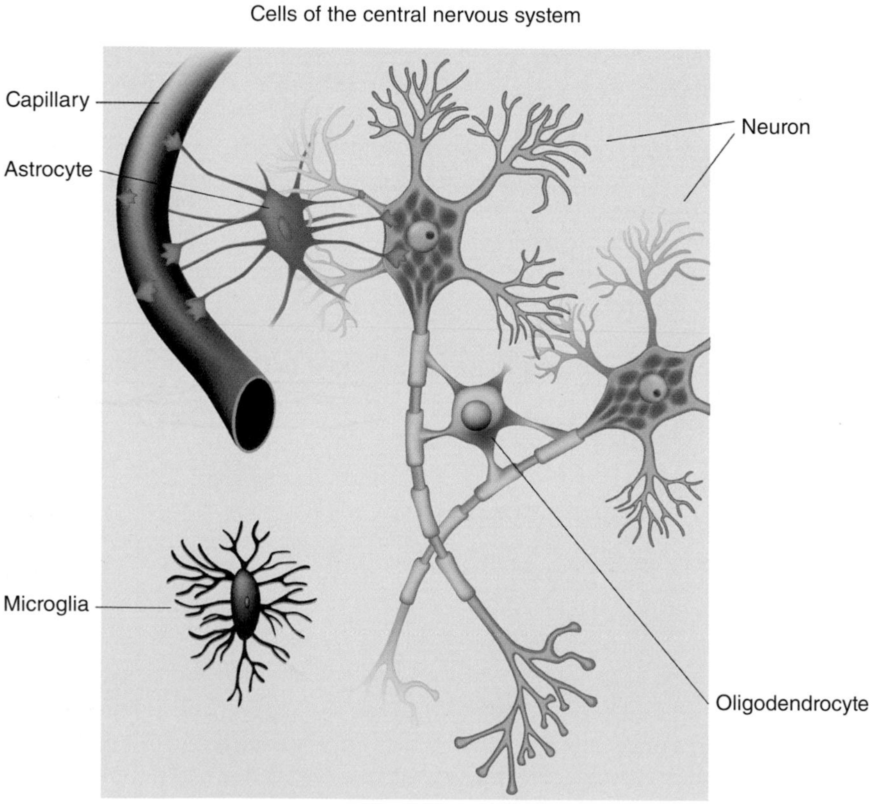

Figure 12.3   Neuroglial cells. Courtesy of shutterstock/Alila Sao Mai.

Microglial cells	Phagocytic cells which protect the nervous system from infection.
Oligodendroglial cells	Cells that form the myelin around the axon of the nerve cell.
Ependymal cells	Cells that line the ventricles of the brain and surround the spinal cord. They produce cerebrospinal fluid that circulates around the brain and spinal cord.
Schwann cells	Dual-action cells that form myelin around the axon and act as phagocytes against foreign organisms.

TECH TIP 12.1 Essentials and Accessories

Tissue that is essential to a system is termed **parenchymal** tissue. Tissue that is supportive to the essential tissue is called **stromal** tissue.

In the case of the nervous system, a neuron is an example of parenchymal tissue and glial cells are classified as stromal tissue.

Divisions of the Nervous System

The nervous system is divided into two portions, the central nervous system and the peripheral nervous system (Figure 12.4). The central nervous system consists of the brain and spinal cord. The peripheral nervous system is made up of cranial nerves, spinal nerves, and the autonomic nervous system.

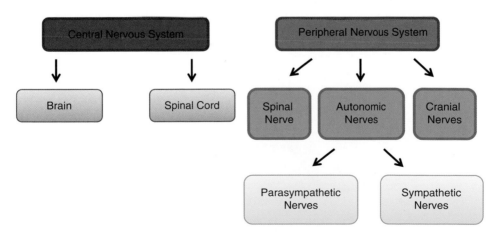

Figure 12.4   Divisions of the nervous system.

The Central Nervous System

Both the brain and spinal cord are a collection of nervous tissue. If cross-sectioned, both have a gray layer and a white layer. The gray layer is made up of nerve cell bodies and the white layer is made up of the axons and myelin sheaths. Therefore, the white matter is the conducting portion of both organs.

The brain and spinal cord are also surrounded by three layers of membranes called meninges. The protective layers, in order from superficial to deep, are listed in Table 12.3.

The spaces between the meninges are named based on their location (Figure 12.5).

Table 12.3   Meninges.

Dura mater	Tough, outermost layer of the meninges. Blood can enter brain tissue through this layer.
Arachnoid membrane	Middle layer of the meninges. Also known as the **arachnoid mater**.
Pia mater	Innermost, delicate layer of the meninges which adheres to the brain and spinal cord.

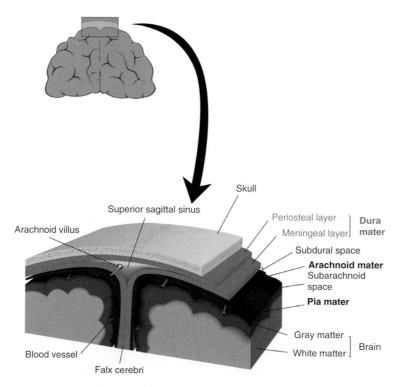

Figure 12.5   The meninges. Courtesy of shutterstock/Alila Sao Mai.

Epidural space   Space above the dura mater.
Subdural space   Space below the dura mater.
Subarachnoid space   Space below the subarachnoid membrane, where
                           cerebrospinal fluid can be found.

Cerebrospinal fluid (CSF) is a transparent fluid that circulates throughout the brain and spinal cord. It is produced by the choroid plexus to help nourish the brain and spinal cord. The choroid plexus is a group of blood vessels in the pia mater of the brain.

The Brain

The brain lies in the skull and is the control center of the body. There are three main sections of the brain: the cerebrum, the cerebellum, and the brainstem (Figure 12.6).

The cerebrum is the largest part of the brain and is responsible for memory, speech, movement, hearing, vision, and smell. Sensory impulses from the afferent nerves are received by the cerebrum and motor impulses are to the efferent nerves. The outer section of the cerebrum, the cerebral cortex, is made up of gray matter that is arranged in folds called gyri. The grooves in between the gyri are called sulci (Figure 12.7). White matter and ventricles, the spaces within the brain, can be found in the

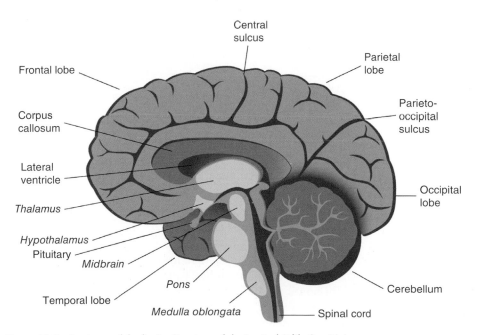

Median section of the brain

Central
sulcus

Parietal
lobe

Frontal lobe

Parieto-
occipital
sulcus

Corpus
callosum

Lateral
ventricle

Occipital
lobe

Thalamus

Hypothalamus
Pituitary

Midbrain

Pons

Temporal lobe

Medulla oblongata

Cerebellum

Spinal cord

Figure 12.6   Anatomy of the brain. Courtesy of shutterstock/Alila Sao Mai.

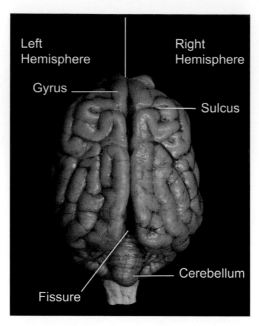

Figure 12.7 Dorsal view of a dog's brain. Courtesy of shutterstock/vetpathologist.

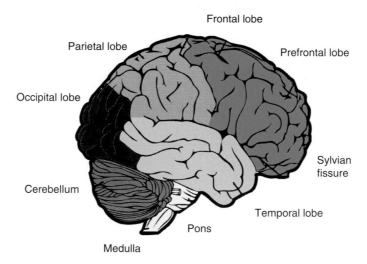

Figure 12.8 Lobes of the brain. Courtesy of shutterstock/MikiR.

inner section of the brain. The cerebrum is divided into a right side and a left side, called the cerebral hemispheres. Within each hemisphere are four lobes which are named based on the skull bones that protect them (Figure 12.8).

The cerebellum is the second largest portion of the brain and is commonly referred to as the "body's gyroscope." It is the cerebellum that helps the body maintain balance and coordinate voluntary movements.

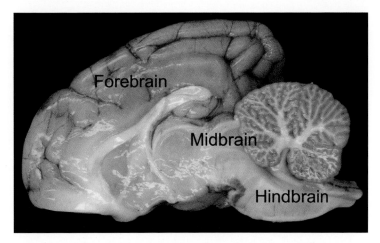

Figure 12.9   Lateral view of a dog's brain. Courtesy of shutterstock/vetpathologist.

The brainstem is the stem-like portion of the brain that connects the cerebrum to the spinal cord. It is made up of the midbrain, interbrain, pons, and medulla oblongata.

The interbrain includes the thalamus and hypothalamus. The thalamus is a relay point of the brain where sensory and motor impulses are received and then redirected to the appropriate part of the cerebrum. The hypothalamus lies just beneath the thalamus and controls the pituitary gland, body temperature, emotions, sleep, thirst, and hunger.

The midbrain is rostral to the pons and contains nerve fibers that allow communication between the cerebral hemispheres (Figure 12.9). This portion of the brain is responsible for reflexes of the eyes, ears, and head.

The pons, or bridge, contains nerve fibers that allow the cerebrum and cerebellum to communicate with each other.

The medulla oblongata is a stem-like structure connecting the brain to the spinal cord. Essential life functions such as breathing, heart function, and blood pressure are controlled by the medulla oblongata. This portion is also responsible for the communication between one side of the body and the opposite side of the brain. When damaged in animals, symptoms include head tilt and circling.

The Spinal Cord

The spinal cord is the highway from the brain to the rest of the body. It carries impulses to and from the brain and carries all the nerves to the limbs (Figure 12.10). The spinal cord runs from the medulla oblongata to the lumbar or sacral vertebrae, depending on the species. When the spinal cord ends, the nerve endings of the cord branch out, thus forming the cauda equina (horse's tail). The name comes from the appearance of the nerves due to their fanned-out appearance.

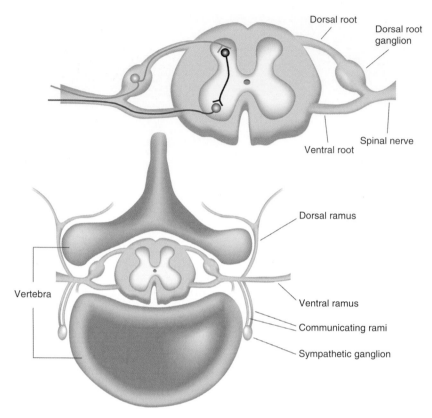

Figure 12.10   Cross-section of the spinal cord. Courtesy of shutterstock/Alila Sao Mai.

The Peripheral Nervous System

Cranial Nerves

Cranial nerves are attached to the brain and pass through the skull to structures in the head and neck (Figure 12.11). There are twelve pairs of cranial nerves, all named using Roman numerals. The tenth cranial nerve, the vagus nerve, is the exception to the rule in that it also controls functions in the chest and abdomen. Table 12.4 lists the cranial nerves and their functions.

There are many mnemonics to help memorize the cranial nerves, some of them are clean, and some of them dirty. One example of a clean mnemonic is Oh, Oh, Oh, To Touch And Feel Vintage Green Velvet, Simply Heaven.

Spinal Nerves

Spinal nerves carry nervous impulses between the spinal cord and the rest of the body (Figure 12.12). These paired nerves pass between the vertebrae where they eventually branch out to supply the trunk and limbs of the body.

Table 12.4   Cranial Nerves.

Cranial Nerve	Function
I. Olfactory	Smell
II. Optic	Vision
III. Oculomotor	Movement of eyes
IV. Trochlear	Movement of eyes
V. Trigeminal	Three branches (thus the name): Ophthalmic: Corneal senses Maxillary: Upper jaw movement Mandibular: Lower jaw movement
VI. Abducens	Movement of eyes
VII. Facial	Movement of face Taste
VIII. Vestibulocochlear	Hearing and balance
IX. Glossopharyngeal	Tongue taste Throat movement
X. Vagus	Throat Voice box Chest movement Abdominal sensations
XI. Accessory	Neck and shoulder movement; also known as the spinal accessory nerve
XII. Hypoglossal	Tongue movement

The Autonomic Nervous System

Unlike the spinal nerves and cranial nerves, which primarily deal with the voluntary functions of skeletal muscle (Figure 12.13), the autonomic nervous system is responsible for involuntary functions of smooth muscle, cardiac muscle, and gland secretion. The two divisions of the autonomic nervous system are the sympathetic nervous system and the parasympathetic nervous system.

The parasympathetic nervous system is responsible for normal body function. Parasympathetic nerves reduce heart rate, decrease blood pressure, constrict the pupils, decrease respiratory rate, and relax the structures of GI tract. The parasympathetic nervous system is also called the cholinergic pathway because it uses the cholinergic acetylcholine.

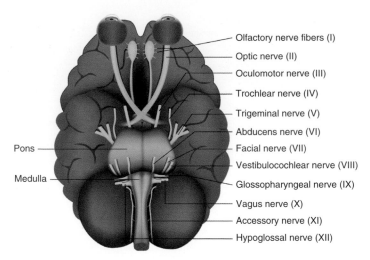

Olfactory nerve fibers (I)
Optic nerve (II)
Oculomotor nerve (III)
Trochlear nerve (IV)
Trigeminal nerve (V)
Abducens nerve (VI)
Pons
Facial nerve (VII)
Vestibulocochlear nerve (VIII)
Medulla
Glossopharyngeal nerve (IX)
Vagus nerve (X)
Accessory nerve (XI)
Hypoglossal nerve (XII)

Figure 12.11   The cranial nerves. Courtesy of shutterstock/Alila Sao Mai.

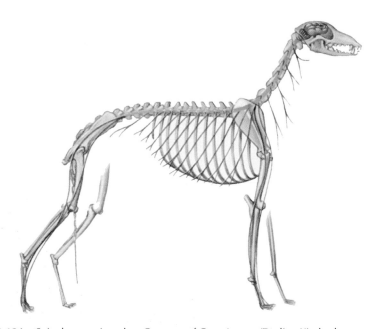

Figure 12.12A   Spinal nerves in a dog. Courtesy of Getty Images/Dorling Kindersley.

The sympathetic nervous system is responsible for the "fight or flight" response is cases of extreme stress. Sympathetic nerves increase heart rate, respiratory rate, and blood pressure. Pupils are dilated and GI function is decreased during this stress response. The sympathetic nervous system is also responsible for stimulating the release of adrenaline from the adrenal glands. The sympathetic

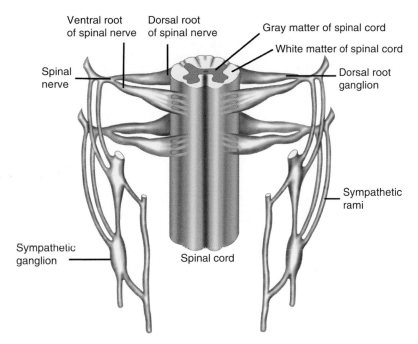

Figure 12.12B   Anatomy of the spinal nerves. Courtesy of shutterstock/Alex Luengo.

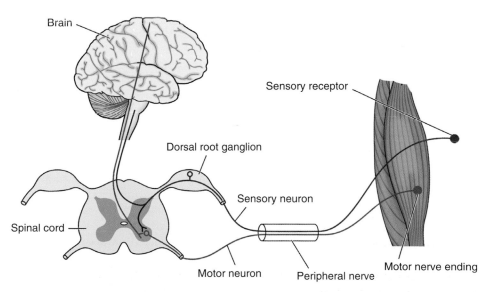

Figure 12.13   Pathways of afferent and efferent nerves through the central and peripheral nervous systems. Courtesy of shutterstock/Annie Potter.

nervous system is also called the adrenergic pathway because it uses the adrenergic epinephrine, or adrenaline.

Ultimately, these two systems oppose each other. Just remember that the parasympathetic nervous system is used to "rest and digest." The sympathetic nervous system is for "fight or flight" and that adrenergic equals adrenaline.

Related Terms

Autonomic nervous system (ANS)	Nerves that control involuntary functions of muscles, glands, and viscera.
Arachnoid membrane	Middle layer of the meninges. Also known as the **arachnoid mater**.
Axon	Fiber that carries the nervous impulse along the nerve cell.
Blood brain barrier (BBB)	Capillaries that allow certain substances to enter the brain while keeping other substances out.
Brainstem	Consists of the pons, medulla oblongata, interbrain, and midbrain. This portion of the brain connects the brain to the spinal cord.
Cauda equina	Nerve roots leaving the caudal end of the spinal cord.
Cell body	Portion of the nerve cell that contains the nucleus.
Central nervous system (CNS)	The brain and spinal cord.
Cerebral cortex	Outer section of the cerebrum.
Cerebrum	Largest part of the brain responsible for voluntary muscle movements, speech, vision, hearing, thought, memory, and taste.
Cerebellum	Second largest part of the brain; responsible for balance and coordination.
Conscious	Awake, alert, aware, responsive.
Cerebrospinal fluid (CSF)	Fluid circulating throughout the brain and spinal cord.
Dendrites	First part of the nerve cell to receive the stimulus.
Dura mater	Tough, outermost layer of the meninges.
Gait	Manner of walking.
Ganglion (Plural: ganglia)	Collection of nerve cell bodies in the peripheral nervous system.
Hippocampus	Portion of the brain responsible for orientation and emotional responses. When an animal is suspected of dying from rabies, this portion of the brain is checked for round, reddish inclusions called Negri bodies (Figure 12.14).

Hypothalamus	Portion of the interbrain that controls the pituitary gland, body temperature, emotions, sleep, thirst, and hunger (Figure 12.14).

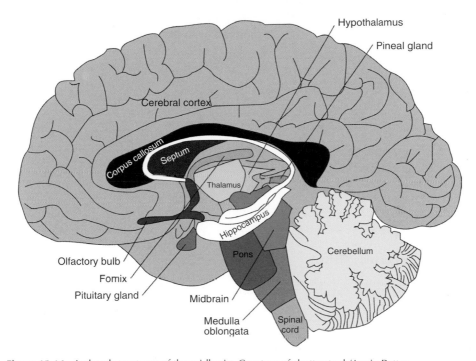

Figure 12.14   Isolated structures of the midbrain. Courtesy of shutterstock/Annie Potter.

Innervation	Supply of nerves to a part of the body.
Medulla oblongata	Stem-like structure of the brainstem connecting the brain to the spinal cord. Responsible for essential life functions such as breathing, heart function, and blood pressure.
Meninges	Three protective layers surrounding the brain and spinal cord.
Motor nerves	Nerves that carry impulses away from the brain and spinal cord. Also known as efferent nerves.
Myelin sheath	Protective, fatty tissue around the axon of a nerve cell.
Nerve	Macroscopic cord-like structure made up of nerve cells.
Neuron	A nerve cell.
Neurotransmitter	Chemical messenger released from a neuron to stimulate or inhibit another nerve or target cell.

Parasympathetic nervous system	Portion of the autonomic nervous system responsible for normal body functions including regulating heart rate and respiratory rate.
Peripheral nervous system	Portion of the nervous system consisting of cranial nerves, spinal nerves, and the autonomic nervous system.
Pia mater	Innermost, delicate layer of the meninges which adheres to the brain and spinal cord.
Plexus	Large, interlacing network of nerves. Named based on where they carry impulses to and from. For example, the **brachial plexus** supply most of the front limbs.
Pons	Contains nerve fibers that allow the cerebrum and cerebellum to communicate with each other. Commonly called the **bridge**.
Proprioception	Knowing where your limbs are in space.
Sensory nerves	Nerves that carry impulses toward the brain and spinal cord. Also known as afferent nerves.
Sympathetic nervous system	Portion of the autonomic nervous system responsible for the "fight or flight" response in cases of extreme stress. Functions include increasing heart rate and respiratory rate.
Thalamus	Relay point of the brain where sensory and motor impulses are received and then redirected to the appropriate part of the cerebrum (Figure 12.15).
Ventricles of the brain	Spaces in the interbrain that contain CSF.

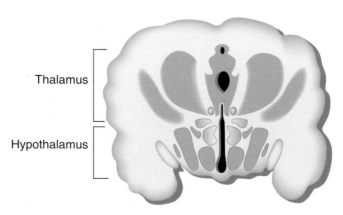

Thalamus

Hypothalamus

Figure 12.15   Location of the thalamus to the hypothalamus. Courtesy of shutterstock/Alila Sao Mai.

Pathology and Procedures

Aneurysm	Localized widening of a blood vessel.
Ataxia	Lack of coordination.
Bovine spongiform encephalopathy (BSE)	Spongy degeneration of the brain and spinal cord causing ataxia, anorexia, aggression, and eventually death. Commonly called **mad cow disease**.
Caprine arthritis encephalitis (CAE)	Multisystem viral disease causing ataxia, paralysis, arthritis, and pneumonia.
Cataplexy	Idiopathic condition causing sudden loss of skeletal muscle function due to extreme excitement, sexual activity, or vigorous exercise.
Cerebellar hypoplasia	Degeneration or loss of cells in the cerebellum causing ataxia.
Cerebrovascular accident	Disruption in the normal blood supply to the brain; **stroke** (Figure 12.16).

Hemorrhagic stroke

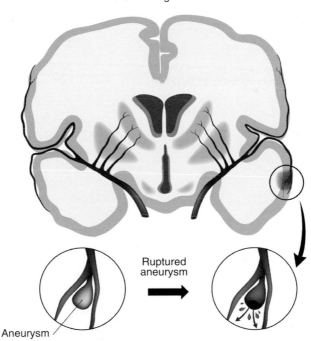

Ruptured aneurysm

Aneurysm

Figure 12.16   Mechanism of a stroke. Courtesy of shutterstock/Alila Sao Mai.

Coma	Deep state of unconsciousness. Also called **comatose**.

Concussion	Violent shaking of the brain.
Contusion	A bruise; injury to tissue without breaking the skin. Characterized by pain, swelling, and tenderness due to broken blood vessels.
CSF analysis	Laboratory examination of CSF to diagnose tumors and infections.
CSF tap	Surgical puncture to remove CSF. Sometimes called a **lumbar or spinal puncture** (Figure 12.17).

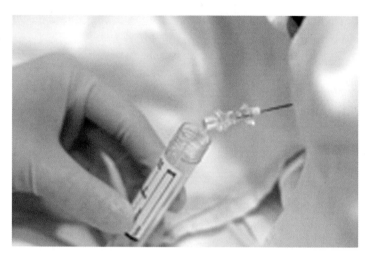

Figure 12.17   CSF tap. Courtesy of shutterstock/Li Wa.

Computed tomography (CT or CAT) of the brain	Radiographic imaging technique showing computerized cross-sections of the brain and spinal cord.
Contraindication	Any condition that renders a particular treatment undesirable.
Epilepsy	Idiopathic brain disorder characterized by recurrent seizures.
Horner's syndrome	Neurological disorder caused by paralysis of the cervical sympathetic nerve supply. Disease is characterized by sunken eyes, drooping of the upper eyelid, slight elevation of the lower eyelid, constriction of the pupils, and a prolapsed third eyelid (Figure 12.18).
Hydrocephalus	Abnormal accumulation of CSF in the ventricles of the brain. Also called **water on the brain**.
Lethargy	Condition of drowsiness or indifference.

(A)

(B)

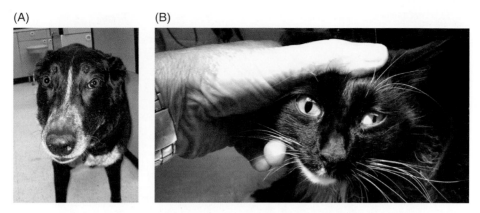

Figure 12.18   Horner's syndrome. (A) Courtesy of AK Traylor, DVM; Microscopy Learning Systems. (B) Courtesy of Greg Martinez, DVM; www.youtube.com/drgregdvm.

Magnetic resonance image (MRI) of the brain	Radiographic imaging technique showing a three-dimensional image of the brain.
Myasthenia gravis	Neuromuscular disorder characterized by weakness of the skeletal muscles.
Narcolepsy	Condition causing sudden, uncontrollable sleep episodes. Can be seen in dogs and Shetland ponies.
Palliative	Relieving symptoms, but not curing. For example, patients with epilepsy can be given drugs to decrease the frequency of seizures, but the drugs can't cure the disease itself.
Paralysis	Loss of motor function. Patients may have partial or complete paralysis. Also called **Palsy** (Figure 12.19).
Positron emission tomography (PET) scan	Radiographic imaging technique in which images are produced after injection of a radioactive substance.
Seizure	Sudden, involuntary contractions of voluntary muscles; also called **convulsions, grand mal, or tonic clonic**.
Spasticity	Increased muscle tone.
Spina bifida	Congenital anomaly in which the spinal canal fails to close around the spinal cord.
Stupor	Partial unconsciousness and decreased response to stimuli.
Syncope	Fainting or temporary loss of consciousness.

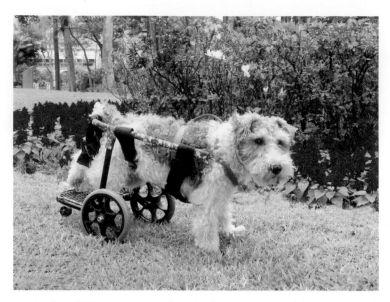

Figure 12.19   Paralyzed Wire Fox Terrier with a wheelchair. Courtesy of shutterstock/pixshots.

Thromboembolic meningoencephalitis (TEME)	Systemic disease in cattle causing blindness, weakness, ataxia, recumbency, and eventually death.
Tremor	Repetitive twitching of skeletal muscle.
Vestibular disease	Idiopathic neurological disorder characterized by head tilt, circling, and rapid back-and-forth movement of the eyes. Generally seen in older dogs (Figure 12.20).

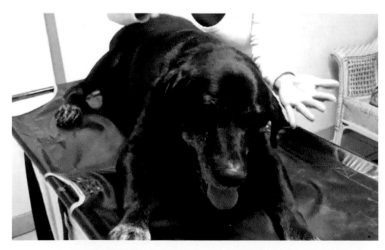

Figure 12.20   Black Lab with vestibular disease. Note the slight head tilt and imbalance on the table. Courtesy of Greg Martinez, DVM; www.youtube.com/drgregdvm.

> **TECH TIP 12.2 Strokes vs. Vestibular Disease**
>
> Although strokes are very rare in veterinary medicine, cases have been documented. The more commonly seen disorder of older dogs is vestibular disease. It presents similarly to a stroke; however, the symptoms begin to subside after a few days and medication can help take the edge off the more severe symptoms.

Building the Terms

Table 12.5   Chapter 12 Combining Forms.

Combining Forms	Definition	Combining Forms	Definition
Alges/o	Sensitivity to pain	Encephal/o	Brain
Arachn/o	Arachnoid membrane	Esthesi/o	Nervous sensation
Astr/o	Star	Gangli/o	Ganglion; collection of nerve cell bodies
Ax/o	Axis; main stem	Ganglion/o	Ganglion; collection of nerve cell bodies
Caus/o	Burning	Gli/o	Neuroglial tissue; glue
Caust/o	Burning	Gyr/o	Folding
Cephal/o	Head	Hemat/o	Blood
Cerebell/o	Cerebellum	Hydr/o	Fluid; water
Cerebr/o	Cerebrum	Kines/o	Movement
Comat/o	Deep sleep; coma	Mening/o	Meninges
Concuss/o	Shaken together violently	Meningi/o	Meninges
Contus/o	Bruise	My/o	Muscle
Crani/o	Skull; cranium	Myel/o	Spinal cord; bone marrow
Dendr/o	Dendrite	Narc/o	Sleep; stupor; numbness
Dur/o	Dura mater	Neur/o	Nerve
Electr/o	Electricity	Plex/o	Plexus; network of nerves

(Continued)

Table 12.5 (*Continued*).

Combining Forms	Definition	Combining Forms	Definition
Pont/o	Pons	**Syncop/o**	To cut off; cut short; fainting
Radicul/o	Nerve root	**Tax/o**	Coordination; order
Spin/o	Spine	**Thalam/o**	Thalamus
Sulc/o	Groove	**Thec/o**	Sheath
Synaps/o	Synapse	**Vag/o**	Vagus nerve
Synapt/o	Synapse	**Vertebr/o**	Vertebrae

Table 12.6 Chapter 12 Prefixes.

Prefix	Definition	Prefix	Definition
a-, an-	no, not, without	**micro-**	small
brady-	slow	**mono-**	one
cata-	down	**oligo-**	scanty
epi-	above; upon; on	**par-**	other than; abnormal
eu-	good; normal; true	**para-**	near; beside; abnormal; apart from; along the side of
hemi-	half	**polio-**	gray matter
hyper-	increased; excessive; above	**poly-**	many; much
hypo-	deficient; below; under	**quadri-**	four
inter-	between	**sub-**	under; below
intra-	within; into	**tetra-**	four
macro-	large		

Table 12.7   Chapter 12 Suffixes.

Suffix	Definition	Suffix	Definition
-al, -ar, -ic	pertaining to	-lepsy	seizure
-algesia	sensitivity to pain	-malacia	softening
-algia	pain	-oma	tumor; mass; collection of fluid
-cele	hernia	-ose	pertaining to; full of; sugar
-cyte	cell	-paresis	slight paralysis
-ectomy	removal; excision; resection	-pathy	disease condition
-esthesia	nervous sensation	-phoria	feeling; to bear; carry
-graphy	process of recording	-plegia	paralysis; palsy
-ia	condition	-plasia	development; formation; growth
-itis	inflammation	-rrhaphy	suture
-kinesia	movement	-sthenia	strength
-kinesis	movement	-tomy	incision; process of cutting
-kinetic	movement	-y	condition; process

Now it's time to put these word parts together. If you memorize the meaning of the combining forms, prefixes, and suffixes, then this will get easier each time. Remember your five basic rules to medical terminology when building and defining these terms. You'll notice some word parts are repeated from the previous chapters.

Parts			Medical Term	Definition
an-	+ -algesia		= Analgesia	:_____
an-	+ -esthesia		= Anesthesia	:_____
hyper-	+ -esthesia		= Hyperesthesia	:_____
par-	+ -esthesia		= paresthesia	:_____
macro-	+ Cephal/o	+ -y	= Macrocephaly	:_____
micro-	+ Cephal/o	+ -y	= Microcephaly	:_____
Cerebell/o	+ -ar		= Cerebellar	:_____

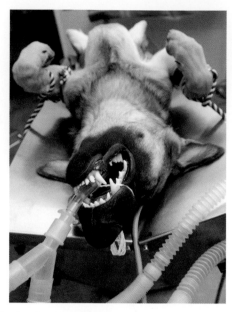

Figure 12.21   German Shepherd under anesthesia. Courtesy of shutterstock/CREATISTA.

TECH TIP 12.3 Analgesia vs. Anesthesia

These terms sound awfully similar and appear similar on paper. Be careful! Analgesia reduces pain. Anesthesia means without pain sensation. Technically it is a loss of all sensations, including pain, heat, cold, etc.

Cerebr/o	+ -al	= Cerebral	:_____
Comat/o	+ -ose	= Comatose	:_____
intra-	+ Crani/o + -al	= Intracranial	:_____
polio-	+ Encephal/o + -malacia	= Polioencephalomalacia	:_____
polio-	+ Encephal/o + Myel/o + -itis	= Polioencephalomyelitis	:_____
Electr/o	+ Encephal/o + -gram	= Electroencephalogram	:_____
Encephal/o + -itis		= Encephalitis	:_____
Encephal/o + -cele		= Encephalocele	:_____
Encephal/o + -pathy		= Encephalopathy	:_____
Encephal/o + Myel/o + -itis		= Encephalomyelitis	:_____

Because myel/o is attached to the combining form for brain, the definition for myel/o is generally the spinal cord.

Hemat/o	+ -oma	= Hematoma	:_____
eu-	+ -phoria	= Euphoria	:_____
a-	+ -kinetic	= akinetic	:_____

brady-	+ -kinesia		= Bradykinesia	:_____
hyper-	+ -kinesis		= hyperkinesis	:_____
Mening/o	+ -eal		= Meningeal	:_____
Meningi/o	+ -oma		= Meningioma	:_____
Mening/o	+ -itis		= Meningitis	:_____
Mening/o	+ Myel/o	+ -cele	= Meningomyelocele	:_____

Because myel/o is attached to the combining form for meninges, the definition for myel/o is generally the spinal cord instead of bone marrow.

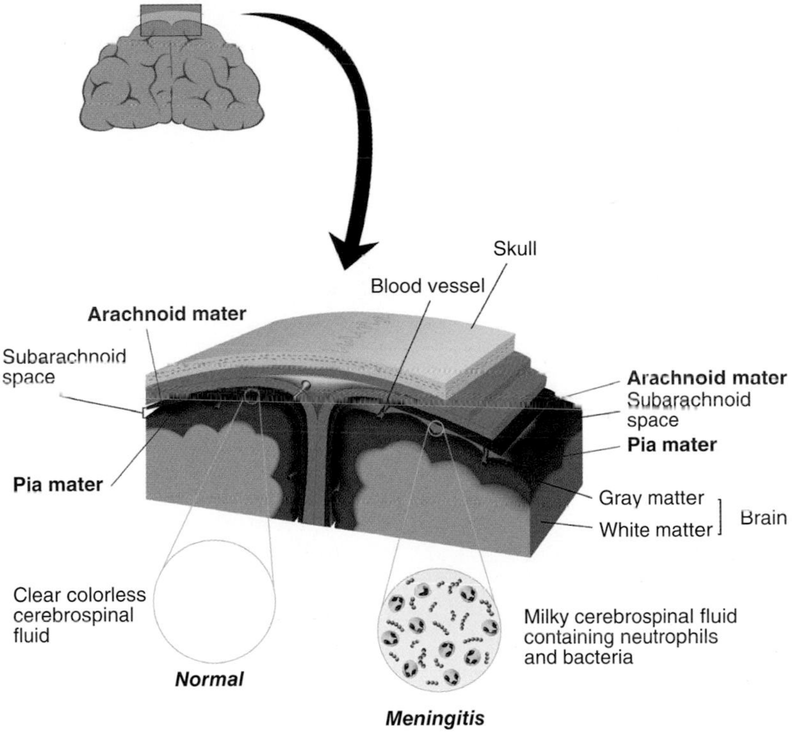

Figure 12.22   Meningitis and a comparison between normal and abnormal CSF. Courtesy of shutterstock/Alila Sao Mai.

Myel/o	+ -gram		= Myelogram	:_____
Myel/o	+ -oma		= Myeloma	:_____
polio-	+ Myel/o	+ -itis	= Polymyelitis	:_____
My/o	+ Neur/o	+ -al	= Myoneural	:_____
My/o	+ -paresis		= Myoparesis	:_____
Neur/o	+ -algia		= Neuralgia	:_____
Neur/o	+ -asthenia		= Neurasthenia	:_____

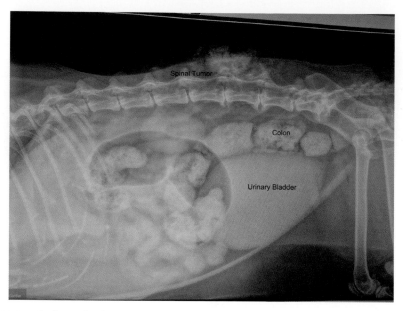

Figure 12.23 Radiograph of a myeloma in a dog. Note the urine retention in the urinary bladder. Courtesy of Beth Romano, AAS, CVT.

Neur/o	+ -ectomy		= Neurectomy	:_____
Neur/o	+ -itis		= Neuritis	:_____
Neur/o	+ -pathy		= Neuropathy	:_____
Neur/o	+ -plasty		= Neuroplasty	:_____
Neur/o	+ -rrhaphy		= Neurorrhaphy	:_____
Neur/o	+ -tomy		= Neurotomy	:_____
poly-	+ Neur/o	+ -itis	= Polyneuritis	:_____
hemi-	+ -paresis		= hemiparesis	:_____
mono-	+ -paresis		= monoparesis	:_____
para-	+ -paresis		= paraparesis	:_____
quadri-	+ -paresis		= quadriparesis	:_____
tetra-	+ -paresis		= tetraparesis	:_____

TECH TIP 12.4 Para vs. Hemi

When using "para-" and "hemi-" on terms related to weakness or paralysis of the body, "para" refers to the hind limb (rear legs) of the body. "Hemi" refers to one side of the body, specifically the right or left side.

---

hemi-	+ -plegia	= hemiplegia	:_____
mono-	+ -plegia	= monoplegia	:_____
para-	+ -plegia	= paraplegia	:_____

quadri-	+ -plegia	= quadriplegia	:_____
tetra-	+ -plegia	= tetraplegia	:_____
Radicul/o	+ -pathy	= Radiculopathy	:_____
Radicul/o	+ -itis	= Radiculitis	:_____
Syncop/o	+ -al	= Syncopal	:_____
Thalam/o	+ -ic	= Thalamic	:_____
Vag/o	+ -al	= Vagal	:_____

Abbreviations

Table 12.8   Chapter 12 Abbreviations.

Abbreviation	Definition
ANS	Autonomic nervous system
BBB	Blood brain barrier
BSE	Bovine spongiform encephalopathy (mad cow disease)
CAE	Caprine arthritis encephalitis virus
CNS	Central nervous system
CSF	Cerebrospinal fluid
CT, CAT scan	Computed tomography
CVA	Cerebrovascular accident (stroke)
EEG	Elecroencephalogram
ICP	Intracranial pressure
LP	Lumbar puncture
MG	Myasthenia gravis
MRI	Magnetic resonance imaging
PEM	Polioencephalomalacia
PET	Positron emission tomography
PNS	Peripheral nervous system
Sz	Seizure
TEME, TME	Thromboembolic meningoencephalitis

Case Study: Define the terms and abbreviations in bold print

A 12-year-old **M/N** Irish Setter named Laddie is rushed into the clinic with bouts of **syncope**, **convulsions**, and **tremors**. The owners are inconsolable after staying up with their dog all night. **Phlebotomy** is performed to run lab work. Muscle enzymes are elevated, but otherwise the labs are unremarkable. The vet orders an **EEG** and **MRI**. No **extracranial** or **intracranial** abnormalities are found. Laddie is diagnosed with **epilepsy** and placed on the drug phenobarbital to help decrease the frequency of the **seizures**. When seen for a follow-up visit the following week, Laddie is **BAR** and the owners are pleased with Laddie's steady improvement.

1. Laddie's treatment with the drug phenobarbital is considered:
   a. A cure
   b. Purulent
   c. Idiopathic
   d. Palliative

Exercises

12-A Give the term for the following definitions of the nervous system.

1. _____: Manner of walking.
2. _____: Condition of drowsiness.
3. _____: Nerve roots leaving the caudal end of the spinal cord that look like a horse's tail.
4. _____: Network of nerves.
5. _____: A nerve cell.
6. _____: Three protective layers of the brain and spinal cord.
7. _____: Largest part of the brain.
8. _____: The body's gyroscope.
9. _____: Tough, outermost layer of meninges.
10. _____: Localized widening of a blood vessel.

12-B: Define the following terms.

1. Encephalomalacia _____
2. Analgesia _____
3. Bradykinesia _____
4. Hematoma _____
5. Neuropathy _____
6. Hemiplegia _____
7. Paraparesis _____
8. Meningitis _____
9. Comatose _____
10. Poliomyelitis _____

12-C: Circle the correct term in parentheses:

1. Knowing where your limbs are in space. (palliative, proprioception, stupor)
2. Protective, fatty tissue around the axon of a nerve cell. (axon, dendrite, myelin sheath)
3. Nerves that carry impulses toward the brain and spinal cord. (afferent, efferent, motor)
4. Capillaries that allow certain substances to enter the brain. (BBB, PET, CSF)
5. The brain and spinal cord. (ANS, CNS, PNS)
6. Mad cow disease. (BSE, CAE, TME)
7. Increased muscle tone. (tremor, seizure, spasticity)
8. Sudden compulsion to sleep. (cataplexy, epilepsy, narcolepsy)
9. Imaging technique showing cross-section of the brain. (CT, MRI, PET)
10. Shaking of the brain. (contusion, concussion, coma)
11. System responsible for "fight or flight." (central, parasympathetic, sympathetic)
12. Chemical messenger released by a neuron. (dendrite, neurotransmitter, terminal end fibers)
13. Supply of nerves to a part of the body. (innervation, plexus, gyri)
14. Hernia of the brain. (cephalocele, encephalocele, myelocele)
15. Contains the pons, medulla oblongata and midbrain. (cerebrum, cerebellum, brainstem)

12-D: Define the following abbreviations.

1. _____ : BSE
2. _____ : LP
3. _____ : ICP
4. _____ : BBB
5. _____ : CAE

6. _____ : TEME
7. _____ : MG
8. _____ : CNS
9. _____ : CSF
10. _____ : Sz

12-E: Match the following disorders with their descriptions.

1. _____ Degeneration or loss of cells in the cerebellum causing ataxia.
2. _____ Neuromuscular disorder characterized by weakness of the skeletal muscles.
3. _____ Neurological disorder caused by paralysis of the cervical sympathetic nerve supply.
4. _____ Abnormal accumulation of CSF in the ventricles of the brain.
5. _____ Idiopathic neurological disorder characterized by head tilt, circling, and rapid back-and-forth movement of the eyes. Generally seen in older dogs.

A. Cerebellar hypoplasia

B. Horner's syndrome

C. Hydrocephalus

D. Myasthenia gravis

E. Vestibular disease

Answers can be found starting on page 571.

Go to www.wiley.com/go/taibo/terminology to find additional learning materials for this chapter:

- A crossword puzzle
- Flashcards
- Audio clips to show how to pronounce terms
- Case studies
- Review questions
- The figures from the chapter in PowerPoint

Chapter 13

The Eyes and Ears

The eye is a sensory organ used for vision. The ear is also a sensory organ; it is used for hearing and equilibrium. These two sensory organs take light and sound and convert those stimuli to nervous impulses to send to the brain to interpret.

The Eye

Using Table 13.1, label parts of the eye on Figure 13.1.

The Layers

The eyeball is protected by several structures. The dorsal aspect of the eyeball is protected by the orbital bones of the skull and the anterior portion of the eye is protected by conjunctiva. Conjunctiva is a thin membrane that covers the anterior eye and lines the eyelids. A group of structures around the eye produce tears to keep the eye lubricated and remove any foreign debris. This grouping is called the lacrimal apparatus. On the edge of the eyelids are tiny cilia called eyelashes which protect the anterior eye from foreign material.

The eyeball is made up of three layers. The tough, white, outer layer of the eye is called the sclera (Figure 13.2).

The middle, vascular layer is called the choroid; it contains the blood vessels that supply the eye. Within a portion of the choroid is an iridescent layer of epithelium called the tapetum lucidum that gives the eye the property of shining in the dark. This layer aids in night vision.

The retina is the light-sensitive nervous tissue that makes up the inner layer of the eye. Lining the retina are specialized photoreceptor cells called rods and cones (Figure 13.3), which share the function of transforming light into a nervous impulse. Rods function best in dim light and aid in night vision and peripheral

Veterinary Medical Terminology Guide and Workbook, First Edition. Angela Taibo.
© 2014 John Wiley & Sons, Inc. Published 2014 by John Wiley & Sons, Inc.
Companion website: www.wiley.com/go/taibo/terminology

Table 13.1 Anatomy of the Eye.

Pupil (1)	Dark opening of the eye where light passes through.
Iris (2)	Muscle around the pupil that controls the amount of light that enters the pupil. When light is bright, the iris constricts to limit light entry. In dim light, the iris dilates to allow for more light entry.
Cornea (3)	Transparent layer of tissue that covers the anterior eyeball.
Lens (4)	Transparent, biconvex structure behind the pupil.
Anterior chamber (A)	Portion of the eyeball between the cornea and iris. This chamber contains a fluid called **aqueous humor**.
Ciliary body (5)	Muscle on each side of the lens that adjusts the shape of the lens.
Vitreous chamber (V)	Area behind the lens containing a jelly-like fluid called **vitreous humor** which maintains the shape of the eyeball.
Sclera (6)	White, outer coat of the eyeball.
Choroid (7)	Middle, vascular coat of the eyeball.
Retina (8)	Light-sensitive innermost layer of the eyeball.
Macula (9)	Small, yellowish area above the optic disc containing the fovea centralis.
Fovea centralis (10)	Central depression of the retina containing a high concentration of cones.
Optic disc (11)	Commonly called the blind spot, this is the portion of the eye where the retina meets the optic nerve.
Optic nerve (12)	Cranial nerve that carries impulses from the eye to the brain.

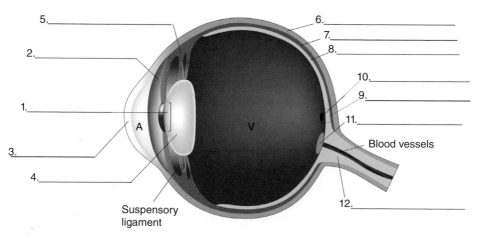

Figure 13.1 Anatomy of the eye. Courtesy of shutterstock/Alila Sao Mai.

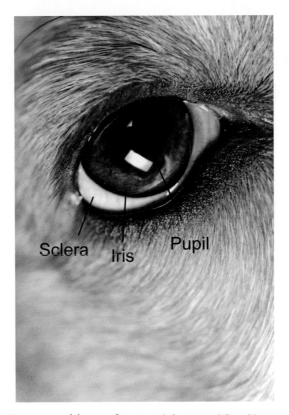

Figure 13.2   External structures of the eye. Courtesy of shutterstock/Igor Normann.

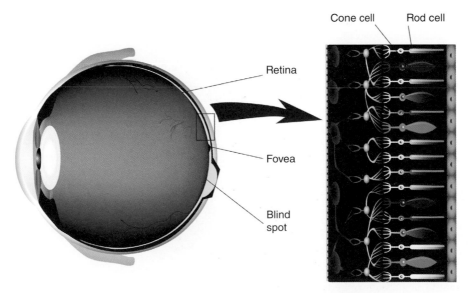

Figure 13.3   Photoreceptor cells of the retina. Courtesy of shutterstock/Zhabska Tetyana.

vision. Cones function best in bright light and are responsible for color vision and central vision. Rods are more numerous along the retina, whereas cones are most concentrated in the fovea centralis.

The Path of Light

Light rays pass through the cornea where they are refracted, or bent, so that they focus toward the receptor cells along the retina. After passing through the cornea, the light rays pass through the pupil. The muscular structure around the pupil, called the iris, dilates and constricts to control how much light can pass through the pupil. From the pupil, the light rays hit the lens of the eye where they are refracted once again (Figure 13.4).

As light passes through the lens, a group of muscles reshapes the lens based on the distance between the animal and the object on which it is focusing. The adjustment in lens shape is referred to as accommodation. The muscles are controlled by the ciliary body of the eye.

The anterior chamber is the section of the eye between the cornea and the iris. The posterior chamber is caudal to the iris and cranial to the lens. Within these two chambers is a thin, watery fluid called aqueous humor which is produced by the ciliary body. The aqueous humor helps to maintain the shape of the anterior eye and helps to nourish the structures of the anterior eye.

From the anterior chamber, light rays hit the receptor cells along the retina. At this point, the light is now in the vitreous chamber of the eye. Within the vitreous chamber is a jelly-like fluid called vitreous humor which helps to maintain the shape of the eyeball.

After light rays activate the photoreceptor cells of the retina, they convert this stimulus into a nervous impulse which is carried to the brain via the optic nerve. The area in which the optic nerve attaches to the retina is called the optic disc. The optic disc does not have rods or cones so it's commonly called the "blind spot" of the eye.

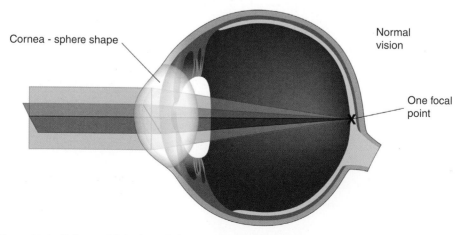

Figure 13.4   Pathway of light through the eye. Courtesy of shutterstock/Alila Medical Images.

Ophthalmology Terms

Accommodation	Adjustment of the eye from various distances.
Acuity	Sharpness or clearness of vision.
Anterior chamber	Portion of the eye between the cornea and iris; contains aqueous humor.
Aqueous humor	Thin, watery fluid produced by the ciliary body and located within the anterior chamber of the eye. Used the nourish the lens and maintain ocular pressure.
Canthus	The corner of the eye
Choroid	Middle, vascular layer of the eye located between the sclera and retina.
Ciliary body	Portion of the eye that connects the choroid to the iris. Contains ciliary muscles which control the shape of the lens.
Cones	Photoreceptor cells of the retina responsible for color and central vision.
Conjunctiva	Thin, delicate mucous membrane lining the eyelids and anterior eyeball.
Cornea	Transparent layer of tissue covering the anterior eyeball.
Fovea centralis	Depression in the macula that is concentrated with cones. This is the area of clearest vision.
Fundus of the eye	Posterior portion of the inner eyeball that can be visualized with an ophthalmoscope.
Intraocular pressure	Pressure exerted against the outer coats of the eyeball.
Iris	Muscle that dilates and constricts to control light entry to the pupil. The colored portion of the eye.
Lens	Transparent, biconvex structure behind the pupil.
Macula	Small, yellowish area above the optic disc containing the fovea centralis.
Nasolacrimal duct	Duct that runs from the lacrimal (tear) sac to the nose.
Nictitating membrane	Third eyelid; piece of conjunctiva reinforced by cartilage that protects the eye (Figure 13.5).
Optic disc	Portion in the posterior eyeball where the retina and optic nerve meet. Commonly called the blind spot.
Optic nerve	Cranial nerve that carries nervous impulses from the eye to the brain.
Orbit	Bony cavity of the skull containing the eyeball.
Palpebra	Eyelid.
Pupil	Dark opening of the eye through which light passes.
Refraction	The bending of light rays.
Retina	Light-sensitive innermost layer of the eyeball that contains rods and cones.

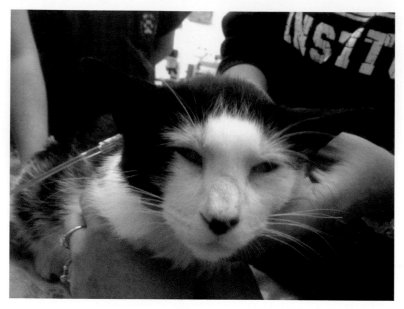

Figure 13.5   Pronounced nictitating membranes in a cat with feline infectious peritonitis (FIP). Courtesy of Amy Johnson, BS, CVT, RLATG.

Rods	Photoreceptor cells of the retina responsible for night and peripheral vision.
Sclera	The tough, white, outer coat of the eyeball.
Tapetum lucidum	Iridescent layer of epithelium that gives the eye the property of shining in the dark; helps to improve night vision (Figure 13.7).
Uvea	Vascular layer of the eye made up of the iris, choroid, and ciliary body.
Vitreous chamber	Posterior chamber of the eyeball containing vitreous humor.
Vitreous humor	Clear, jelly-like fluid in the vitreous chamber that gives the eyeball its shape.

Pathology and Procedures

Anophthalmos	Congenital anomaly in which the animal lacks one or both eyes. Most commonly seen in pigs and sheep.
Blindness	Inability to see.
Cataract	Clouding of the lens leading to decreased vision. Commonly seen in older dogs (Figure 13.6).
Chalazion	Granuloma of the eyelid due to obstructed sebaceous gland.

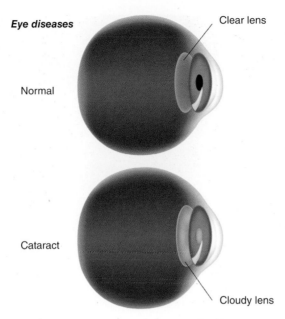

Figure 13.6A   Illustration of a cataract. Courtesy of shutterstock/Alila Sao Mai.

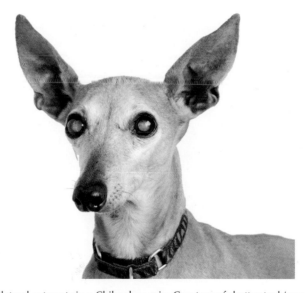

Figure 13.6B   Bilateral cataracts in a Chihuahua mix. Courtesy of shutterstock/marekuliasz.

Corneal ulcer	Erosion of the corneal epithelium.
Distichiasis	Double row of eyelashes causing irritation to the conjunctiva.
Ectropion	Turning outward of the eyelid.
Entropion	Turning inward of the eyelid (Figure 13.7).

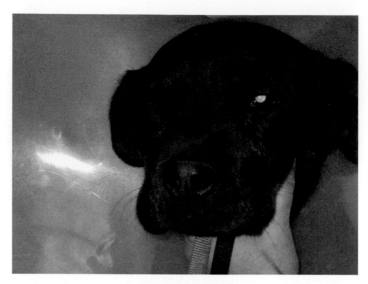

Figure 13.7   Black Lab puppy with entropion. Note the green glow of the left eye from the tapetum lucidum. Courtesy of AK Traylor, DVM; Microscopy Learning Systems.

Enucleation   Removal of the eyeball (Figure 13.8).

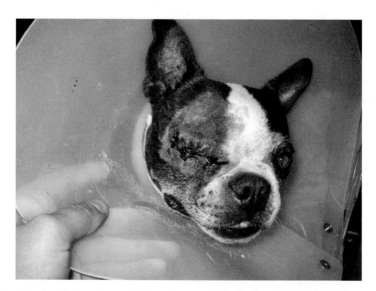

Figure 13.8   Enucleation in a Boston Terrier. Courtesy of AK Traylor, DVM; Microscopy Learning Systems.

Epiphora   Overflow of tears due to an obstructed lacrimal
                                   (tear) duct.
Esotropia   Crosseyed. Commonly seen in Siamese cats
                                   (Figure 13.9).

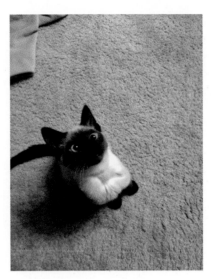

Figure 13.9   Esotropia in a Siamese kitten. Courtesy of Amy Johnson, BS, CVT, RLATG.

Exophthalmos	Forward protrusion of the eyeballs. Brachycephalic breeds normally have exophthalmos, but it can also be a symptom of various conditions.
Exotropia	Deviation of one eye outward.
Floaters	Particles in the vitreous fluid that cast shadows on the retina. Also called **vitreous floaters**. Can lead to a behavior called "fly biting."
Fluorescein stain	Dye used to stain the cornea to help visualize injury.
Follicular ophthalmitis	Hypertrophy and prolapse of the nictitating membrane. Commonly called "**cherry eye**" (Figure 13.10).

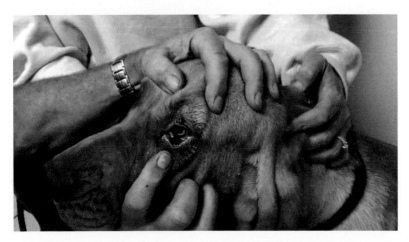

Figure 13.10   Cherry eye in a bloodhound. Courtesy of Greg Martinez, DVM; www.youtube.com/drgregdvm.

Glaucoma | Increased intraocular pressure resulting in damage to the eye (Figure 13.11).
Goniotomy | Incision into the anterior chamber to treat glaucoma.
Hordeolum | Inflammation of the sebaceous glands in the eyelid.

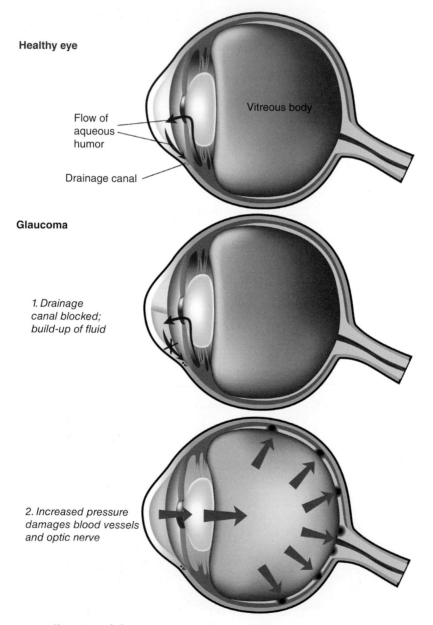

Healthy eye

Flow of aqueous humor

Vitreous body

Drainage canal

Glaucoma

1. Drainage canal blocked; build-up of fluid

2. Increased pressure damages blood vessels and optic nerve

Figure 13.11   Illustration of glaucoma compared to a normal eye. Courtesy of shutterstock/Alila Sao Mai.

(A)

(B)

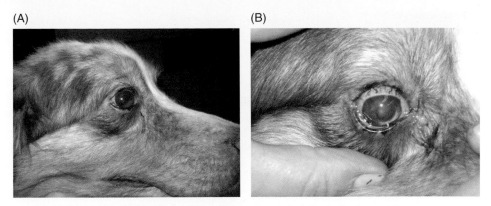

Figure 13.12A,B   Australian Shepherd with glaucoma. Note the scleral injection (red eyes) and aqueous flare. Courtesy of AK Traylor, DVM; Microscopy Learning Systems.

Hypertropia	Condition in which one eye deviates upward.
Hypopyon	Pus in the anterior chamber of the eye.
Hypotropia	Condition in which one eye deviates downward.
Macrophthalmia	Abnormal enlargement of the eye.
Macular degeneration	Degeneration of the macula causing loss of central vision.
Microphthalmia	Abnormally small eyes.
Miosis	Abnormal contraction of the pupils.
Mydriasis	Abnormal dilation of the pupils.
Nuclear sclerosis	Drying out of the lens with age.
Nyctalopia	Night blindness.
Nystagmus	Rhythmic, rapid, back and forth movement of the eyes.
Ocular dermoid	Mass in the eye containing elements found in skin tissue such as epithelial cells and hair. Typically found in the corner of the eye around the conjunctiva, eyelid, or cornea (Figure 13.13).

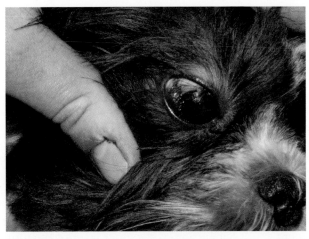

Figure 13.13   Ocular (conjunctival) dermoid in a Shih Tzu. Courtesy of AK Traylor, DVM; Microscopy Learning Systems.

Palpebral reflex	Blink reflex when the eyelids are touched.
Papilledema	Swelling of the optic disc due to intracranial pressure.
Photophobia	Sensitivity or visual intolerance to light.
Proptosis	Forward displacement of the eye from its orbit (socket).

(A)   (B)

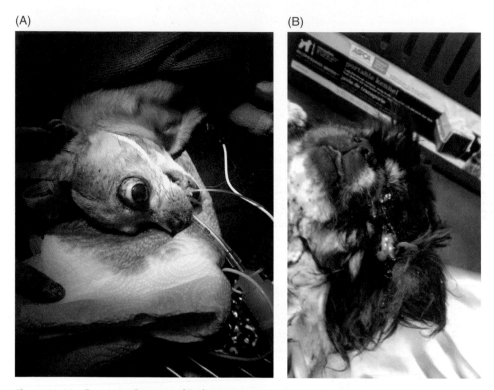

Figure 13.14   Proptosis. Courtesy of Beth Romano, AAS, CVT. (A) Chihuahua. (B) Shih-tzu.

TECH TIP 13.1 Proptosis vs. Exophthalmos

The definitions of proptosis and exophthalmos are very similar, but the difference is in the placement. In exophthalmos, the eyes are still intact in the skull. In proptosis, the eyes have "popped out" of the head. Proptosis is often seen in brachycephalic breeds that normally have exophthalmos. Causes include trauma or excessive restraint.

Pupillary light reflex (PLR)	Constriction of the pupils in response to light and dilation of the pupils when the light is removed.
Retinal detachment	Separation of the inner layer of the retina from the other layers of the eyeball (Figure 13.15).

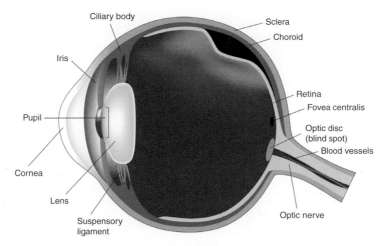

Figure 13.15   Illustration of retinal detachment. Courtesy of shutterstock/Alila Sao Mai.

Schirmer tear test	Test to measure secretions from the lacrimal (tear) duct. A strip of filter paper is placed just inside the conjunctiva of the lower eyelid for a short period of time (Figure 13.16).

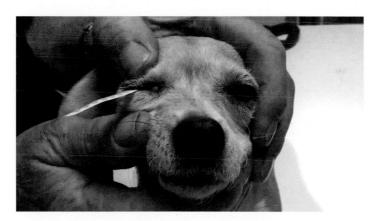

Figure 13.16   Schirmer tear test being performed on a mixed breed dog. Courtesy of Greg Martinez, DVM; www.youtube.com/drgregdvm.

Strabismus	Deviation of one or both eyes. Examples include esotropia and exotropia.
Tonometer	Instrument to measure intraocular pressure (Figure 13.17).
Tonometry	Measurement of intraocular pressure (Figure 13.17).

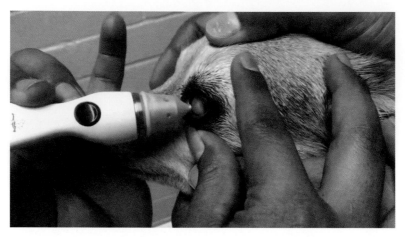

Figure 13.17   Tonometry on a Chihuahua to measure intraocular pressure. Courtesy of Greg Martinez, DVM; www.youtube.com/drgregdvm.

Building the Terms

Table 13.2   Chapter 13 Combining Forms for the Eye.

Combining Forms	Definition	Combining Forms	Definition
Ambly/o	Dim; dull	Dacry/o	Tear
Anis/o	Unequal	Dacryoaden/o	Tear gland; tear duct
Aque/o	Water	Dacryocyst/o	Tear sac; lacrimal sac
Blephar/o	Eyelid	Dipl/o	Double
Canth/o	Corner of the eye or eyelid	Electr/o	Electricity
Choroid/o	Choroid layer of the eye	Glauc/o	Gray
Conjunctiv/o	Conjunctiva	Goni/o	Seed; angle
Cor/o	Pupil	Ir/i	Iris
Core/o	Pupil	Ir/o	Iris
Corne/o	Cornea	Irid/o	Iris
Cycl/o	Ciliary body of the eye; cycle; circle	Kerat/o	Cornea; horny; hard

Table 13.2   (Continued).

Combining Forms	Definition	Combining Forms	Definition
Lacrim/o	Tear; tear duct; lacrimal duct	**Palpebr/o**	Eyelid
Mi/o	Smaller; less	**Phac/o**	Lens of the eye
Mydr/o	Wide	**Phot/o**	Light
Nas/o	Nose	**Pupill/o**	Pupil
Nyct/o	Night	**Retin/o**	Retina
Ocul/o	Eye	**Scler/o**	Sclera
Ophthalm/o	Eye	**Tars/o**	Edge of eyelid; tarsus
Opt/i	Eye; vision	**Uve/o**	Uvea
Opt/o	Eye; vision	**Vitre/o**	Glassy
Optic/o	Eye; vision	**Vitr/o**	Vitreous body

Table 13.3   Chapter 13 Prefixes for the Eye.

Prefix	Definition	Prefix	Definition
an-	no, not, without	**extra-**	outside
bi-	two	**hyper-**	increased; excessive; above
bini-	double	**hypo-**	deficient; below; under; less than normal
ec-	out; outside	**intra-**	within; into
en-	in; within	**micro-**	small
epi-	above; upon; on	**mono-**	one
eso-	inward	**pan-**	all
exo-	out; away from	**peri-**	surrounding; around

Table 13.4   Chapter 13 Suffixes for the Eye.

Suffix	Definition	Suffix	Definition
-al, -ar, -ic	pertaining to	**-pathy**	disease condition
-ation	process; condition	**-phobia**	fear
-centesis	surgical puncture to remove fluid	**-plegia**	paralysis; palsy
-graphy	process of recording	**-ptosis**	drooping; sagging; prolapse
-ia	condition	**-rrhaphy**	suture
-iasis	abnormal condition	**-scope**	instrument for visual examination
-ist	specialist	**-scopy**	visual examination
-itis	inflammation	**-spasm**	sudden, involuntary contraction of muscles
-logy	study of	**-tomy**	incision; process of cutting into
-metry	measurement	**-tropia**	to turn
-opia	vision		

Now it's time to put these word parts together. If you memorize the meaning of the combining forms, prefixes, and suffixes, then this will get easier each time. Remember your five basic rules to medical terminology when building and defining these terms. You'll notice some word parts are repeated from the previous chapters.

Parts		Medical Term	Definition
Ambly/o	+ -opia	= Amblyopia	: _____
Blephar/o	+ -ectomy	= Blepharectomy	: _____
Blephar/o	+ -itis	= Blepharitis	: _____
Blephar/o	+ -plasty	= Blepharoplasty	: _____
Blephar/o	+ -ptosis	= Blepharoptosis	: _____
Blephar/o	+ -rrhaphy	= Blepharorrhaphy	: _____
Blephar/o	+ -spasm	= Blepharospasm	: _____
Blephar/o	+ -tomy	= Blepharotomy	: _____
Canth/o	+ -ectomy	= Canthectomy	: _____
Canth/o	+ -tomy	= Canthotomy	: _____
Conjunctiv/o	+ -al	= Conjunctival	: _____
Conjunctiv/o	+ -itis	= Conjunctivitis	: _____
Conjunctiv/o	+ -plasty	= Conjunctivoplasty	: _____

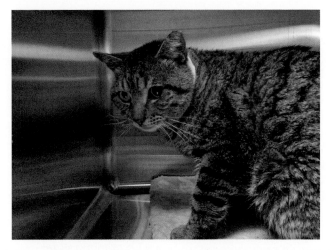

Figure 13.18   Anisocoria in a Domestic Shorthair cat. Courtesy of Amy Johnson, BS, CVT, RLATG.

aniso-	+ Core/o	+ -ia	=	Anisocoria	: _____
Corne/o	+ -al		=	Corneal	: _____
Corne/o	+ Scler/o	+ -al	=	Corneoscleral	: _____
Dacryoaden/o	+ -itis		=	Dacryoadenitis	: _____
Dacryocyst/o	+ -ectomy		=	Dacryocystectomy	: _____
Dacryocyst/o	+ -itis		=	Dacryocystitis	: _____
Dacryocyst/o	+ -tomy		=	Dacryocystotomy	: _____
Irid/o	+ -ectomy		=	Iridectomy	: _____
Irid/o	+ -ic		–	Iridic	: _____
Ir/o	+ -itis		=	Iritis	: _____
Kerat/o	+ -ectomy		=	Keratectomy	: _____
Kerat/o	+ -itis		=	Keratitis	: _____
Kerat/o	+ -centesis		=	Keratocentesis	: _____
Kerat/o	+ Conjunctiv/o	+ -itis	=	Keratoconjunctivitis	: _____

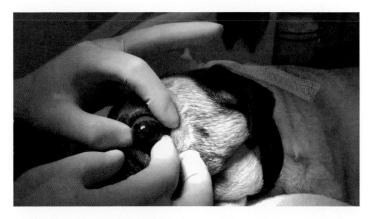

Figure 13.19   Keratoconjunctivitis in a Pug about to have an enucleation. Courtesy of Greg Martinez, DVM; www.youtube.com/drgregdvm.

Kerat/o	+ -plasty		=	Keratoplasty	: _____
Kerat/o	+ -tomy		=	Keratotomy	: _____
Lacrim/o	+ -al		=	Lacrimal	: _____
Lacrim/o	+ -ation		=	Lacrimation	: _____
Nas/o	+ Lacrim/o	+ -al	=	Nasolacrimal	: _____
Lens/o	+ -ectomy		=	Lensectomy	: _____
Ocul/o	+ -ar		=	Ocular	: _____
bini-	+ Ocul/o	+ -ar	=	Binocular	: _____
extra-	+ Ocul/o	+ -ar	=	Extraocular	: _____
intra-	+ Ocul/o	+ -ar	=	Intraocular	: _____
peri-	+ Ocul/o	+ -ar	=	Periocular	: _____
Ophthalm/o	+ -ic		=	Ophthalmic	: _____
Ophthalm/o	+ -logy	+ -ist	=	Ophthalmologist	: _____
Ophthalm/o	+ -plegia		=	Ophthalmoplegia	: _____
Ophthalm/o	+ -scope		=	Ophthalmoscope	: _____
Ophthalm/o	+ -scopy		=	Ophthalmoscopy	: _____
pan-	+ Ophthalm/o + -itis		=	Panophthalmitis	: _____
Opt/o	+ -ic		=	Optic	: _____
Palpebr/o	+ -al		=	Palpebral	: _____
Pupill/o	+ -ary		=	Pupillary	: _____
Electr/o	+ Retin/o	+ -graphy	=	Electroretinography	: _____
Retin/o	+ -itis		=	Retinitis	: _____
Retin/o	+ -pathy		=	Retinopathy	: _____
Scler/o	+ -itis		=	Scleritis	: _____

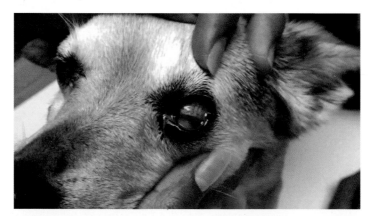

Figure 13.20   Scleritis in a Chihuahua. Courtesy of Greg Martinez, DVM; www.youtube.com/drgregdvm.

Tars/o	+ -ectomy	=	Tarsectomy	: _____
Tars/o	+ rrhaphy	=	Tarsorrhaphy	: _____
Uve/o	+ itis	=	Uveitis	: _____

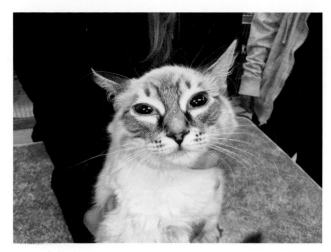

Figure 13.21   Uremic uveitis in a cat. Courtesy of Amy Johnson, BS, CVT, RLATG.

The Ear

Using Table 13.5, label the parts of the ear on Figure 13.22.

Table 13.5   Anatomy of the Ear.

Auricle (1)	Flap of the ear; also known as the pinna.
Auditory canal (2)	Tube from the auricle to the eardrum. Also called the external auditory canal or external auditory meatus. A **meatus** is a passage. Glands along this tube secrete **cerumen**, or ear wax.
Tympanic membrane (3)	Eardrum; membrane between the outer and middle ear.
Malleus (4)	First ossicle of the middle ear. Malleus means hammer.
Incus (5)	Second ossicle of the middle ear. Incus means anvil.
Stapes (6)	Third ossicle of the middle ear. Stapes means stirrup.
Oval window (7)	Membrane between the middle and inner ear.
Eustachian tube (8)	Channel that connects the middle ear to the pharynx.
Cochlea (9)	Spiral, snail-shaped tube filled with fluid that is essential for hearing.
Vestibule (10)	Oval cavity connecting the cochlea to the semicircular canals.
Semicircular canals (11)	Passages containing fluid and sensitive hairs. Their function is to maintain balance during movement.

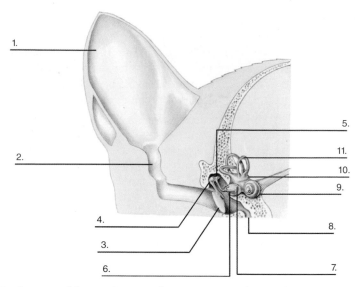

Figure 13.22   Anatomy of the ear. Courtesy of Getty Images/Dorling Kindersley.

The ear is most often associated with hearing, but it also is used to help maintain balance. There are three sections of the ear: the outer ear, middle ear, and inner ear. When sound is produced, the sound waves travel through all three sections and then are converted to nervous impulses that travel to the brain.

The Outer Ear

The ear flap, or auricle, is the first structure to pick up a sound wave. That sound wave then travels from the auricle through the auditory canal where it hits the tympanic membrane, or eardrum. Along the external auditory canal are sebaceous glands that produce a waxy substance called cerumen, or ear wax, which helps protect and lubricate the canal. Cerumen acts as an insect repellent and can protect the ear from water.

The Middle Ear

When a sound wave hits the tympanic membrane, the membrane vibrates and transmits the sound to the ossicles just behind it. Ossicles are small bones in the middle ear that vibrate to transmit the sound waves to the inner ear. The ossicles, in order of occurrence, are the malleus, incus, and stapes. They are named based on their shape. Sound waves from the ossicles travel to the oval window which is a membrane separating the middle and inner ear. Between the ossicles and oval window is an auditory tube called a Eustachian tube which maintains equilibrium. This tube opens upon deglutition to help equalize the air pressure in the middle ear to match the air pressure in the outside environment.

The Inner Ear

The inner ear is the most intricate portion of the ear. In fact, the inner ear is commonly called the labyrinth due to its maze-like anatomy. The bony labyrinth is made up of the cochlea, semicircular canals, and vestibule (Figure 13.23). From the oval window, sound waves enter a structure called the cochlea which gets its name because of its snail shape (cochlea means snail in Latin). Within the cochlea are two types of fluid called perilymph and endolymph, which transmit sound vibrations. From the two fluids, sound waves pass through the spiral-shaped portion of the cochlea called the organ of Corti, which contains sensitive hairs that transmit the sound waves to the auditory nerves. The auditory nerves convert the sound waves into nervous impulses that travel to the brain to be interpreted.

Next to the oval window is a cavity called the vestibule which connects the cochlea to the semicircular canals. Within the vestibule are specialized receptors which aid in balance. The semicircular canals are actually three tubes containing endolymph and sensory hair-like structures that aid in balance while the animal is moving. The three canals, called the anterior, lateral, and posterior canals, are located at right angles to each other. When the animal moves its head, the fluid in the canals begins to shift. This shift causes the fluid to press against the sensitive hair-like receptors. The receptors convert this response to a nervous impulse that is sent to the brain. The fluid shifting in the semicircular canals after movement is what causes dizziness and vertigo. Animals riding in the car or on an airplane can experience motion sickness due to the fluid shifts after they move their head.

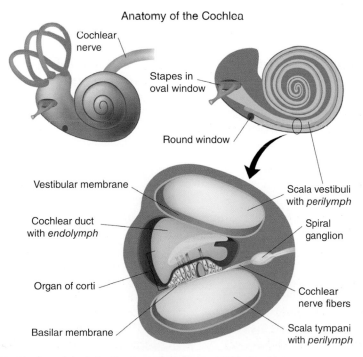

Figure 13.23   The bony labyrinth. Courtesy of shutterstock/Alila Sao Mai.

Otology Terms

Auditory canal	Tube from the auricle to the tympanic membrane (eardrum).
Auricle	Flap of the ear; also known as the **pinna**.
Cerumen	Waxy substance secreted by the sebaceous glands in the auditory canal. Commonly called **ear wax**.
Cochlea	Spiral, snail-shaped tube in the inner ear containing fluid that is essential for hearing.
Endolymph	Fluid within the inner ear.
Eustachian tube	Channel that connects the middle ear to the pharynx.
Incus	Second ossicle of the inner ear. Incus means anvil in Latin.
Labyrinth	Maze-like structure of the inner ear consisting of the vestibule, cochlea, and semicircular canals. Also known as the bony labyrinth.
Organ of Corti	Sensitive receptor area in the cochlea.
Ossicles	Small bones of the inner ear: the malleus, incus, and stapes.
Oval window	Membrane between the middle and inner ear.
Perilymph	Fluid within the inner ear.
Semicircular canals	Three tubes of the inner ear used to maintain equilibrium.
Stapes	Third ossicle of the inner ear. Stapes means stirrup in Latin.
Tympanic membrane	Eardrum; membrane between the outer and middle ear.
Vestibule	Cavity connecting the cochlea to the semicircular canals. The vestibule is associated with balance.

Pathology and Procedures

Ablation	Separation, detachment, or removal by cutting. Most often associated with removal of the external ear canal in cases of neoplasia or chronic otitis.
Aural hematoma	Mass or collection of blood in the ear flap. Also known as an **auricular hematoma** (Figure 13.24).
Deafness	Loss of hearing.

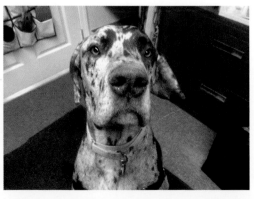

Figure 13.24　Aural hematoma in a Great Dane. Courtesy of Amy Johnson, BS, CVT, RLATG.

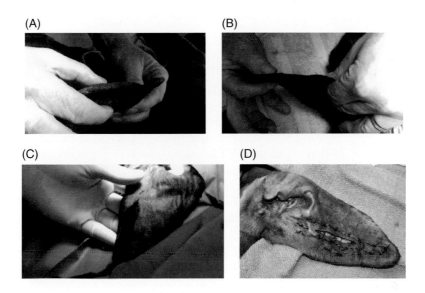

Figure 13.25   Stages of treatment for aural hematoma. Courtesy of Greg Martinez, DVM; www. youtube.com/drgregdvm. (A) Aural hematoma in a black lab. (B) The normal other ear of the black lab for comparison. (C) Draining the hematoma. (D) Surgical repair of the aural hematoma.

Ear docking	Cosmetic procedure in which a portion of the auricle is removed and the remainder is set in a brace to stand erect. In the United States, this is a common practice in breeds such as Dobermans, Great Danes, Schnauzers, and Boxers. In Great Britain, the procedure is considered inhumane (Figure 13.26).
Otitis externa	Inflammation of the external ear.
Otitis media	Inflammation of the middle ear.
Otitis interna	Inflammation of the inner ear.
Vertigo	Sense of dizziness.

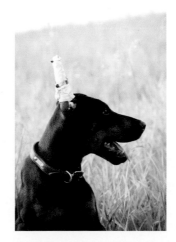

Figure 13.26   Ear docking on a Doberman. Courtesy of shutterstock/mmaxer.

Table 13.6   Chapter 13 Prefixes for the Ear.

Combining Forms	Definition	Combining Forms	Definition
Acoust/o	Hearing	**Laryng/o**	Voice box; larynx
Audi/o	Ear; hearing	**Myc/o**	Fungus
Audit/o	Hearing	**Myring/o**	Tympanic membrane; eardrum
Auricul/o	Ear	**Ot/o**	Ear
Aur/i	Ear	**Pinn/i**	External ear
Aur/o	Ear	**Py/o**	Pus
Hemat/o	Blood	**Tympan/o**	Tympanic membrane; eardrum
Labyrinth/o	Maze		

Table 13.7   Chapter 13 Prefixes for the Ear.

Prefix	Definition	Prefix	Definition
macro-	large	**pan-**	all
micro-	small	**post-**	after; behind

Table 13.8   Chapter 13 Suffixes for the Ear.

Suffix	Definition	Suffix	Definition
-al, -ar, -eal, -ic, -ory	pertaining to	**-osis**	abnormal condition
-algia	pain	**-otia**	ear condition
-ectomy	removal; excision; resection	**-pathy**	disease condition
-itis	inflammation	**-plasty**	surgical repair
-logy	study of	**-rrhea**	flow; discharge
-metry	measurement	**-scope**	instrument for visual examination
-oma	tumor; mass; collection	**-scopy**	visual examination

Building the Terms

Now it's time to put these word parts together. If you memorize the meaning of the combining forms, prefixes, and suffixes, then this will get easier each time. Remember your five basic rules to medical terminology when building and defining these terms. You'll notice some word parts are repeated from the previous chapters.

Parts		Medical Term	Definition
Audi/o + -metry	=	Audiometry	:_____
Audit/o + -ory	=	Auditory	:_____
Aur/o + -al	=	Aural	:_____
Auricul/o + -ar	=	Auricular	:_____
post- + Auricul/o + -ar	=	Postauricular	:_____
Myring/o + -ectomy	=	Myringectomy	:_____
Myring/o + -itis	=	Myringitis	:_____
macro- + -otia	=	Macrotia	:_____
micro- + -otia	=	Microtia	:_____
Ot/o + -algia	=	Otalgia	:_____
Ot/o + -ic	=	Otic	:_____
Ot/o + -itis	=	Otitis	:_____
Ot/o + Laryng/o + -logy	=	Otolaryngology	:_____
Ot/o + Myc/o + -osis	=	Oto mycosis	:_____
Ot/o + -pathy	=	Otopathy	:_____
Ot/o + Py/o + -rrhea	=	Otopyorrhea	:_____
Ot/o + -rrhea	=	Otorrhea	:_____
Ot/o + -scope	=	Otoscope	:_____
Ot/o + -scopy	=	Otoscopy	:_____
pan- + Ot/o + -itis	=	Panotitis	:_____
Tympan/o + -plasty	=	Tympanoplasty	:_____

Abbreviations

Table 13.9   Chapter 13 Abbreviations.

Abbreviation	Definition
AD	Right ear
AS	Left ear
AU	Both ears

(Continued)

Table 13.9   (*Continued*)

Abbreviation	Definition
IOP	Intraocular pressure
OD	Right eye
OS	Left eye
OU	Both eyes
PLR	Pupillary light reflex
VA	Visual acuity

Case Study

A Cocker Spaniel named Lady has come to the clinic with swelling on the flap of her ear. The owner found blood splatter on her walls when she got home from work. Lady has a PPH of chronic otitis externa and otomycosis. Using an otoscope, the veterinarian noted myringitis. Lady was diagnosed with an aural hematoma and surgery was ordered. The hematoma was drained and lady was sent home with ear cleaner and medications. Because Lady has frequent issues with her ears, the veterinarian has recommended an ear resection to prevent future ear infections. Ear infections cause chronic head shaking in dogs, which can lead to hematoma from the ruptured blood vessels in the ear flaps.

1. In which part of the ear had the hematoma formed?
   a. Pinna
   b. Eardrum
   c. Ear canal
   d. Cochlea
2. What is the veterinarian's recommendation for prevention?
   a. Remove the ear
   b. Cut the opening of the ear back
   c. Remove the ear flap
   d. Remove the ear canal
3. Which of the following describes Lady's PPH?
   a. External ear infection
   b. Internal ear infection
   c. Middle ear infection
   d. None of the above

Exercises

13-A: Give the term for the following definitions of structures.

1. _____: Colored portion of the eye
2. _____: Eardrum
3. _____: Ear wax
4. _____: White of the eye
5. _____: Blind spot of the eye
6. _____: Dark opening of the eye
7. _____: Vascular layer of the eye containing the iris
8. _____: The corner of the eye
9. _____: Ear flap; pinna
10. _____: Small bones of the inner ear
11. _____: Third eyelid.
12. _____: Innermost layer of the eyeball.

13-B: Define the following terms.

1. Tympanoplasty _____
2. Blepharoptosis _____
3. Conjunctivits _____
4. Postauricular _____
5. Keratitis _____
6. Lacrimation _____
7. Otorrhea _____
8. Ophthalmology _____
9. Otoscope _____
10. Macrotia _____

13-C: Circle the correct term in parentheses:

1. Clouding of the lens. (cataract, glaucoma, chalazion)
2. Forward displacement of the eye. (anophthalmos, exophthalmos, proptosis)
3. Rapid, back and forth movements of the eyes. (ectropion, hypertropia, nystagmus)
4. Snail-shaped structure of the inner ear. (cochlea, incus, stapes)
5. Removal of the eyeball. (anophthalmos, enucleation, proptosis)
6. Jelly-like substance in the posterior eye chamber. (aqueous humor, floaters, vitreous humor)
7. Abnormal dilation of the pupils. (miosis, mydriasis, nyctalopia)
8. Iridescent layer of the retina. (conjunctiva, nictitating membrane, tapetum lucidum)
9. Crosseyed. (ectropion, entropion, esotropia)
10. Sensitivity to light. (photophobia, strabismus, tonometry)

13-D: Define the following abbreviations.

1. _____: OD
2. _____: AU
3. _____: IOP
4. _____: OU
5. _____: AD
6. _____: PLR
7. _____: OS
8. _____: AS

13-E: Match the following with their descriptions.

1. _____ Drying out of the lens   A.   Ablation
   with age.

2. _____ Inflammation of the   B.   Eustachian tube
   sebaceous glands in the eyelid.

3. _____ Channel that connects the   C.   Hordeolum
   middle ear to the pharynx.

4. _____ Separation, detachment,   D.   Nuclear sclerosis
   or removal by cutting.

5. _____ Swelling of the optic disc   E.   Papilledema
   due to intracranial pressure.

Answers can be found starting on page 571.

Go to www.wiley.com/go/taibo/terminology to find additional learning materials for this chapter:

* A crossword puzzle
* Flashcards
* Audio clips to show how to pronounce terms
* Case studies
* Review questions
* The figures from the chapter in PowerPoint

The Urinary System

The urinary system is made up of the kidneys, ureters, urinary bladder, and urethra (Figure 14.1). All four organs work together to eliminate waste products from the body; however, the kidney has additional and more specialized functions.

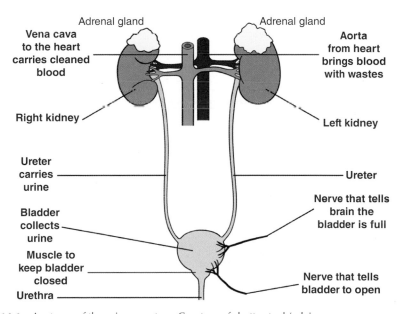

Figure 14.1   Anatomy of the urinary system. Courtesy of shutterstock/udaix.

Veterinary Medical Terminology Guide and Workbook, First Edition. Angela Taibo.
© 2014 John Wiley & Sons, Inc. Published 2014 by John Wiley & Sons, Inc.
Companion website: www.wiley.com/go/taibo/terminology

Anatomy of the Urinary System

The urinary system begins with the kidneys which are located retroperitonealy on either side of the lumbar spine. Generally the right kidney lies slightly more cranial than the left kidney. It may help to remember that "right is tight." The kidney is divided into three sections: the renal cortex (outer section), renal medulla (inner section), and renal pelvis (central section).

Once urine has been produced by the kidneys, it travels to the urinary bladder via the ureters, a pair of tubes that carry urine from the kidneys to the urinary bladder by peristalsis. The point at which the ureters enter the urinary bladder is called the trigone, which translates to triangle in Greek. The function of the urinary bladder is to temporarily store urine.

From the urinary bladder, urine travels through the urethra to the outside of the body. The function of the urethra varies depending on the sex of the animal. In females, the urethra carries urine from the urinary bladder to the outside of the body. In males, the urethra carries both urine and semen to the outside of the body. The external opening of the urethra in both sexes is called the urinary meatus. When the animal excretes urine to the outside of the body, it is termed urination or micturition.

The Kidney

The kidney is made up of three basic sections: the cortex, the medulla, and the renal pelvis (Figure 14.2). The indentation in the center of the kidney is referred to as the hilus. There are three steps of urine formation: filtration, reabsorption, and excretion. These steps take place in the functional unit of the kidney called the nephron. The number of nephrons varies in each kidney depending on the species (Figure 14.3).

TECH TIP 14.1 **How Many Nephrons Are in the Kidney?**

The number of nephrons in the kidney varies depending on the species. Cats have roughly 200,000 nephrons in each kidney. Dogs have approximately 400,000 nephrons in each kidney.

Filtration

Renal circulation begins at the aorta, where the blood then travels to the renal arteries (Figure 14.3). From there the blood continues to the renal arterioles, which enter the renal cortex. The renal arterioles become a collection of capillaries called a glomerulus (Figure 14.4). The number of glomeruli varies depending on the species. Cats have approximately 200,000 glomeruli, whereas dogs have roughly 400,000 glomeruli. Filtration of substances occurs from the glomerulus to Bowman's capsule, a cup-shaped capsule that encloses each glomerulus. Substances

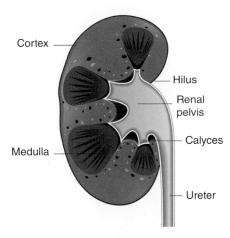

Figure 14.2A   Anatomy of the kidney. Courtesy of shutterstock/Maxi_m.

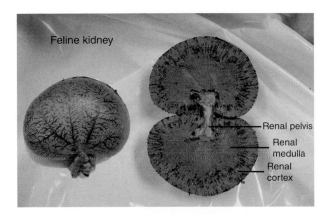

Figure 14.2B   Feline kidney from a dissected cat. The kidney was injected with a blue latex dye to designate venous flow. The vessels on the surface of the kidney are sometimes referred to as "arbor vitae," which translates to "tree of life" in Latin. The branching of the vessels looks similar to the branches of a tree.

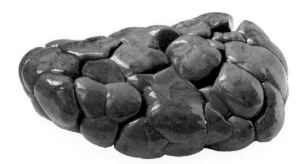

Figure 14.2C   Bovine kidney. Courtesy of shutterstock/llepet.

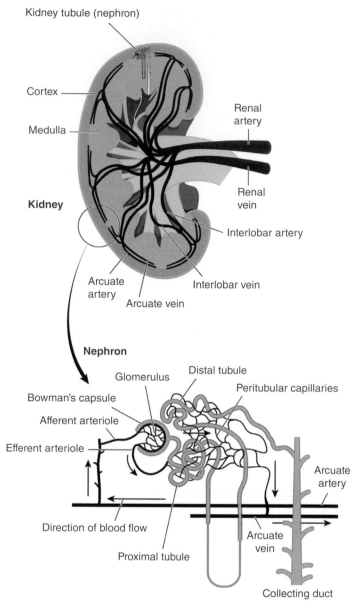

Figure 14.3   The kidney and nephron in relation. Courtesy of shutterstock/blamb.

that are filtered into the nephron are termed freely filtered substances. These substances follow the laws of diffusion in that they move from a high concentration to a low concentration. Examples of freely filtered substances include water, electrolytes, nitrogenous wastes, and glucose.

Filtration depends on blood pressure, the size of the molecules, and the actual amount of blood that reaches the glomerulus. If an animal has hypotension (decreased blood pressure), then the degree of filtration is decreased. When this

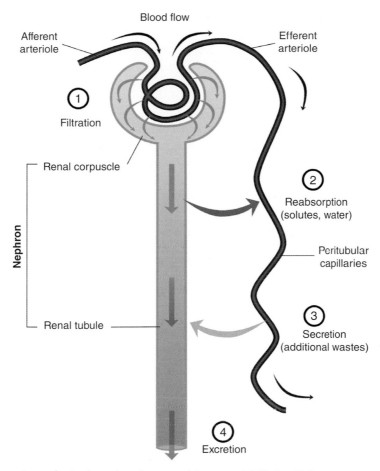

Figure 14.4   Steps of urine formation. Courtesy of shutterstock/Alila Sao Mai.

occurs, the kidneys secrete an enzyme called renin to increase the blood pressure. If an animal goes into shock, then the blood pools in the capillaries to increase their blood volume. As a result, decreased amounts of blood reach the glomerulus and the degree of filtration is decreased.

Reabsorption

Substances in Bowman's capsule then move to the renal tubules where they are either reabsorbed back into the bloodstream or carried further in the nephron to become urine. Reabsorption is controlled by hormones in the body such as antidiuretic hormone (ADH) and aldosterone. ADH is responsible for the reabsorption of water from the renal tubules to the bloodstream. Aldosterone controls the reabsorption of sodium and excretion of potassium. Reabsorption is affected if these hormone levels change. For example, an animal with diabetes insipidus (DI) lacks the hormone ADH which means its kidneys can't reabsorb water. The water in the kidneys is all excreted in the urine; thus, the animal feels dehydrated.

Feeling dehydrated causes the animal to drink more water, which in turn causes it to urinate more frequently.

Certain substances that were filtered into the nephron are reabsorbed back into the bloodstream because the concentration of those substances is lower in the blood than in the kidney. Again, this follows the laws of diffusion. For example, all glucose that was filtered into the nephron should be reabsorbed by the renal tubules back into the bloodstream because the blood glucose of the animal is less than the concentration of the glucose in the kidneys. If an animal has hyperglycemia, such as a dog with diabetes mellitus, then the glucose in the renal tubules will not be reabsorbed back into the blood. Instead, it will be excreted in the urine, causing glucosuria.

After reabsorption occurs, waste products in the blood such as drugs are secreted into the renal tubules where they will join with the remaining glomerular filtrate to form urine. The renal tubules lead to two collecting tubules that carry urine to the renal pelvis. The renal pelvis is the central collecting region in the kidney. Within the renal pelvis are cup-like spaces called calyces which temporarily collect and store the urine before it moves to the ureters.

Storage and Excretion

Urine travels to the urinary bladder via the ureters. Once in the urinary bladder, the urine is temporarily stored until the sphincters relax to allow for the passage of urine into the urethra. Sphincters are groups of ring-like muscles that can contract in diameter. When an animal urinates, it voluntarily relaxes its sphincters to allow for the excretion of urine. The urine then travels through the urethra to the outside of the body.

Related Terms

Antidiuretic hormone	Hormone produced in the pituitary gland to control the reabsorption of water by the renal tubules.
Aldosterone	Hormone produced by the adrenals to control sodium reabsorption and potassium excretion.
Bowman's capsule	Cup-like capsule enclosing each glomerulus.
Capillaries	Smallest blood vessels.
Creatinine	Non-protein nitrogenous waste produced by muscle cell metabolism.
Electrolytes	Chemical substance that carries an electrical charge.
Erythropoietin (EPO)	Hormone produced by the kidney to stimulate the production of red blood cells in the bone marrow.
Filtration	Passage of substances from the glomerulus to Bowman's capsule.
Glomerulus	Collection of capillaries in the renal cortex where filtration takes place.

Kidney	Pair of retroperitoneal bean-shaped organs where urine is formed.
Nephron	The functional unit of the kidney.
Nitrogen	Electrolyte component of protein and amino acids.
Nitrogenous wastes	Waste product of protein metabolism; excreted in urine.
Potassium	Electrolyte secreted from the bloodstream to the renal tubules and then excreted in the urine.
Reabsorption	Substances return to the bloodstream from the renal tubules.
Renal cortex	Outer section of the kidney.
Renal medulla	Inner section of the kidney.
Renal pelvis	Central collecting region of the kidney.
Renal tubules	Small tubes in the kidney where reabsorption takes place.
Renin	Proteolytic enzyme produced by the kidney to regulate blood pressure.
Sodium	Electrolyte in the blood and urine; regulated by the kidneys.
Urea (BUN)	Non-protein nitrogenous waste that results from protein breakdown. When the body breaks down protein, it is converted to ammonia. Ammonia is then sent to the liver to be converted to urea which is then excreted in the urine.
Ureter	Tube that carries urine from the kidneys to the urinary bladder.
Urethra	Tube that carries urine from the urinary bladder to the outside of the body.
Uric acid	Metabolic byproduct produced by the liver; excreted in the urine.

TECH TIP 14.2 Dalmatians and Uric Acid

Uric acid is a byproduct produced by the liver, filtered into the kidneys, and then reabsorbed into the bloodstream. In Dalmatians, this is not the case. Dalmatians have an increased excretion of uric acid in their urine; therefore, uric acid crystals are a common and normal finding in Dalmatians. In most other breeds, it's an indication of liver disease or portosystemic shunt.

Urinary bladder	Sac that temporarily stores urine.
Urinary catheterization	Catheter placed in the urethra to the urinary bladder to obtain a urine sample or relieve a urinary obstruction (Figure 14.5).

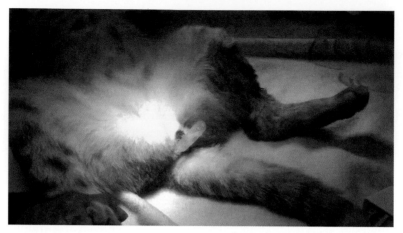

Figure 14.5   Urinary catheter in a male cat to relieve a urinary obstruction. Courtesy of Greg Martinez, DVM; www.youtube.com/drgregdvm.

Urine	Water and waste products produced by the kidneys and stored in the urinary bladder.
Voiding	Emptying or urine from the urinary bladder. Also called micturition or urination.

Pathology and Procedures

Azotemia	Increase in non-protein nitrogenous wastes in the blood. Also called **Uremia**.
Calculus (plural: calculi)	Another name for a stone. Calculus is most often used to describe the small sedimentary particles in urine (Figure 14.6).

TECH TIP 14.3 **What is a Stone?**

Urinary stones are formed from high concentrations of minerals and crystals in the urinary tract.

Stone formation can be caused by the following:

Adequate pH: Some stones require acidic or alkaline urine to form. Urinary pH can be altered by changing the animal's diet.

Increased urine concentration: Urine concentration can be altered by giving the animal more access to water and by changing its diet. Foods advertised as low ash have low mineral content. Canned food has a higher water concentration than dry food.

Adequate time in the urinary tract: Animals have an increased likelihood of stone formation if they have to hold their bladders for an extended period of time.

A nidus: A nidus is something upon which a stone can form. Examples include crystals, suture material, polyps, and bacteria.

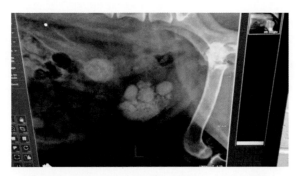

Figure 14.6A Radiograph from a dog with urinary stones. Courtesy of Greg Martinez, DVM; www.youtube.com/drgregdvm.

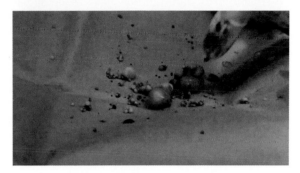

Figure 14.6B Stones that have been removed from the dog in Figure 14.6A.

| Dialysis | Separation of waste products from the bloodstream. |

TECH TIP 14.4 Do Animals Receive Dialysis or Kidney Transplants?

Renal failure creates a build-up of waste products in the blood due to a lack of glomerular filtration. Humans in renal failure receive dialysis from a machine called a hemodialyser. The machine removes the patient's blood, separates and removes the waste products, and then gives the "clean" blood back to the patient.

In animals, hemodialysers are far too expensive for most owners and clinics. Instead, the most common practice is to administer subcutaneous (SQ) fluids to the animal to increase the filtration of waste products across the glomerulus. Animals may be required to receive SQ fluids weekly or bi-weekly depending on the severity of the renal failure.

In intensive care units (ICUs), a common treatment for acute renal failure patients is the administration of continuous abdominal peritoneal dialysis (CAPD).

Kidney transplantation has been performed at various teaching hospitals in the United States.

| Diuresis | Increased excretion of urine. |
| Enuresis | Inability to control excretion; also called **incontinence**. |

| Feline lower urinary tract disease (FLUTD) | Disease with a collection of symptoms including cystitis, urethritis, hematuria, dysuria, and crystalluria. Also known as **feline urological syndrome (FUS)**. |

TECH TIP 14.5 FLUTD vs. FUS

FLUTD is considered the new name for FUS; however, many veterinarians still draw a difference between these two names. In fact, after speaking with five different veterinarians regarding these conditions, I received five different answers.

Some veterinarians see FLUTD as a disease most commonly caused by stress. Male cats begin displaying behavioral issues such as inappropriate urination. When a urinalysis is performed, blood cells are increased, but bacteria are not necessarily present. In essence, the cat has a sterile cystitis, also called feline idiopathic cystitis (FIC). These cats are at risk for urinary stone formation if left untreated. The cause of the stress should be identified and the cats placed on anti-inflammatories. In some cases, the cats may even be placed on anti-anxiety medications such as Prozac®.

These same veterinarians associate FUS with stone formation in cats. The stone formation in this disease is often associated with increased urine concentration or urinary pH changes. These cases are treated similar to other species in that diet is used to change pH or to change mineral content.

| Free catch | Also known as a voided sample, this is the collection of urine into an open container. |
| Perineal urethrostomy | New opening in the area between the anus and scrotum to correct FUS (Figure 14.7). |

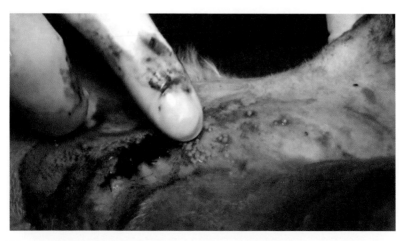

Figure 14.7   Urethrostomy in a dog. Note the stones that have been flushed out once the opening has been made. Courtesy of Greg Martinez, DVM; www.youtube.com/drgregdvm.

TECH TIP 14.6 **Polyuria vs. Pollakiuria**

Pollakiuria is an increase in the frequency of urination. The animal wants to go outside or to the litter box often. Common causes include stress and pregnancy.

Polyuria is an increase in the volume or quantity of urine being excreted. This term is often used with physical conditions such as diabetes mellitus or renal failure.

Pollakiuria	Frequent urination.
Polycystic kidney	Fluid-filled sacs within or upon the kidney; the most common congenital renal defect (Figure 14.8).

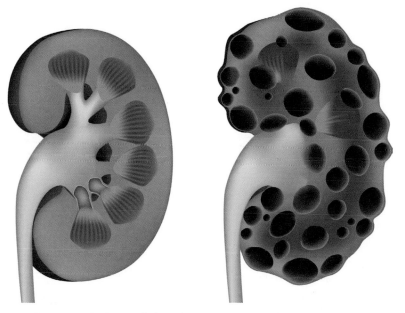

Figure 14.8   Illustration of polycystic kidney disease. Courtesy of shutterstock/Alila Medical Images.

Renal colic	Pain caused by stones in the kidney.
Renal ischemia	Lack of blood flow to the kidneys.
Stranguria	Straining to urinate; slow or painful urination.
Urinalysis (U/A)	Separation of urine into its components.
Urethral stricture	Tightening or narrowing of the urethra.
Urinary retention	Inability to completely empty the bladder.

Building the Terms

Table 14.1   Chapter 14 Combining Forms.

Combining Forms	Definition	Combining Forms	Definition
Albumin/o	Albumin	Ile/o	Ileum
Azot/o	Nitrogen	Ket/o	Ketones; ketone bodies
Bacteri/o	Bacteria	Keton/o	Ketones; ketone bodies
Crystall/o	Crystals	Lith/o	Stone
Cyst/o	Urinary bladder; cyst	Nephr/o	Kidney
Dips/o	Thirst	Olig/o	Scanty
Erythr/o	Red	Protein/o	Protein
Glomerul/o	Glomerulus	Py/o	Pus
Gluc/o	Glucose; sugar	Pyel/o	Renal pelvis
Glyc/o	Glucose; sugar	Ren/o	Kidney
Glucos/o	Glucose; sugar	Ur/o	Urine; urinary tract
Glycos/o	Glucose; sugar	Ureter/o	Ureter
Hemat/o	Blood	Urethr/o	Urethra
Hydr/o	Fluid; water	Urin/o	Urine

Table 14.2   Chapter 14 Prefixes.

Prefix	Definition	Prefix	Definition
an-	no, not, without	dys-	bad; painful; difficult; abnormal
anti-	against	para-	near; beside; abnormal; apart from; along the side of
di-	twice	poly-	many; much

Table 14.3   Chapter 14 Suffixes.

Suffix	Definition	Suffix	Definition
-ar, -ic	pertaining to	**-pathy**	disease condition
-centesis	surgical puncture to remove fluid	**-pexy**	surgical fixation; to put in place
-ectomy	removal; excision; resection	**-plasty**	surgical repair
-emia	blood condition	**-poiesis**	formation
-etic	pertaining to; pertaining to a condition	**-poietin**	substance that forms
-gram	record	**-ptosis**	drooping; sagging; prolapse
-ia	condition	**-sclerosis**	hardening
-iasis	abnormal condition	**-scopy**	visual examination
-itis	inflammation	**-stomy**	new opening
-lithiasis	abnormal condition of stones	**-tomy**	incision; process of cutting
-malacia	softening	**-tripsy**	to crush
-osis	abnormal condition	**-uria**	urination; condition of urine

Now it's time to put these word parts together. If you memorize the meaning of the combining forms, prefixes, and suffixes, then this will get easier each time. Remember your five basic rules to medical terminology when building and defining these terms. You'll notice some word parts are repeated from the previous chapters.

Parts			Medical Term	Definition
Albumin/o	+	-uria	= Albuminuria	: _____
an	+	-uria	= Anuria	: _____
Bacteri/o	+	-uria	= Bacteriuria	: _____
Crystall/o	+	-uria	= Crystalluria	: _____
Cyst/o	+	-ectomy	= Cystectomy	: _____
Cyst/o	+	-itis	= Cystitis	: _____
Cyst/o	+	-centesis	= Cystocentesis	: _____

(A)

(B)

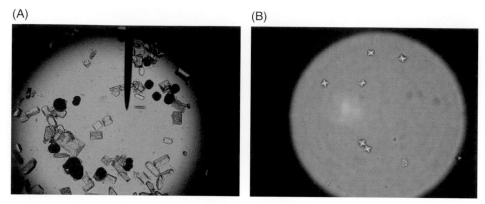

Figure 14.9 Crystalluria in canine urine. (A) Ammonium biurate crystals, struvite crystals, and sperm. (B) Calcium oxalate dihydrate crystals.

Cyst/o	+ -gram	= Cystogram	: _____
Cyst/o	+ -pexy	= Cystopexy	: _____
Cyst/o	+ -scopy	= Cystoscopy	: _____
Cyst/o	+ -stomy	= Cystostomy	: _____

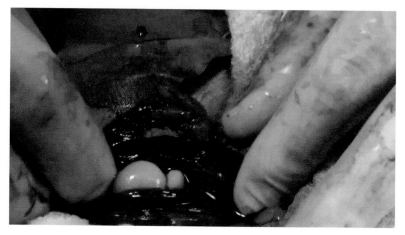

Figure 14.10 Cystotomy to remove stones. Courtesy of Greg Martinez, DVM; www.youtube.com/drgregdvm.

Cyst/o	+ -tomy	= Cystotomy	: _____
dys-	+ -uria	= dysuria	: _____
Erythr/o	+ -poiesis	= Erythropoiesis	: _____
Glomerul/o	+ -ar	= Glomerular	: _____
Glomerul/o	+ Nephr/o + -itis	= Glomerulonephritis	: _____
Glucos/o	+ -uria	= Glucosuria	: _____
Hemat/o	+ -uria	= Hematuria	: _____
Hydr/o	+ Nephr/o + -osis	= Hydronephrosis	: _____

Keton/o + -uria   = Ketonuria   : _____
Ket/o   + -osis   = Ketosis   : _____
Lith/o   + -tripsy   = Lithotripsy   : _____

Also called litholapaxy.

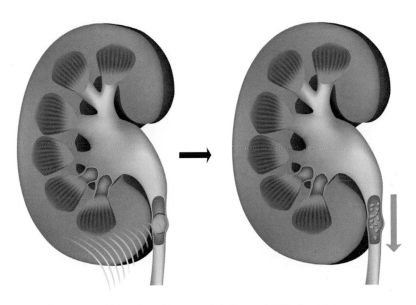

Figure 14.11   Illustration of lithotripsy. Courtesy of shutterstock/Alila Sao Mai.

Neprh/o + -itis   = Nephritis   : _____
Nephr/o + -lithiasis   = Nephrolithiasis   : _____
Nephr/o + Lith/o   + -tomy   = Nephrolithotomy   : _____
Nephr/o + -malacia   = Nephromalacia   : _____
Nephr/o + -pathy   = Nephropathy   : _____
Nephr/o + -ptosis   = Nephroptosis   : _____
Nephr/o + -sclerosis   = Nephrosclerosis   : _____
Nephr/o + -osis   = Nephrosis   : _____
Nephr/o + -stomy   = Nephrostomy   : _____
para-   + Nephr/o   + -ic   = Paranephric   : _____
oligo-   + -uria   = Oliguria   : _____
poly-   + -dipsia   = Polydipsia   : _____

TECH TIP 14.7 Rules for Using the Prefix "poly-"

When "poly-" is attached to a word component that involves an action, then the meaning of "poly-" changes to excessive or frequent. For example, polyphagia is defined as excessive eating instead of many eating or much eating.

poly-	+	-uria	= Polyuria	: _____
Protein/o	+	-uria	= Proteinuria	: _____
Pyel/o	+	-itis	= Pyelitis	: _____
Pyel/o	+	-gram	= Pyelogram	: _____
Pyel/o	+	-Lith/o + -tomy	= Pyelolithotomy	: _____
Pyel/o	+	Nephr/o + -itis	= Pyelonephritis	: _____

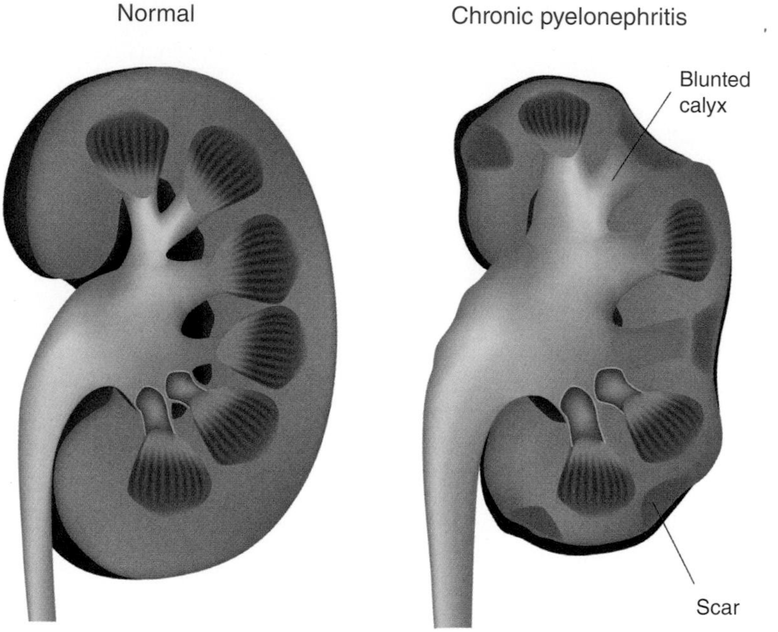

Figure 14.12   Illustration of pyelonephritis. Courtesy of shutterstock/Alila Sao Mai.

| Py/o | + | -uria | = Pyuria | : _____ |
| Ureter/o | + | Ile/o + -stomy | = Ureteroileostomy | : _____ |

Remember the rule for "-stomy" when it is attached to more than one combining form.

Ureter/o	+	Lith/o + -tomy	= Ureterolithotomy	: _____
Ureter/o	+	-plasty	= Ureteroplasty	: _____
Urethr/o	+	-itis	= Urethritis	: _____
Urethr/o	+	-plasty	= Urethroplasty	: _____
Ur/o	+	-lithiasis	= Urolithiasis	: _____
Ur/o	+	-poiesis	= Uropoiesis	: _____

Abbreviations

Table 14.4   Chapter 14 Abbreviations.

Abbreviation	Definition
ADH	Antidiuretic hormone
Bili	Bilirubin
BUN	Blood urea nitrogen
Cl⁻	Chloride
Creat	Creatinine
CRF	Chronic renal failure
Cysto	Cystocentesis
FLUTD	Feline lower urinary tract disease
FUS	Feline urological syndrome
IVP	Intravenous pyelogram
K⁺	Potassium
Na⁺	Sodium
PU	Perineal urethrostomy
sp. gr	Specific gravity
U/A	Urinalysis
USG	Urine specific gravity
UTI	Urinary tract infection

Case Study

Hershey, a 12-year-old Dalmatian, presents to your clinic with hematuria and dysuria. On macroscopic examination, the urine is dark red and cloudy. Microscopic evaluation reveals crystalluria and bacteriuria. After taking radiographs, two stones are discovered in the urinary bladder. Hershey will require surgery to remove the stones.

1. Which term is used in the diagnosis?
   a. Cholelithiasis
   b. Urolithiasis
   c. Choledocholithiasis
2. Which type of surgery will be performed?
   a. Cystectomy
   b. Cystotomy
   c. Cystostomy
3. The symptoms that Hershey presented with include:
   a. Bloody urine, frequent urination
   b. Bilirubin in urine, difficulty urinating
   c. Bloody urine, straining to urinate

Exercises

14-A: Give the term for the following definitions of structures.

1. _____: Functional unit of the kidney.
2. _____: Nitrogenous waste of muscle cell metabolism.
3. _____: Tube from the kidney to the urinary bladder.
4. _____: Outer region of the kidney.
5. _____: Collection of capillaries where filtration takes place.
6. _____: Tube from the urinary bladder to the outside of the body.
7. _____: Hormone responsible for the reabsorption of water in the renal tubules.
8. _____: Cup-like capsule enclosing the glomerulus.
9. _____: Tubes in the kidney where reabsorption takes place.
10. _____: Synonymous term for urination and voiding.

14-B: Define the following terms.

1. Lithotripsy_____
2. Nephrosclerosis _____
3. Pyelonephritis _____
4. Cystocentesis _____
5. Erythropoiesis _____
6. Anuria _____
7. Polyuria _____
8. Urethritis _____
9. Ketosis _____
10. Glomerular_____

14-C: Circle the correct term in parentheses:

1. Enzyme produced by the kidney to regulate blood pressure. (EPO, renin, sodium)
2. Scanty urine. (anuria, oliguria, pyuria)
3. Plasma protein that maintains oncotic pressure found in the urine. (albuminuria, ketonuria, proteinuria)
4. Incision into the kidney to remove a stone. (pyelolithotomy, nephrolithotomy, cystotomy)
5. Increased excretion of urine. (azotemia, diuresis, enuresis)
6. Lack of blood flow to the kidney. (renal hypoxia, renal colic, renal ischemia)
7. Passage of substances from the glomerulus to Bowman's capsule. (filtration, reabsorption, excretion)
8. Electrolyte reabsorbed by the renal tubules due to aldosterone. (chloride, potassium, sodium)
9. Nitrogenous waste that results from protein breakdown. (BUN, creatinine, ketones)
10. Increase in non-protein nitrogenous wastes in the blood. (azotemia, diuresis, enuresis)

14-D: Define the following abbreviations.

1. _____ : ADH
2. _____ : PU
3. _____ : Na⁺
4. _____ : Cysto
5. _____ : UTI
6. _____ : USG
7. _____ : FLUTD
8. _____ : FUS
9. _____ : BUN
10. _____ : U/A

14-E: Match the following with their descriptions.

1. _____ Excessive thirst.
2. _____ Abnormal accumulation of fluid in the kidney.
3. _____ Pertaining to near the kidney.
4. _____ Frequent urination.
5. _____ Incontinence.

A. Enuresis
B. Hydronephrosis
C. Paranephric
D. Pollakiuria
E. Polydipsia

Answers can be found starting on page 571.

Go to www.wiley.com/go/taibo/terminology to find additional learning materials for this chapter:

- A crossword puzzle
- Flashcards
- Audio clips to show how to pronounce terms
- Case studies
- Review questions
- The figures from the chapter in PowerPoint

Chapter 15

The Horse

Now that you have a good foundation for medical terminology and the basics with regard to anatomy, we can introduce more species of animals. This chapter introduces terms common to equine medicine.

Equine Anatomy

The horse's internal and external anatomy are different from those of dogs and cats. While the majority of bones are similar to small animals, the external terminology is considerably different.

Equine Skeleton

The equine skeleton is similar to that of small animals, but there are some differences in the distal limbs. The differences begin with the front limb (Figure 15.1).

TECH TIP 15.1 How to Remember the Joint Names

Joints are named based on the bones that comprise them. The common name of the proximal interphalangeal joint, the pastern, is made up of the long pastern and short pastern. The common name of the distal interphalangeal joint is the coffin, which is made up of P2 and the coffin bone.

The Front Limb

The scapula, commonly called the shoulder blade, connects to the humerus, the long bone of the upper arm. The elbow joint of the horse is still medically called the humeroradioulnar joint. From the elbow, the anatomical changes begin.

Veterinary Medical Terminology Guide and Workbook, First Edition. Angela Taibo.
© 2014 John Wiley & Sons, Inc. Published 2014 by John Wiley & Sons, Inc.
Companion website: www.wiley.com/go/taibo/terminology

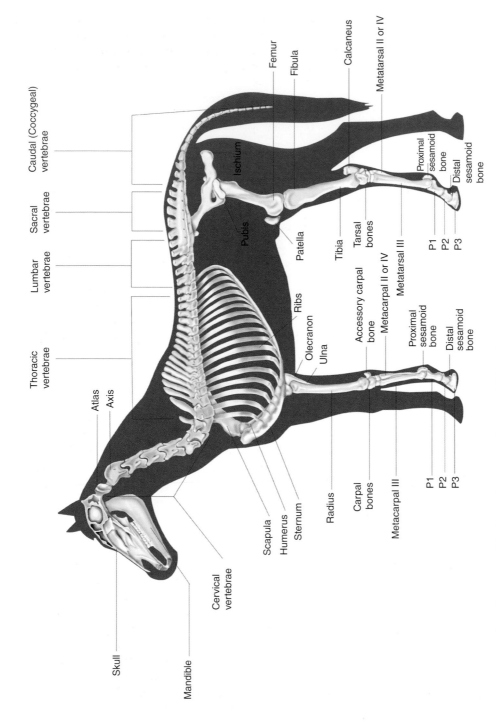

Figure 15.1 Skeletal anatomy of the horse. Courtesy of shutterstock/Alexonline.

The radius and ulna of the horse are fused. The radius sits cranial to the ulna and the ulna still has a process on the proximal aspect called the olecranon.

The carpal bones make up the joint known as the carpus. In horses, this joint is commonly called the knee. Distal to the carpus are the metacarpals. Horses lack metacarpals I and V. Because the metacarpals are counted from medial to lateral, the first metacarpal in the horse is metacarpal II, commonly called the medial splint bone. Metacarpal III is the largest of the metacarpals and is commonly called the cannon bone. Lastly, metacarpal IV is commonly called the lateral splint bone. Metacarpals II and IV do not articulate with the phalanges as they do in other species.

The point at which the metacarpals meet the phalanges is called the fetlock. The medical name for the fetlock is the metacarpophalangeal joint.

Horses only have one "finger," the middle finger. This phalanx, or digit, is made up of three bones that are named proximally to distally. The proximal phalanx, or P1, is commonly known as the long pastern. The second bone of the phalanx is the middle phalanx, or P2, commonly called the short pastern. The last phalanx, called the distal phalanx, or P3, is commonly called the coffin bone.

An interphalangeal joint is located between each phalanx. The joint between P1 and P2 is known as the proximal interphalangeal joint, or pastern. The joint between P2 and P3 is the distal interphalangeal joint, or coffin joint.

Horses have proximal sesamoid bones, which are caudal to their fetlock joint. The distal sesamoid bone, or navicular, is caudal to the coffin joint.

The Rear Limb

The rear limb begins the same as in the small animals. The pelvis meets the femur to create the coxofemoral joint, or hip. The femur, the long bone of the upper rear limb, leads to the femorotibial joint, or stifle. The sesamoid bone just cranial to the stifle joint is the patella. The tibia is the largest bone of the lower rear limb and is used for weight bearing. In horses, the fibula is a reduced bone. The shaft of the horse's fibula is vestigial, or not present, and the ends are fused with the tibia. The tarsal bones make up the tarsus joint, commonly called the hock.

The remaining bones are almost identical to the front limb. Horses lack metatarsals I and V and the remaining metatarsals are still counted from medial to lateral. Metatarsal II is commonly known as the medial splint bone, metatarsal III is commonly known as the cannon bone, and metatarsal IV is commonly known as the lateral splint bone. The joint between the metatarsals and phalanges is the metatarsophalangeal joint, commonly called the fetlock.

The medical names and common names of the phalanges in the rear limb are identical to those of the front limb, as are those of the interphalangeal joints. Horses also have proximal sesamoid bones caudal to the fetlock in their rear limbs and a navicular caudal to the coffin joint in their rear limbs.

Hoof Anatomy

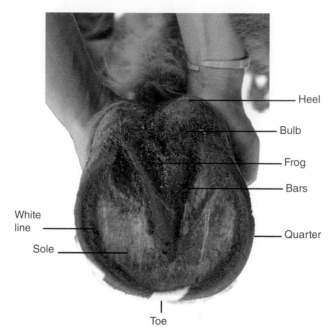

Figure 15.2   Anatomy of the hoof.

Bars	V-shaped depression on the distal surface of the hoof.
Frog	V-shaped pad of soft horn between the bars on the sole of the hoof.
Heel bulb	Swollen part of the hoof wall and adjacent soft tissue at the back of the hoof.
Hoof	Hard, horny covering of the digit of **ungulates** (hooved animals).
Hoof wall	Hard, horny covering of the hoof.
Lamina	Sensitive tissue that attaches the hoof wall to the underlying foot structures.
Quarter	Medial and lateral aspects of the hoof.
Sole	Palmar and plantar surfaces of the hoof.
Toe	Cranial aspect of the hoof.
White line	The fusion between the wall and the sole of the hoof.

External Landmarks and Terminology

Barrel	The trunk of the horse; determined largely by the chest's capacity.

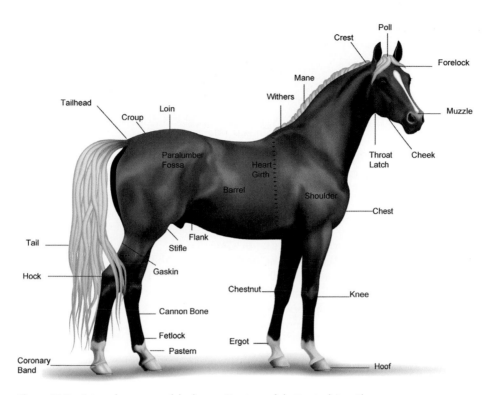

Figure 15.3   External anatomy of the horse. Courtesy of shutterstock/IronFlame.

Cheek	Fleshy portion on either side of the face, forming the sides of the mouth and continuing rostrally to the lips.
Chest	Part of the body between the neck and abdomen; also called the thorax.
Chestnuts	Flattened, oval masses or horny tissue on the medial surface near the knee and hock.
Corners	Common name for the third incisors.
Coronary band	Junction between the skin and the horny tissue of the hoof.
Crest	Root of the mane.
Croup	Muscular area around and above the base of the tail.
Cutters	Common name for the second incisors.
Dock	Solid portion of the tail.
Ergot	Small mass of horny tissue in a small bunch of hair on the palmar and plantar aspects of the fetlock.
Forelock	Cranial aspect of the mane hanging down between the ears and onto the forehead.
Gaskin	Muscular portion of the hindleg between the hock and stifle.

Heart girth	Greatest circumference of the chest behind the withers, shoulders, and elbows.
Loin	Lumbar region of the back between the thorax and pelvis.
Mane	Region of long, course hair at the dorsal border of the neck and terminating at the poll.
Muzzle	Skin, muscles, and fascia of the upper and lower lip and including the nasal bones.
Nippers	Common name for the central incisors.
Paralumbar fossa	Hollow of the flank between the transverse process of the lumber vertebrae, the last rib, and the thigh muscles.
Poll	Top of the head; also known as the **occiput**.
Tail head	Base of the tail that connects to the trunk of the body.
Teat	Nipple of the mammary gland.
Udder	Mammary gland.
Withers	Region of the backline where the neck meets the thorax and where the dorsal margins of the scapula lie just below the skin.
Wolf teeth	First upper premolars that are usually shed when the horse matures.

Mobility

Horses are used for working, recreation, competition, and transportation. Therefore, there are a variety of terms used to describe their gait, or manner of walking. This chapter merely introduces basic terms used to describe the gait and will not go into more specific terminology that relates to their jobs.

Beat	Time when the foot touches the ground.
Canter	Galloping at an easy pace. This stride involves a three-beat rhythm in which two diagonal legs are paired.
Gallop	Fastest gait of the horse in which all four limbs are off the ground at one point. This stride involves a four-beat rhythm; also known as a **run**.
Jog	Slow trot.
Lame	Unable to walk; deviation from the normal gait.
Pace	Fast, two-beat rhythm similar to a trot except that the front and rear limbs on each side move in unison instead (Figure 15.4).
Stride	A single, coordinated movement of all four legs until they return to their normal position.
Trot	Two-beat rhythm gait in which diagonal limbs take off at the same time (Figure 15.5).
Walk	Slow, four-beat rhythm in which all four limbs take off at separate times.

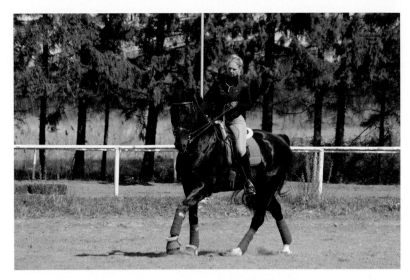

Figure 15.4   Pace. Courtesy of shutterstock/Anastasija Popova.

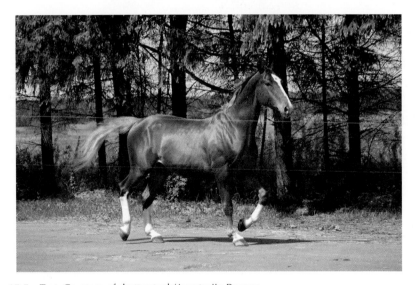

Figure 15.5   Trot. Courtesy of shutterstock/Anastasija Popova.

Types of Horses and Their Markings

Horses are divided into categories based on their common characteristics. There are hundreds of horse breeds, so this book focuses on the groups into which the various breeds are categorized.

Regardless of the breed of horse, the terminology for markings is always the same.

Table 15.1 Types of Horses.

Draft horses	Breeds with large muscular and bone structure. These breeds are commonly used as work horses because of their powerful bodies. Draft horses are generally 18 hands or greater. Examples of draft horses include the Clydesdale and the Belgian.
Gaited horses	Breeds with a smooth, easy gait commonly used for transportation and show. These breeds are typically 14 to 16 hands. Examples include the Tennessee Walker and American Saddlebred.
Horses of color	Breeds with uniquely spotted patterns. These breeds are typically 14 to 16 hands. Some horses of color are also classified as light horses. Examples include the Pinto and Appaloosa.
Light horses	Breeds that are 14 to 16 hands. Like the gaited horse, these breeds are typically used for transportation and show. Examples include the Arabian and the Thoroughbred.
Ponies	Breeds that are less than 14 hands. These breeds are often used for recreation and show. Examples include the Shetland Pony and the Welsh Pony.

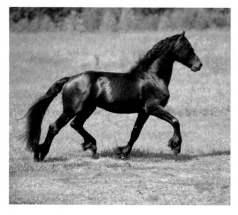

Figure 15.6A Friesian, which is a type of draft horse. Courtesy of shutterstock/Makarova Viktoria (Vikarus).

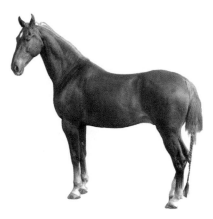

Figure 15.6B American Saddlebred. Courtesy of shutterstock/Jeff Banke.

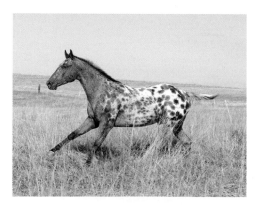

Figure 15.6C Appaloosa. Courtesy of shutterstock/Zuzule.

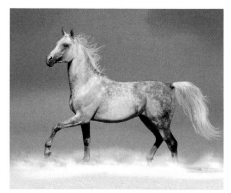

Figure 15.6D Arabian. Courtesy of shutterstock/Olga_i.

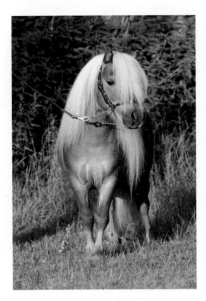

Figure 15.6E   Shetland Pony. Courtesy of shutterstock/Vera Zinkova.

TECH TIP 15.2   What's a Hand?

A hand is a unit of measurement for the height of a horse. One hand = 4 inches = 10.16 centimeters.

The Face

(A)   (B)

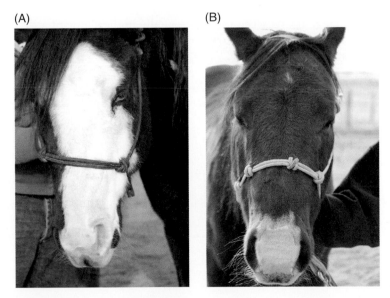

Figure 15.7   Facial markings. (A) Bald. (B) Snip.

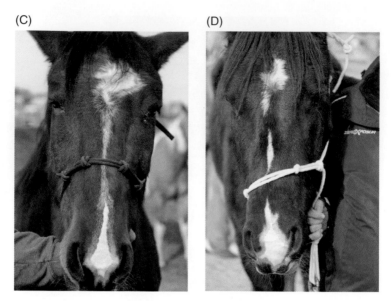

Figure 15.7   Facial markings. (C) Star and stripe. (D) Star, stripe, and snip.

Bald	White face; face with a blaze and a snip that extends beyond the eyes and nostrils.
Blaze	White stripe on the face.
Chin spot	White spot on the chin.
Snip	White marking on the muzzle.
Spot	White mark on the face.
Star	White mark between the eyes, usually in the shape of a diamond.
Stripe	Long, narrow, white mark down the nose; also called a **strip** or **race**.

TECH TIP 15.3   Half Markings

Markings that only span half of their area have the word "half" in front of their term. For example, a half stocking has a white marking from the coronet to the middle of the cannon. A half pastern has a white marking from the coronet to the middle of the pastern.

The Legs

(A)

(B)

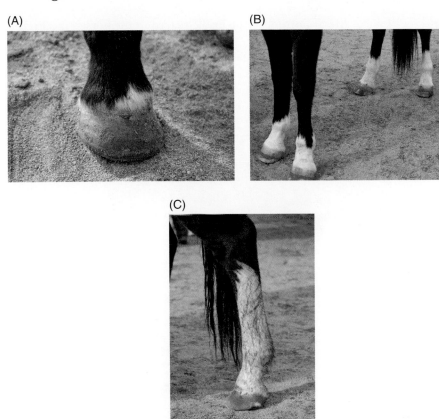

(C)

Figure 15.8   Leg markings. (A) Coronet. (B) Pastern markings on the front legs, socks on the rear legs. (C) Stocking.

Ankle	White marking from the fetlock down to the coronet; also called a **sock**.
Coronet	White marking covering the coronary band.
Heel	White marking on the heel.
Pastern	White marking from the pastern to the coronet.
Stocking	White mark from the coronet to the knee.

Equine Husbandry

The care and management of horses involves various equipment and housing tools not used in small animal medicine.

Equipment

Bit	Metal portion of the bridle placed in the horse's mouth to control it.
Bridle	Headgear made up of a bit, reins, and straps to control the horse.

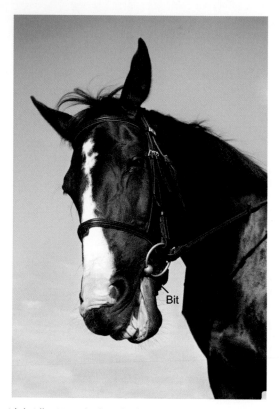

Figure 15.9 Horse with bridle. Note the bit which is part of the bridle. Courtesy of shutterstock/ Inara Prusakova.

Cradle	Barred restraining device on the horse that prevents it from biting an injured area.
Halter	Head restraint for a horse used to guide and tie a horse.
Hobble	Leather straps fastened around the front and hind feet of the horse to restrain it from moving.

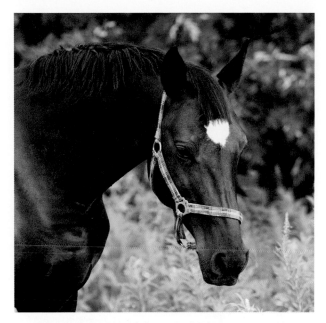

Figure 15.10   Horse with halter. Courtesy of shutterstock/Edoma.

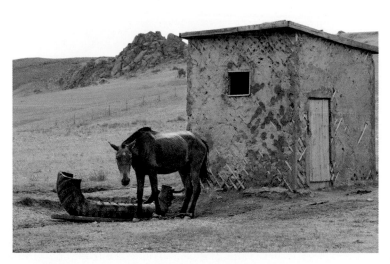

Figure 15.11   Hobbled horse. Courtesy of shutterstock/withGod.

Hoof pick   Instrument to remove debris from the crevices of the hoof.
Hoof tester   Instrument shaped like a pair of pincers used to test the
                   sensitivity of the hoof.
Rasp   Instrument used for fine trimming of the hoof.

(A)

(B)

(C)

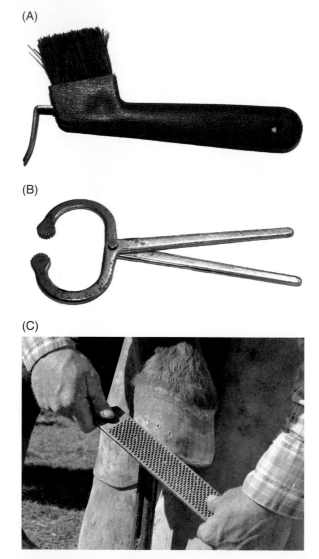

Figure 15.12　Hoof tools. (A) Hoof pick. (B) Hoof tester. (C) Rasp. Courtesy of shutterstock/Terrance Emerson.

Shoe   Steel or aluminum plate nailed to the planter and palmar
                   aspects of the hoof for protection.
Tack   Equipment used for riding and care of the horse; also
                   known as tackle.

Care and Management

Bolt	Startle.
Box stall	Enclosed area where the horse can stay and move around.
Cast	A horse that lies down and is unable to rise into sternal recumbency.
Casting	Method of restraint in horses to pull them down for surgical procedures.
Cribbing	Habit in which the horse grasps an object with its incisors and applies pressure as it swallows air. Commonly called wind-sucking, this habit can be acquired or a neurosis. It can cause the teeth to erode and can cause severe weight loss with abdominal distention.

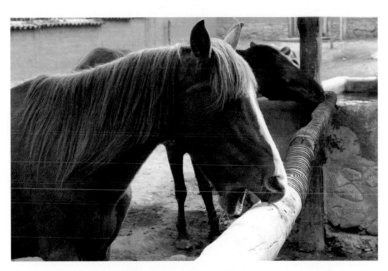

Figure 15.13   Cribbing. Courtesy of shutterstock/Thomas Barrat.

Cross tie	Restraint method in which the horse is tied to two pillars on each side. This method is commonly used for simple procedures such as grooming.
Farrier	Person skilled in the making, fitting, and remodeling of horseshoes.
Firing	Method used on lower limbs to encourage healing of tendons or ligaments in lame horses. A red hot iron is place on an anesthetized area of skin to promote healing and rest. The iron may be placed deep or superficial depending on the desired effect.
Flighty	Nervous.
Floating	Filing of teeth using a dental float. Sometimes called **rasping**.

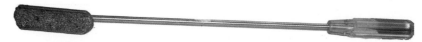

Figure 15.14   Dental float.

> **TECH TIP 15.4   Why is Floating Necessary?**
>
> Equine dentistry is a critical part of horse maintenance because occlusions are critical to proper mastication. Horses can develop high and low points on their teeth which interfere with two surfaces rubbing together.

Grade	Animal that results from the mating of purebred and crossbred animals.
Lather	The common name for sweat that develops on a horse's body.
Lunging	Exercising a horse by having it circle at the end of a long lead.
Near side	Left side of the horse.
Off side	Right side of the horse.
Paddock	Small, fenced-in field or enclosure; also called a **corral**.
Pasture	Land area for animals to graze where grasses grow.
Pasture breeding	Males are placed in a pasture with many females for natural mating.
Pasture rotation	Movement of animals from pasture to pasture to decrease the incidence of parasites.
Quick release knot	Knot that unties easily.
Saddle	Tack placed on the back of the horse for riding. There are two types; the Western saddle and English saddle.

(A)   (B)

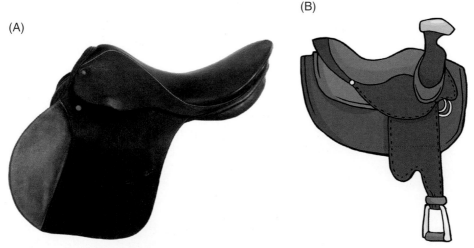

Figure 15.15   Saddles. (A) English saddle. Courtesy of shutterstock/marekuliasz. (B) Western saddle. Courtesy of shutterstock/HitToon.Co.

Tease	Parading a male in front of a female to determine if she is in heat.
Teaser	Male used to sexually tease a female to determine if she is in heat.
Twitch	Restraint method in which a device is used to twist the upper lip of the horse.
Waxing	Waxy covering derived from colostrum that accumulates on the teats and signals foaling.

Age and Sex

Colt	Intact male horse 4 years old or younger.
Filly	Intact female horse 4 years old or younger.
Foal	Young horse less than a year old.
Foaling	Giving birth.
Gelding	Castrated male horse.
Herd	Group of horses
Mare	Intact female horse 4 years or older.

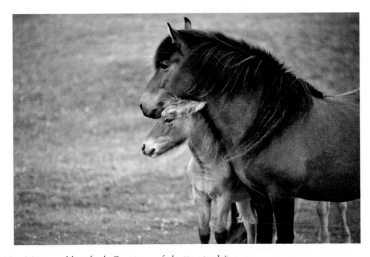

Figure 15.16   Mare and her foal. Courtesy of shutterstock/topora.

TECH TIP 15.5   Different Types of Mares

Mares are further classified based on their status.

Agalactic mare	Intact female horse that is not producing milk.
Barren mare	Intact female horse that did not conceive in the previous breeding season; also known as an open mare.
Brood mare	Breeding female horse.
Maiden mare	Intact female horse that has never been bred.
Wet mare	Intact female horse that has been bred and has foaled in the current breeding season.

Ridgeling	Cryptorchid male horse.
Stallion	Intact male horse 4 years or older.
Weanling	A foal that has been weaned and is less than a year old.
Yearling	Young horse between the ages of 1 and 2 years.
Jack	Intact male donkey; also known as a **jack ass**.
Jenny	Intact female donkey.

Physiology and Pathology and Procedures

Soundness is the ability of the horse to perform the function required of it, including the ability to compete or work. An animal that is classified as unsound has been found to be unsatisfactory.

Bishoping	Altering of the teeth to make the horse appear younger.
Bog spavin	Chronic synovitis of the tibiotarsal joint causing distention of the joint capsule. **Spavin** means inflammation.
Bone spavin	Periosteitis of the bones of the hock.
Bowed tendons	Chronic tendinitis of the superficial flexor tendons causing enlargement of the tendons and lameness.
Capped hock	Accumulation of fluid in a bursa near the hock.
Check ligament	One of two ligaments to the digital flexors that help maintain the limbs in an extended position when standing. Also known as **suspensory ligaments**, they help suspend the sesamoid bones behind the fetlock.
Clostridium tetani	Bacteria that causes tetanus characterized by hyperesthesia, convulsions, and eventually death; commonly called **lockjaw**.
Cracks	Commonly known as **sandcracks**, these defects form in the hoof at the coronet due to injury or extension of the sole.
Curb	Thickening of the plantar tarsal ligament in the hock.
Dental star	Mark on the occlusal surface of the incisors that develops as the tooth wears. These marks begin as narrow yellow lines and develop into dark circles.
Equine ehrlichiosis	Infectious disease caused by the genus Ehrlichia; causes fever, ataxia, anorexia, and edema of extremities; commonly called **Potomac horse fever**.

Equine infectious anemia (EIA)	Anemia caused by a retrovirus leading to jaundice, petechiae, weakness, and emaciation.
Equine influenza (EI)	Upper respiratory infection caused by an influenza A virus. Symptoms include a mild fever and persistent cough.
Equine protozoal myeloencephalitis (EPM)	Condition caused by the parasite Sarcocystis neurona manifested by ataxia, weakness, recumbency, and eventually death.
Equine viral arteritis (EVA)	Virus caused by the genus Pestivirus. Symptoms include upper respiratory infection and lesions on the arteries.
Equine viral encephalomyelitis	Encephalomyelitis caused by the genus Alphavirus and transmitted by mosquitos. Symptoms include excitement, tremors, circling, paralysis, and recumbency. Three strains include Easter (**EEE**), Venezuelan (**VEE**), and Western (**WEE**).
Equine viral rhinopneumonitis (EVR)	Virus caused by the Herpesvirus 4 leading to abortions, coughing, fever, and nasal discharge.
Fistulous withers	Inflammation of the withers causing a discharge at the withers.
Flehmen's response	Reaction in males after sniffing the urine or perineum of females. The nostrils dilate and upper lip curls.
Flexor tendon	Tendon that causes the fetlock to flex.
Foal heat	The first heat cycle of the foal.
Full-mouthed	Horse with all permanent teeth present.
Galvayne's groove	Vertical groove on the labial surface of a horse's tooth used to determine its age.
Greasy heel	Dermatitis of the back of the pastern commonly seen in horses in wet standing areas; commonly called **scratches**.
Guttural pouch	Large air-filled sac that develops in the Eustachian tube of horses.

TECH TIP 15.6 How To Determine Age

The Galvayne's groove appears on the gingival margin at 10 years of age. At 15 years of age, the groove extends halfway to the end of the tooth. Around 20 years of age, the groove reaches the end of the tooth. The groove disappears at the top of the tooth around 25 years of age and completely disappears around 30 years of age.

Hindgut	The small intestine, cecum, and large intestine, collectively.
Laminitis	Inflammation of the lamina causing lameness; commonly called **founder**.
Monkey mouth	Condition in which the mandible is longer than the maxilla.
Osselets	Periosteitis of the cranial aspect of the fetlock joint.
Parrot mouth	Condition in which the maxilla in longer than the mandible.

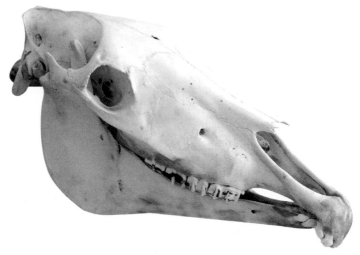

Figure 15.17   Skull of a horse with parrot mouth. Courtesy of shutterstock/Margo Harrison.

Quidding	Condition in which the horse drops food from its mouth during mastication. Commonly seen in cases of stomatitis and bad teeth. Horses with this condition are called **quiddors**.
Quittor	Chronic inflammation of the lateral cartilage of P3 causing a purulent discharge at the coronet and lameness.
Ringbone	Osteoarthritis or periosteitis of P1 and P2, creating a bony prominence at the pastern or coffin joint.
Smooth mouth	Condition in which the molars are worn so that the dentin and enamel are even.
Splints	Inflammation of the interosseous ligament between the splint bones and cannon bone.

Stay apparatus	Anatomical mechanism in the limbs that enables the horse to stand with little or no muscular effort. Involves the participation of many tendons, muscles, and ligaments.
Streptococcus equi	Bacterial infection causing high fever, purulent nasal discharge, anorexia, pharyngitis, laryngitis, and swollen lymph nodes. Disease is commonly called **Strangles**.
Sweeney	Paralysis of the scapular muscles.
Thoroughpin	Tenosynovitis of the sheath of the deep flexor tendon of the hindleg. Though it causes swelling, there is no lameness.
Vesicular stomatitis	Inflammation of the mouth characterized by ulcers that rupture and become necrotic.
West Nile virus	Mosquito-transmitted virus causing ataxia, head tilt, seizures, paralysis, and eventually death.
Winking	Quick, uncontrolled opening of the vulva when a mare is in heat.

Abbreviations

Table 15.2   Chapter 15 Abbreviations.

Abbreviation	Definition
EEE	Eastern equine encephalitis
EI	Equine influenza
EIA	Equine infectious anemia
EPM	Equine protozoal myeloencephalitis
EVA	Equine viral arteritis
EVR	Equine viral rhinopneumonitis
KBH	Kicked by horse
LA	Large animal
TEME/TME	Transmissible gastroenteritis
VEE	Venezuelan equine encephalitis
VS	Vesicular stomatitis
WEE	Western equine encephalitis

Exercises

15-A: Give the term for the following definitions of structures.

1. _____: Common name of P3.
2. _____: Medical name of the long pastern.
3. _____: Common name of the carpus in horses.
4. _____: Common name of the distal sesamoid bone.
5. _____: Common name of the metacarpophalangeal joint.
6. _____: Medical name of the coffin joint.
7. _____: Common name of the metatarsal III.
8. _____: Top of the head.
9. _____: Mammary gland.
10. _____: First upper premolars shed at maturity.

15-B: Define the following terms.

1. Ergot_____
2. Chestnuts _____
3. Lame_____
4. Canter_____
5. Mare _____
6. Gelding_____
7. Hindgut _____
8. Parrot mouth _____
9. Laminitis _____
10. Cribbing _____

15-C: Circle the correct term in parenthesis:

1. V-shaped pad of soft horn between the bars on the sole of the hoof. (bar, frog, bulb)
2. Head restraint used to guide and tie a horse. (bridle, halter, harness)
3. Solid portion of the tail. (mane, tail head, dock)
4. Breeds with large muscular and bone structure, over 18 hands. (draft, gaited, pony)
5. Muscular area around and above the base of the tail. (croup, occiput, withers)
6. White stripe on the face. (blaze, snip, stripe)
7. Instrument used for fine trimming of the hoof. (dental float, hobble, rasp)
8. Exercising a horse by having it circle at the end of a long lead. (firing, blistering, lunging)
9. White marking covering the coronary band. (coronet, pastern, heel)
10. Region of the backline where the neck meets the thorax and where the dorsal margins of the scapula lie just below the skin. (croup, occiput, withers)

15-D: Define the following abbreviations.

1. _____: EEE
2. _____: EIA
3. _____: TEME
4. _____: VS
5. _____: KBH
6. _____: VEE
7. _____: WEE
8. _____: EPM
9. _____: LA
10. _____: EI

15-E: Match the following diseases with their causes.

1. _____ Equine ehrlichiosis   A. Tetanus
2. _____ Clostridium equi   B. Strangles
3. _____ Laminitis   C. Potomac horse fever
4. _____ Clostridium tetani   D. Founder
5. _____ Sarcocystis neurona   E. EPM

Answers can be found starting on page 571.

Go to www.wiley.com/go/taibo/terminology to find additional learning materials for this chapter:

- A crossword puzzle
- Flashcards
- Audio clips to show how to pronounce terms
- Case studies
- Review questions
- The figures from the chapter in PowerPoint

Chapter 16

Ruminants

As introduced in Chapter 4, ruminants are a group of animals with a more specialized stomach that contains four compartments. The parts of the ruminant stomach include the rumen, reticulum, omasum, and abomasum. Ruminants regurgitate their food (cud), chew it, and then swallow it again. Cattle, sheep, goats, llamas, and alpacas are all ruminants.

Cattle

Cattle play a large role in the food industry. They can be divided into two basic types: dairy cattle and beef cattle (Figure 16.1). The hides of some cattle are also valuable. Terminology for the care and use of cattle will be discussed in this chapter; basic anatomy has been discussed previously.

External Terminology

The terminology used to describe the external anatomy of cattle is similar to that of other animals (Figure 16.2). Therefore, the only terms listed here are those that may be new compared to those of other species. Terms such as elbow and hock are still labeled on the diagrams, but will not be discussed.

Brisket	Mass of connective tissue and fat covering the cranial aspect of the chest.
Crest	Dorsocranial margin of the neck.
Dewclaw	Accessory claw in ruminants.
Dewlap	Loose skin under the throat and neck which may be pendulous in some breeds.
Flank	Side of the body between the ribs and the ilium.

Veterinary Medical Terminology Guide and Workbook, First Edition. Angela Taibo.
© 2014 John Wiley & Sons, Inc. Published 2014 by John Wiley & Sons, Inc.
Companion website: www.wiley.com/go/taibo/terminology

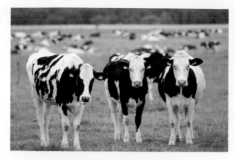

Figure 16.1A Dairy cattle. Courtesy of shutterstock/tarczas.

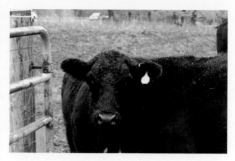

Figure 16.1B Angus beef cattle. Courtesy of shutterstock/operative401.

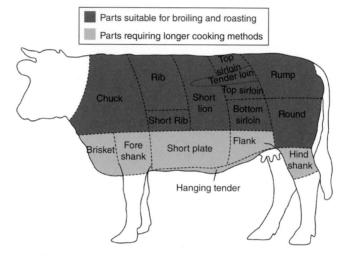

Figure 16.1C Meat diagram of a cow. Courtesy of shutterstock/life_is_fantastic.

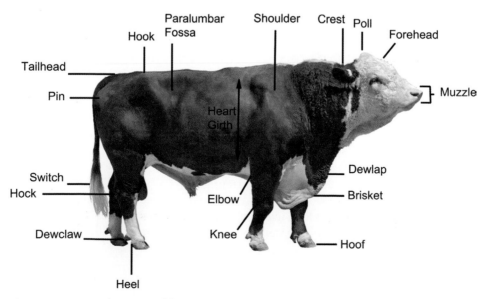

Figure 16.2 External anatomy of the cow. Courtesy of shutterstock/Rey Kamensky.

420

Heart girth	Circumference of the chest just caudal to the shoulders.
Heel	Area at the rear of the hoof or claw where horn and skin meet and where the hoof wall becomes the sole.
Hide	Skin of cattle.
Hooks	Bony protrusion of the wing of the ilium dorsolaterally.
Loin	Lumber region of the back, between the thorax and pelvis.
Muzzle	Skin, muscles, and fascia of the upper and lower lip, including the nasal bones.
Paralumbar fossa	Hollow of the flank between the transverse process of the lumber vertebrae,the last rib, and the thigh muscles.
Pin	Bony protrusion of the ischium lateral to the tail base.

TECH TIP 16.1 Hooks and Pins

Hooks and pins are used for body condition scoring (BCS).

Poll	Top of the heads; also called the **nuchal crest**.
Rump	The gluteal region; region around the pelvis, hindquarters, and buttocks.
Sole	Palmar and plantar surfaces of the hoof.
Switch	Hairy portion at the end of the tail.
Teat	Nipple of the mammary gland.
Toe	Cranial aspect of the hoof.
Udder	Mammary gland.

Bovine Husbandry

The care and management of cattle involves various equipment, housing tools, and techniques not used in small animal medicine.

Balling gun	Instrument to administer bolus to livestock (Figure 16.3).

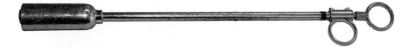

Figure 16.3   Balling gun.

Bolus	Mass of food or medication to be swallowed.
Brand	Mark put on the skin as a means of identification (Figure 16.4).

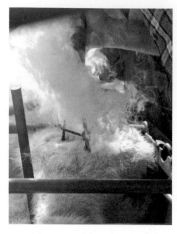

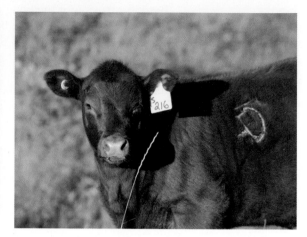

Figure 16.4A Cow branding. Courtesy of shutterstock/sursad.

Figure 16.4B Cow with brand and ear tag. Courtesy of shutterstock/BG Smith.

Calving interval	Average time between successive calves.
Carcass	Body of the animal after slaughter.
Casting	Method of restraint to pull the cow down to lateral recumbency.
Chute	Small stall used as a restraint device for the animal to be examined and treated (Figure 16.5).

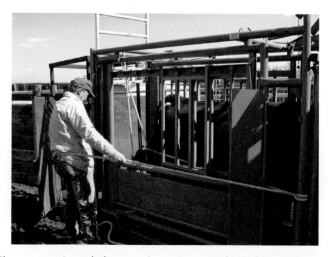

Figure 16.5 Chute to restrain cattle for procedures. Courtesy of Patrick Hemming, DVM.

Cull	Removal of an animal from a herd. Culling can be due to disease, age, or a failure to reproduce.
Dehorning	Removal of horns when the animal is young for the safety of the other animals in the herd. Methods of dehorning include electrocautery or use of a caustic paste (Figure 16.6).

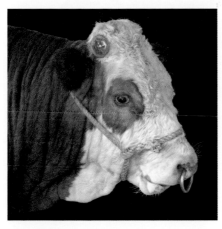

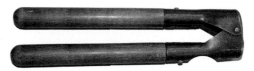

Figure 16.6A   Dehorned bull. Courtesy of shutterstock/Margo Harrison.

Figure 16.6B   Barnes dehorner.

Dual purpose	Cattle that can be used for both dairy and beef production.
Ear tagging	Placement of tags in the ear for identification of the animals (Figure 16.4).
Emasculotome	Instrument used for a bloodless castration. The procedure is commonly referred to as a **pinch**. Other commonly used instruments for castration include the **emasculator** and the **elastrator** (Figure 16.7).

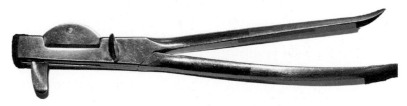

Figure 16.7A   Instruments used for castration. Emasculator is used to sever the spermatic cord with minimal bleeding.

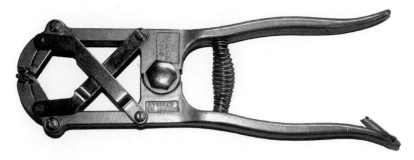

Figure 16.7B Instruments used for castration. Elastrator is used to place a rubber band around the neck of the scrotum.

Feedlot	Confined area where animals are fed and "fattened up" before going to slaughter.
Flushing	Increase in nutrition to promote ovulation and conception in females and improve semen characteristics in males.
Free stall	Stall in which the cow is not tied and is free to move around or lie down.
Halter	Head restraint for a cow used to guide and tie a cow.
Hutch	Housing area for calves.
Hybrid	Offspring that results from the mating of two different breeds.
Hybrid vigor	Increased productivity and performance in the first generation of crossbred animals produced by the mating of dissimilar breeds.
Inbred	Offspring produced by inbreeding; the result of the mating of closely related animals.
Marbling	Intermixing of fat and muscle fibers in beef.
Offal	Non-edible products from slaughter.
Rendering	The melting of fatty tissue.
Rumination	The act of regurgitation, remastication, and reswallowing; **chewing cud.**
Scurs	Vestigial (underdeveloped) horns not attached to the skull.
Springing	Heifer in the last one to two weeks before parturition.
Stall	Small compartment to house an animal.
Stanchion	Device used to restrain the neck of cattle for procedures such as milking or administration of medicine (Figure 16.8).
Standing heat	Stage of estrus in which the female stands to be mounted by a bull.

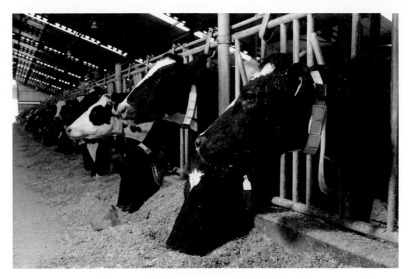

Figure 16.8   Stanchion. Courtesy of shutterstock/polat.

Tailing	Restraint method in which the tail is grabbed and raised vertically; also known as **tail jacking**.
Tankage	Heat-digested animal residues left over after fat has been rendered in slaughter. Commonly called **meat meal**, these residues can be used as fertilizer or feed due to their high protein content.
Tattooing	Permanent identification method in which ink is introduced via skin punctures. These identification numbers are typically placed inside the pinna on cattle.
Tie-stall	Stall just large enough for one animal, which is generally tied in by a neck chain.
Veal	Calves fed only milk to produce tender meat.

Age and Sex

Bull	Intact male bovine of breeding age; generally older than 1 year of age.
Calf	Bovine less than a year old.
Calving	Giving birth in a bovine.
Cow	Female bovine that has given birth.
Freemartin	Sterile female that was born as a twin with a male.
Heifer	Female bovine that has never given birth.

Herd	Group of cattle.
Teaser bull	Bull used to detect females in heat; also known as a **gomer bull**.

Bovine Pathology

Bovine mastitis	Inflammation of the mammary glands due to *Staphylococcus aureus*.
Bovine respiratory syncytial virus (BRSV)	Virus caused by the genus Pneumovirus. Symptoms include dyspnea and pneumonia with a high mortality rate.
Bovine viral diarrhea (BVD)	Virus caused by the genus Pestivirus manifested in young cattle. Symptoms include diarrhea, stomatitis, and rhinitis.
Brucellosis	Infection caused by *Brucella abortus* characterized by abortions in late pregnancy.
Clostridium	Genus of bacteria which causes various conditions depending on the species involved.
Clostridium tetani	Bacteria that causes tetanus characterized by hyperesthesia, convulsions, and eventually death; commonly called **lockjaw**.
Coronavirus	Ribonucleic acid (RNA) virus that causes enteritis in calves.
Hemophilosis	Endometritis and purulent cervicitis caused by a bacterial infection of *Hemophilus somnus*.
Infectious bovine rhinotracheaitis (IBR)	Herpesvirus infection causing fever, rhinitis, tracheitis, and pneumonia.
Leptospirosis	Infectious disease causing fever, hemolytic anemia, jaundice, nephritis, and abortion.
Parainfluenzavirus (PI3)	Virus causing fever and cough; part of complex etiology of **shipping fever**.
Pasteurellosis	Bacterial infection of *Pasteurella multocida* which causes hemorrhagic septicemia; *Pasteurella hemolytica* causes septicemia and respiratory disease.
Rotavirus	Virus causing diarrhea in young cattle.
Tritrichomoniasis	Infestation of the protozoan *Tritrichomonas foetus* leading to embryonic death and infertility.
Vibriosis	Venereal disease of cattle caused by *Campylobacter fetus* leading to embryonic death and infertility.

Sheep

Sheep are important for their wool and their meat. The skeletal system of sheep is not much different from that of cattle and horses, so we will focus here on external landmarks.

External Terminology

The external landmarks in sheep are very similar to those of cattle. Joints that have been covered previously are still labeled, but will not be discussed (Figure 16.9).

Brisket   Mass of connective tissue and fat covering the cranial
                                   aspect of the chest.
Crest   Dorsocranial margin of the neck.
Dewclaw   Accessory claw in ruminants.

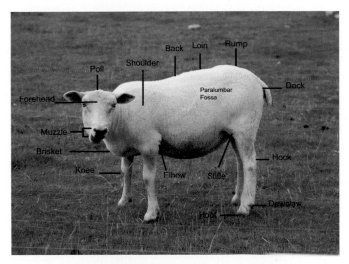

Figure 16.9A   External anatomy of sheep. Courtesy of shutterstock/ShaunWilkinson.

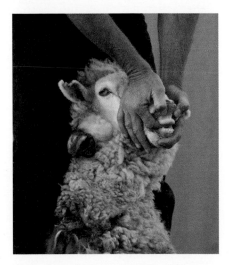

Figure 16.9B   Figure showing the absence of upper teeth in sheep. Courtesy of shutterstock/Margo Harrison.

Flank	Side of the body between the ribs and the ilium.
Heart girth	Circumference of the chest just caudal to the shoulders.
Heel	Area at the rear of the hoof or claw where horn and skin meet and where the hoof wall becomes the sole.
Loin	Lumbar region of the back, between the thorax and pelvis.
Muzzle	Skin, muscles, and fascia of the upper and lower lip and including the nasal bones.
Paralumbar fossa	Hollow of the flank between the transverse process of the lumber vertebrae,the last rib, and the thigh muscles.
Poll	Top of the heads; also called the **nuchal crest**.
Rump	The gluteal region; region around the pelvis, hind-quarters, and buttocks.
Sole	Palmar and plantar surfaces of the hoof.
Switch	Hairy portion at the end of the tail.
Teat	Nipple of the mammary gland.
Toe	Cranial aspect of the hoof.
Udder	Mammary gland.

Ovine Husbandry

The care and management of sheep involves various equipment, housing tools, and techniques not used in small animal medicine.

Clip	Removing the wool of sheep; total wool produced by a flock at one shearing.
Combing	Long-fibered wool processed in a combing machine that separates longer and shorter fibers and then arranges them.
Crimp	Regular wave formation in wool.
Crutching	Shearing of wool from the perianal region to prevent fly strike.
Docking	Tail amputation.
Felting	Property of wool fibers interlocking and forming a compact mass.
Fleece	Wool.
Lanolin	Commonly called wool fat or wool grease, this is the fatty substance produced by the sebaceous glands of sheep.
Mutton	Meat obtained from adult sheep.
Rumping	Restraint method in which sheep are placed in a seated position and their front legs are elevated; also known as **tipping**.

Age and Sex

Band	Large group of range sheep; usually 1,000 or more.
Ewe	Intact female sheep.
Lamb	Young sheep less than 4 months of age.
Lambing	Giving birth in the ewe.
Flock	Group of sheep.
Ram	Intact male sheep.
Wether	Castrated male sheep.
Yearling	Sheep between 1 and 2 years of age.

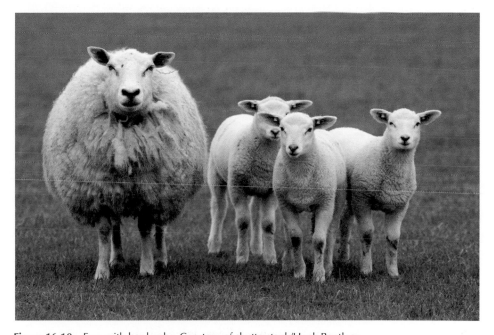

Figure 16.10   Ewe with her lambs. Courtesy of shutterstock/Henk Bentlage.

TECH TIP 16.2 Twins?

Sheep typically give birth to twins. When they give birth to one lamb that lamb is referred to as a singleton.

Goats

Goats are raised for their milk, meat, and wool. Most of the terminology that has been discussed under cattle and sheep is also commonly used with goats.

External Terminology

The external landmarks in goats are very similar to those of sheep and cattle. Joints that have been previously discussed are still labeled but are not discussed (Figure 16.11).

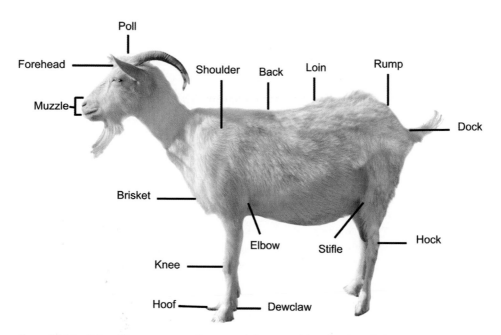

Figure 16.11 External goat anatomy. Courtesy of shutterstock/Vasyl Helevachuk.

Brisket	Mass of connective tissue and fat covering the cranial aspect of the chest.
Chine	Thoracic region of the back.
Crest	Dorsocranial margin of the neck.
Dewclaw	Accessory claw in ruminants.
Flank	Side of the body between the ribs and the ilium.
Heart girth	Circumference of the chest just caudal to the shoulders.
Heel	Area at the rear of the hoof or claw where horn and skin meet and where the hoof wall becomes the sole.

Hook	Bony protrusion of the wing of the ilium dorsolaterally.
Loin	Lumbar region of the back, between the thorax and pelvis.
Muzzle	Skin, muscles, and fascia of the upper and lower lip, including the nasal bones.
Paralumbar fossa	Hollow of the flank between the transverse process of the lumbar vertebrae,the last rib, and the thigh muscles.
Pins	Bony protrusions of the ischium lateral to the tail base.
Poll	Top of the heads; also called the **nuchal crest**.
Rump	The gluteal region; region around the pelvis, hindquarters, and buttocks.
Sole	Palmar and plantar surfaces of the hoof.
Switch	Hairy portion at the end of the tail.
Teat	Nipple of the mammary gland.
Toe	Cranial aspect of the hoof.
Udder	Mammary gland.
Wattle	Appendage suspended by the mandibular area (Figure 16.12); also called **tassel**.

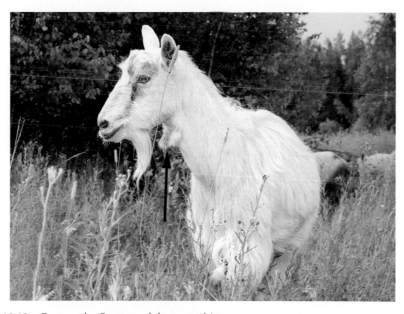

Figure 16.12   Goat wattle. Courtesy of shutterstock/everst.

Withers	Region of the backline where the neck meets the thorax and where the dorsal margins of the scapula lie just below the skin.

Caprine Husbandry

Because most of the ruminant terminology has already been discussed, only new terminology is introduced in this section.

Cabrito   Meat from a young goat.
Cashmere   Fine wool from the Kashmiri goat.
Chevon   Meat from an adult goat.
Clip   Total wool produced from one animal at one shearing.
Disbudding   Removal of the immature horns in young ruminants.

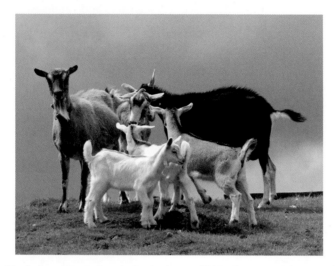

Figure 16.13   Herd of goats including the buck, doe, and kids. Courtesy of shutterstock/ Maria Gaellman.

Age and Sex

Buck   Intact male goat.
Doe   Intact female goat.
Herd   Group of goats.
Kid   Young goat.
Kidding   Giving birth in the doe.
Wether   Castrated male goat.

Camelids

Camelids are mammals that fall in the camel family. These mammals have two toes and a three-compartment stomach. Therefore, they are not considered true ruminants; instead, they are termed pseudoruminants. Their stomach consists of a reticulum, omasum, and abomasum. The llama and alpaca are popular domesticated camelids which are commonly used for their very soft, lanolin-free wool.

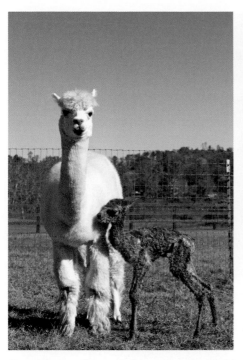

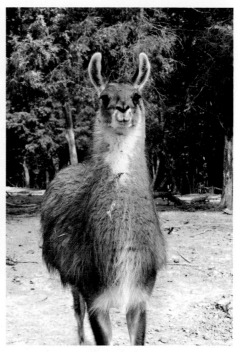

Figure 16.14   Alpacas. Courtesy of shutterstock/ David Kay.

Figure 16.15   Llama. Courtesy of shutterstock/ Don Fink.

Camelid Husbandry

Because most of ruminant terminology has already been discussed, only new terminology is introduced in this section.

Banana ears	Terminology used to describe the orientation of the ears turning inwards.
Berserk male syndrome	Aggressive behavior of males that have improperly imprinted on humans.
Fighting teeth	Set of six modified canine and incisor teeth (Figure 16.16).
Fleece	Another name for the wool from a llama.
Harem breeding	Male is left with the females most of the year.
Kush	The act of lying in sternal recumbency. Most often used to describe the female lying down in the mating ritual.
Spitting	The spitting of saliva to establish dominance or as a defense mechanism.

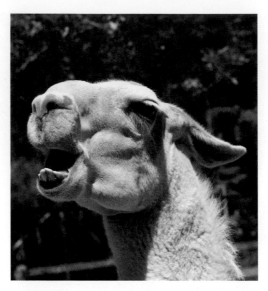

Figure 16.16   Llama teeth. Courtesy of shutterstock/Joy Brown.

Age and Sex

Bull	Intact male llama; also called a **stallion** or **herdsire**.
Cow	Intact female llama; also called a **dam**.
Cria	Young llama.
Gelding	Castrated male llama.
Herd	Group of llamas.
Yearling	Llama between 1 and 2 years of age.

Abbreviations

Table 16.1   Chapter 16 Abbreviations.

Abbreviation	Definition
BRSV	Bovine respiratory syncytial virus
BVD	Bovine viral diarrhea
IBR	Infectious bovine rhinotracheitis
PI3	Parainfluenzavirus 3

Exercises

16-A: Give the term for the following definitions of structures.

1. _____ : Hairy portion at the end of the tail.
2. _____ : Bovine giving birth.
3. _____ : Intact female goat.
4. _____ : Castrated male sheep.
5. _____ : Intermixing of fat and muscle fibers in beef.
6. _____ : Circumference of the chest just caudal to the shoulders.
7. _____ : Group of sheep.
8. _____ : Body of the animal after slaughter.
9. _____ : Another name for the nuchal crest.
10. _____ : Head restraint for a cow used to guide and tie a cow

16-B: Define the following terms.

1. Offal _____
2. Feedlot _____
3. Bolus _____
4. Heifer _____
5. Lanolin _____

6. Mutton _____
7. Wattle _____
8. Hooks _____
9. Pins _____
10. Kid _____

16-C: Circle the correct term in parentheses:

1. Lumbar region of the back, between the thorax and pelvis. (rump, loin, crest)
2. Accessory claw in ruminants. (dewclaw, dewlap, cottin)
3. Teaser bull. (gomer, herdsire, wether)
4. The melting of fatty tissue. (spitting, rendering, springing)
5. Tail amputation. (crimp, clipping, docking)
6. Instrument to administer bolus to livestock. (boluser, emasculotome, balling gun)
7. Goat meat from an adult goat. (cabrito, chevon, clip)
8. Side of the body between the ribs and the ilium. (flank, brisket, loin)
9. Thoracic region of the back of the goat. (crest, chine, withers)
10. Removal of an animal from a herd. (casting, cull, crimp)

16-D: Define the following abbreviations.

1. _____ : BRSV
2. _____ : IBR
3. _____ : BVD
4. _____ : PI3

16-E: Match the following diseases with their causes.

1. _____ Complex in shipping fever
2. _____ Brucellosis
3. _____ Hemorrhagic septicemia
4. _____ RNA virus causing enteritis
5. _____ Bovine mastitis

A. *Brucella abortus*
B. Coronavirus
C. Parainfluenzavirus
D. *Staphylococcus aureus*
E. *Pasteurella multicida*

Answers can be found starting on page 571.

Go to www.wiley.com/go/taibo/terminology to find additional learning materials for this chapter:

- A crossword puzzle
- Flashcards
- Audio clips to show how to pronounce terms
- Case studies
- Review questions
- The figures from the chapter in PowerPoint

Chapter 17

Swine

The swine category includes domesticated pigs used for meat and research, potbellied pigs used as pets, and wild pigs such as the wild boar. Basic anatomy has already been discussed in previous chapters, so this chapter focuses on anatomy, physiology, and husbandry related strictly to swine.

Anatomy

The external anatomy of swine is very similar that of other large animals with just a few changes (Figure 17.1).

Dewclaw	Accessory claw in ruminants.
Flank	Side of the body between the ribs and the ilium. Divided into the **fore flank** and **rear flank**.
Ham	Muscular portion of the upper thigh.
Loin	Lumbar region of the back between the thorax and pelvis.
Poll	Top of the head.
Rump	The gluteal region; region around the pelvis, hindquarters, and buttocks.
Snout	Upper lip and apex of the nose; also called the **rostrum**. The bone on the rostral end of the nasal septum of pigs is called the **os rostrale** or **os rostri**.
Teat	Nipple of the mammary gland.
Toe	Cranial aspect of the hoof.

Veterinary Medical Terminology Guide and Workbook, First Edition. Angela Taibo.
© 2014 John Wiley & Sons, Inc. Published 2014 by John Wiley & Sons, Inc.
Companion website: www.wiley.com/go/taibo/terminology

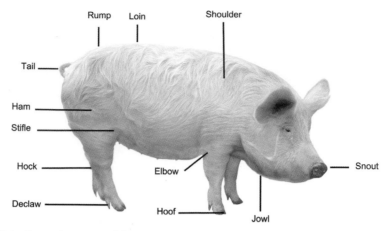

Figure 17.1 External anatomy of the pig. Courtesy of shutterstock/Vasyl Helevachuk.

TECH TIP 17.1 Why Do Pigs Have Curly Tails?

There are several theories as to why pigs have curly tails. The most common theory is that tails became curled for protection. Tail biting is a common problem among pigs, so if the tails are curled, they are more difficult to grab.

The other theory is that early Chinese farmers specifically bred for curly tails in some pigs.

Not all pigs have curly tails. Wild boars and pot-bellied pigs have straight tails.

Age and Sex

Barrow	Castrated, young male pig.
Boar	Intact male pig.
Farrowing	Giving birth in pigs.
Gilt	Female pig that has not yet had a litter of piglets.
Herd	Group of pigs; also called a **drove**.
Piglet	Young pig (Figure 17.2).

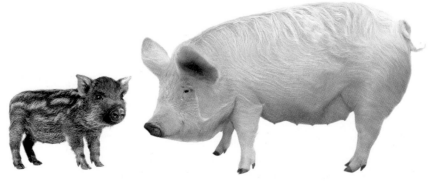

Figure 17.2 Piglet and sow. Courtesy of shutterstock/Vasyl Helevachuk.

Sow	Intact female pig (Figure 17.2).
Stag	Castrated, mature male pig.

Husbandry

The care and management of pigs involves various equipment and housing tools not used in small animal medicine.

Abbatoir	Building used for slaughter; also called a **slaughterhouse**.
Backfat	Thickness of fat along the back of a pig (Figure 17.3).

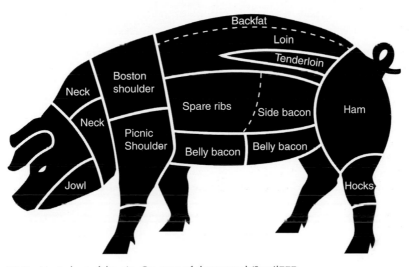

Figure 17.3   Meat chart of the pig. Courtesy of shutterstock/Stanil777.

Backfat probe	Sharp instrument used to measure the thickness of backfat without incising the carcass. Electronic versions of the probe can be used on live animals.
Bacon	Meat from the back and side of a pig (Figure 17.3).
Boar taint	Unpleasant odor or flavor from the meat of an adult boar. The word **taint** describes the unpleasant odor or flavor of meat or milk products that go into human consumption.
Brimming	Time of sexual receptivity when the female accepts the male.
Casting	Method of restraint to pull the pig down to lateral recumbency.
Creep	Area that only young piglets can access.
Creep feeding	Food is placed in an area that only piglets can access.
Dung	Feces; sometimes called manure or droppings.
Dunging pattern	Animal's tendency to defecate in certain areas.

Ear marking   Also called **ear notching;** patterned pieces of cartilage punched out as a means of identification (Figure 17.4).

(A)   (B)

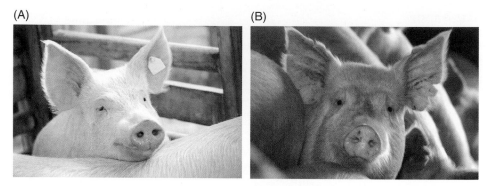

Figure 17.4   Ear marking. (A) Ear tagging. Courtesy of shutterstock/Dmitry Kalinovsky. (B) Ear notching. Courtesy of shutterstock/gudak.

Farrowing crate   Pipework holding pen large enough to hold the sow, but too narrow to allow movement. Farrowing crates prevent crushing losses of the piglets because they allow the piglets to escape (Figure 17.5). Also called a **farrowing pen**.

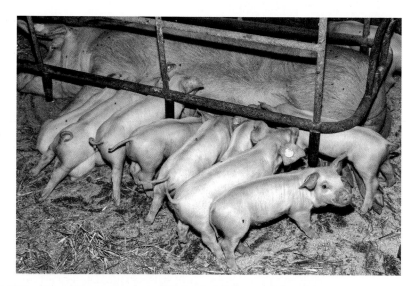

Figure 17.5   Farrowing pen. Courtesy of shutterstock/Edler von Rabenstein.

Finish   Degree of fatness short of obesity.
Hog snare   Wire loop passed over the hog's snout and pulled by a person on the other end as a means of restraint.

Hog tied	All four feet are tied together so that the pig is unable to stand.
In-pig	Terminology for a pregnant sow.
Lard	Pig fat. Once rendered it can be used for cooking.
Needle teeth	Common name for the deciduous incisors and canines of piglets. These teeth are often trimmed at birth to prevent injury to the sow during nursing.
Ringing	Ring placed in the nose of pigs to deter rooting.
Rooting	Turning up of the ground using the snout to look for food.
Slap mark	Tattoo placed on a pig as a means of identification.
Tusk	Well-developed canine tooth in a boar.
Wallow	Area for pigs to rest and cool down; usually contains water or mud.

Pathology and Procedures

Aujeszky's disease	Herpesvirus causing respiratory, reproductive, and neurological signs. Symptoms in piglets include convulsions and recumbency leading to death. Commonly called **pseudorabies** or "**mad itch**."
Bordetella	Bacteria found in the respiratory tract of pigs that can cause **atrophic rhinitis** in pigs.
Clostridium	Bacteria that causes enterotoxemia in pigs.
E. coli	Bacteria causing coliform gastroenteritis in piglets characterized by severe diarrhea and death. In adult pigs, this bacteria can cause colibacillosis, which is characterized by metritis and mastitis in sows and diarrhea, edema, ataxia, and death in all pigs.
Erysipelas	Common infection in pigs causing septicemia, skin lesions, endocarditis, and arthritis.
Glässer's disease	Viral disease caused by a species of *Haemophilus* characterized by polyarthritis, pericarditis, and peritonitis.
Haemophilus influenzae	Commonly called **swine flu**, this disease causes fever, stiffness, recumbency, and dehydration with a high mortality rate.
Leptospirosis	Infectious disease causing abortions, stillbirths, and septicemia in piglets.
Mycoplasma hyopneumoniae	Bacterial infection causing a lethal pneumonia in pigs.

Parvovirus	Viral infection causing abortions, stillbirths, and infertility.
Pasteurella multocida	Bacteria causing hemorrhagic septicemia.
Proliferative hemorrhagic enteropathy	Acute disease of young pigs causing anemia, dysentery, and hemorrhagic lesions in the distal ileum and proximal colon with a high mortality rate.
Proliferative ileitis	Ulceration and thickening of the ileum which may lead to perforation and acute peritonitis.
Porcine respiratory and reproductive syndrome (PRRS)	Viral infection causing stillbirths, abortions, mummified fetuses, and cyanosis of the ear, leading it to commonly be called "**blue-ear pig disease**." In piglets, it causes respiratory disease.
Porcine SMEDI virus	Enterovirus causing stillborn, mummification, embryonic death, and infertility (SMEDI).
Porcine stress syndrome (PSS)	Acute death due to increased stress caused by shipping, fighting, exercise, and increased environmental temperature. Symptoms prior to death include dyspnea, tremors, stiffness, and hyperthermia.
Rotavirus	Virus in piglets causing damage to the small intestine villi, leading to malabsorption and diarrhea.
Streptococcus suis	Bacterial infection causing meningitis in pigs.
Transmissible gastroenteritis (TGE)	Coronavirus of piglets characterized by vomiting, diarrhea, dehydration, and eventually death.

Abbreviations

Table 17.1 Chapter 17 Abbreviations.

Abbreviation	Definition
PRRS	Porcine respiratory and reproductive syndrome
PSS	Porcine stress syndrome
SMEDI	Stillborn, mummification, embryonic death, infertility
TGE	Transmissible gastroenteritis

Exercises

17-A: Give the term for the following definitions of structures.

1. _____ : Intact female pig.
2. _____ : Muscular portion of the upper thigh.
3. _____ : Female pig that has not yet had a litter of piglets.
4. _____ : Well-developed canine tooth in a boar.
5. _____ : Intact male pig.
6. _____ : Upper lip and apex of the nose in pigs.
7. _____ : Giving birth in pigs.
8. _____ : Common name for the deciduous incisors and canines of piglets.
9. _____ : Pig fat.
10. _____ : Unpleasant odor or flavor from the meat of an adult boar

17-B: Define the following terms.

1. Rooting_____
2. Abbatoir _____
3. Creep _____
4. Finish _____
5. Wallow _____
6. Farrowing crate _____
7. Brimming _____
8. Backfat_____
9. Ear marking _____
10. Barrow _____

17-C: Define the following abbreviations.

1. _____ : SMEDI
2. _____ : PRRS
3. _____ : TGE
4. _____ : PSS

17-D: Match the following diseases with their causes.

1. _____ Blue-ear disease
2. _____ Meningitis
3. _____ Pseudorabies
4. _____ Causes polyarthritis, pericarditis, and peritonitis
5. _____ Colibacillosis

A. Aujesky's disease
B. E. coli
C. Glässer's disease
D. PRRS
E. Streptococcus suis

Answers can be found starting on page 571.

Go to www.wiley.com/go/taibo/terminology to find additional learning materials for this chapter:

- A crossword puzzle
- Flashcards
- Audio clips to show how to pronounce terms
- Case studies
- Review questions
- The figures from the chapter in PowerPoint

Chapter 18

Exotics

In veterinary medicine, animals such as birds, reptiles, and amphibians are classified as exotics. These animals are more specialized because of their anatomy and physiology. Veterinarians that are able to examine these animals are commonly called "exotic vets."

Avian

Avian medicine is a broad category which includes birds used as pets such as canaries and parakeets as well as poultry, ratites, and birds of prey. Basic anatomy has been covered in previous chapters so this section will focus on concepts specific to birds (Figure 18.1).

External Anatomy

Beak	Hard, keratin layer that covers the maxilla and mandible.
Breast	Anterior pectoral region of the bird.
Cere	Fleshy part above the beak.

TECH TIP 18.1 Sexing Budgerigars

The color of the cere is an easy means of sexing budgerigars. Male budgies have a blue cere and female budgies have a light brown or tan cere.

Cheek	Area of the face below the eyes.
Comb	Vascular, red cutaneous structure attached in a sagittal plane to the dorsum of the skull of domestic fowl.

Veterinary Medical Terminology Guide and Workbook, First Edition. Angela Taibo.
© 2014 John Wiley & Sons, Inc. Published 2014 by John Wiley & Sons, Inc.
Companion website: www.wiley.com/go/taibo/terminology

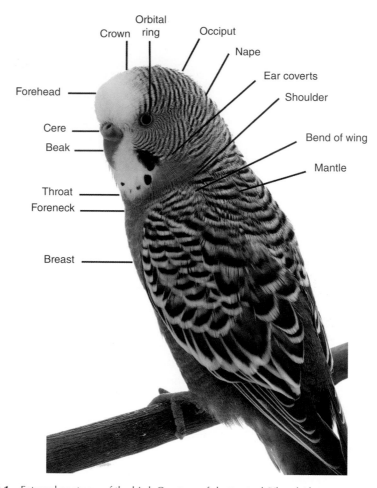

Figure 18.1 External anatomy of the bird. Courtesy of shutterstock/Khmel Alena.

Crown	The top of the head.
Forehead	Portion of the head that is rostral to the eyes.
Foreneck	Cranial aspect of the breast where the clavicle is located.
Frontal process	Cone-shaped mass of red vascular tissue that lies across the base of the turkey's beak; commonly called the **snood** or **nasal comb.**
Lore	Lateral aspect of the face between the eye and rostral aspect of the beak.
Nape	Back of the neck.
Occiput	Back of the head.
Orbital ring	Fleshy, unfeathered ring around the eye.
Rump	Space between the pelvis and tail.
Throat	Space between the head and chest.
Wattle	Double fold of skin suspended from the mandible in chickens and turkeys.

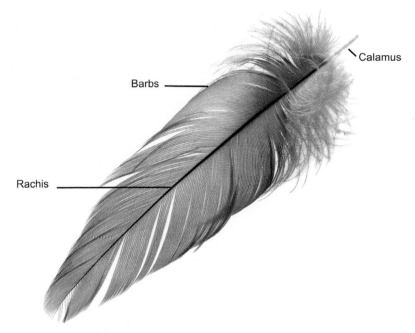

Figure 18.2 Anatomy of a feather. Courtesy of shutterstock/MustafaNC.

Feathers

A feather is a skin appendage of birds (Figure 18.2). Equivalent to hairs in vertebrates, feathers share similar functions. Feathers are used for:

Protection	Feathers have waterproof traits and can be used as camouflage in the wild.
Insulation	Feathers can insulate the body when temperatures are low.
Flight	Certain groups of feathers are used to control flight.
Mating	Feathers can be used as a display in mating rituals.
Nesting	Females pluck their own feathers to create a nest for their young.

Feathers differ depending on the species of bird, but their basic anatomy and terminology is the same (Figure 18.3).

Apterium	Area of the bird's skin carrying no feathers or down.
Barb	Paired delicate filaments projecting from the main shaft of the feather.
Barbule	Hooked processes that fringe from the edges of the barbs.
Calamus	Proximal hollow shaft, or quill, that inserts into the skin.
Coverts	Small feathers that cover other feathers at the base.
Down feathers	Soft, fine feathers found underneath the exterior feathers; also called **plume**.

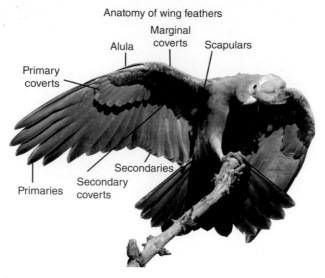

Figure 18.3A The different wing feathers. Courtesy of shutterstock/EcoPrint.

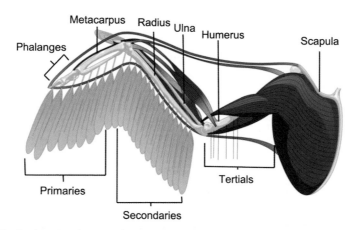

Figure 18.3B Feathers in relation to the skeleton. Courtesy of Getty Images/Dorling Kindersley.

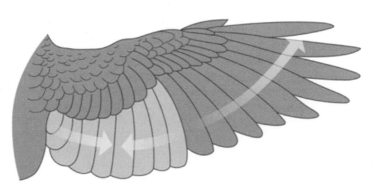

Figure 18.3C Molting pattern of wing feathers. Courtesy of Getty Images/Dorling Kindersley.

Flight feathers	Long, stiff feathers found on the wings and tail to enable flight.
Filoplume	Hair-like feathers that grow along down feathers.
Molt	The shedding and replacement of old feathers with new ones.
Pin feathers	Developing feathers with a blood supply through them; they are commonly called **blood feathers**. Mature feathers lack a blood supply and are in essence dead feathers. After becoming worn, they eventually fall off.
Primary feathers	Flight feathers connected to the metacarpus and phalanges of the wing. These feathers are responsible for thrust.
Pteryla	Feather tracts on the skin of birds.
Rachis	The distal shaft of a feather.
Rectrices	Flight feathers of the tail.
Remiges	Flight feathers of the wing.
Secondary feathers	Short, wide flight feathers connected to the ulna; used for lift.
Shaft	Central part of the feather.
Tertiary feathers	Short feathers connected to the humerus and used to protect the primaries and secondaries. Tertiary feathers are not considered true flight feathers.
Uropygial gland	Bi-lobed sebaceous gland at the base of the tail that secretes an oil to waterproof feathers; commonly called the **preen gland**.

Skeletal System

Columella	Bony structure between the eardrum and perilymph of the inner ear. This structure is the equivalent to the ossicles in mammals.
Coracoid	Bone of the shoulder braced against the sternum.
Furcula	Commonly called the **wishbone**, this bone is the fusion of two clavicles.
Keel	Commonly called the **breastbone**, this is the large surface of the bird's sternum.
Pygostyle	Bony termination of the vertebral column in birds. Also known as the rump post, this is where the tail feathers attach.
Synsacrum	Fused lumbar and sacral vertebrae in birds.
Tarsometatarsus	Fused metatarsal and tarsal bones.
Tibiotarsus	Fused tibia and tarsal bones.

Internal Anatomy

The body systems of birds have much in common with other vertebrates. This section focuses on the structures specific to the bird's organ systems.

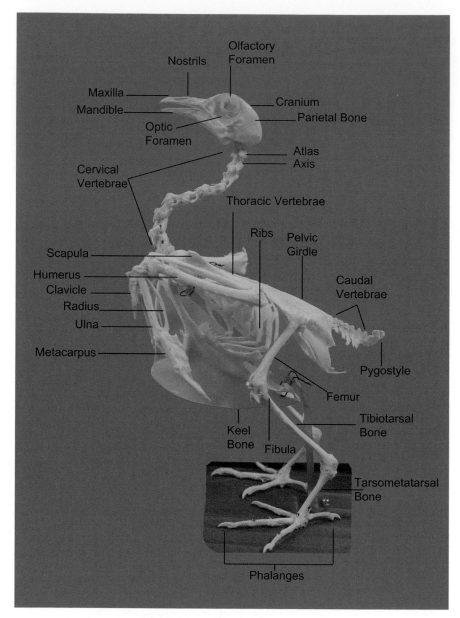

Figure 18.4 Skeletal system of the bird.

Gastrointestinal System

Cloaca	Common passage for fecal, urinary, and reproductive discharge in birds and lower vertebrates.
Crop	Esophageal pouch near the throat to store food temporarily.
Droppings	Term used for the combination of evacuated urine and feces.

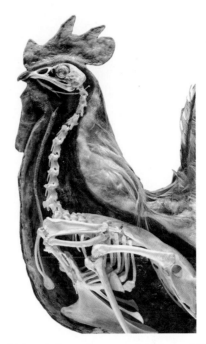

Figure 18.5   Cross section of a chicken skeleton. Courtesy of shutterstock/liubomir.

Proventriculus	Elongated, spindle-shaped, glandular stomach of birds.
Vent	External opening of the cloaca.
Ventriculus	Stomach of birds. Also called the gizzard.

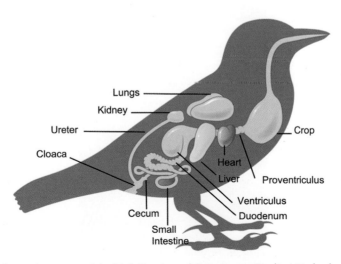

Figure 18.6   Internal anatomy of the bird. Courtesy of Getty Images/Dorling Kindersley.

Respiratory Tract

Air sacs   Thin-walled sacs found in the respiratory tract and bones of
                  birds. Air sacs in the respiratory tract connect to small bronchi
                  in the lungs. The air sacs in bones help make them hollow to
                  allow for gliding in flight (Figure 18.7).

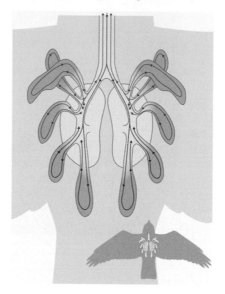

Figure 18.7   Air sacs of the bird showing the air flow. Courtesy of Getty Images/Dorling Kindersley.

Choana   Paired openings between the nasal cavity and nasopharynx
                  (Figure 18.8).

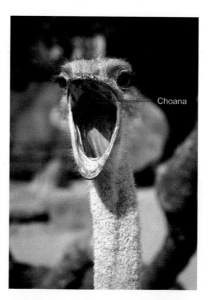

Figure 18.8   Choana in an ostrich. Courtesy of shutterstock/KarSol.

| Parabronchi | Tertiary bronchi; tiny passages where gas exchange occurs. Birds lack alveoli. |
| Syrinx | Vocal organ in birds at the base of the trachea that produces sound. |

Reproductive System

| Infundibulum | Funnel-shaped structure at the top of the oviduct which captures the ova after ovulation. |

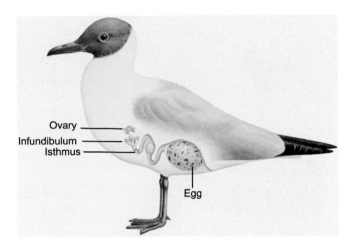

Figure 18.9   Reproductive system of the female bird carrying eggs. Courtesy of Getty Images/Dorling Kindersley.

Isthmus	Short, narrower portion of the oviduct that is farthest from the ovary. The function of this passage is to add the shell membranes.
Magnum	Mid-portion of the oviduct known as the albumen-secreting zone. Albumen is the white of the egg.
Shell gland	Caudal portion of the uterus where the egg is held while the shell is produced.
Sperm nests	"Packages" in the infundibulum where sperm is kept until it can fertilize the egg when released from the ovary; also called **sperm tubules or sperm glands.**
Urodeum	Portion of the cloaca in which the urogenital system opens.
Vagina	Portion of the reproductive tract in which the egg passes into the cloaca.

Egg Terminology

| Albumen | The white of the egg surrounding the yolk and surrounded by the shell. |
| Chalaza | Strands of albumen that suspend the yolk from the poles of the egg. |

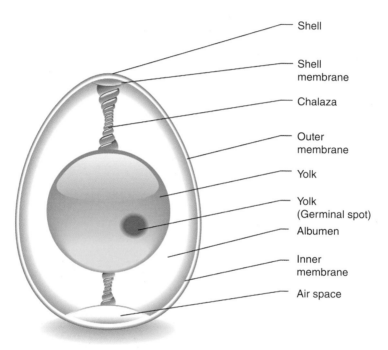

Figure 18.10A Anatomy of an egg. Courtesy of shutterstock/fkdkondmi.

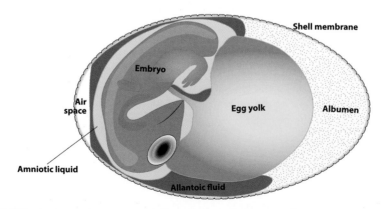

Figure 18.10B Anatomy of an egg containing an embryo. Courtesy of shutterstock/Zhabska Tetyana.

Hatch   Term used for the emergence from an egg.
Incubation   Development of an embryo inside an egg.
Yolk   The yellow portion of the egg where nutrients and antibodies are
             stored for the developing embryo.

Age, Sex, and Type

Anseriformes   Order of birds that includes ducks, geese, and swans;
                 commonly called **Anserines**.
Clutch   Group of eggs.
Columbiformes   Order of birds with short beaks, short legs, small heads, and
                 stout bodies. Examples include pigeons and doves (Figure 18.11).
Fledgling   A young bird whose wing feathers have just come in
                 (Figure 18.12).
Hatchling   Young bird that has recently emerged from the egg
                 (Figure 18.12).
Passeriformes   Order of perching birds including canaries, finches, and
                 sparrows (Figure 18.11).

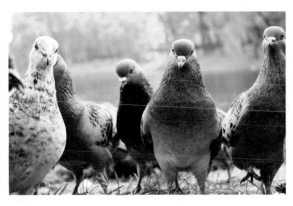

Figure 18.11A   Pigeons are an example of Columbiformes. Courtesy of shutterstock/Denis Omelchenko.

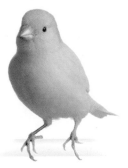

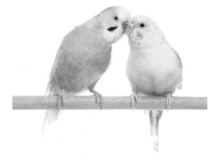

Figure 18.11B   Canaries are an example of
Passeriformes. Courtesy of shutterstock/Eric Isselée.

Figure 18.11C   Budgies are an example of
Psittacines. Courtesy of shutterstock/Jagodka.

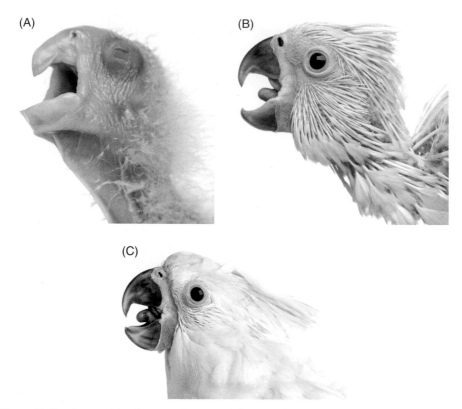

Figure 18.12   Stages of development. Courtesy of shutterstock/Eric Isselée. (A) Sulphur crested cockatoo hatchling, 4 days old. (B) Sulphur crested cockatoo fledgling, 35 days old. (C) Sulphur crested cockatoo, 8 weeks old.

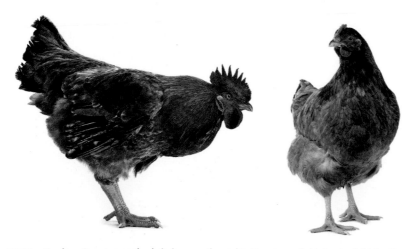

Figure 18.13   Poultry. Rooster on the left, hen on the right. Courtesy of shutterstock/Valentina and shutterstock/Lepas.

Poultry	Farmed, domesticated birds such as fowl, turkey, ducks, and geese (Figure 18.13).

Chicken

Broiler	Young male or female chicken about 8 weeks of age and weighing 1.5 kg.
Brood	Group of young birds produced from one hatching.
Chick	Young chicken.
Cockerel	Young male chicken.
Capon	Castrated male fowl.
Flock	Group of chickens.
Hen	Intact female chicken.
Layer	Commercial fowl that is laying eggs.
Poult	Young chicken.
Pullet	Young female chicken.
Rooster	Intact male chicken; also called **cock**.

Duck

Drake	Intact male duck.
Duck	Intact female duck.
Duckling	Young duck.
Flock	Group of ducks.

Goose

Gander	Intact male goose.
Goose	Intact female goose.
Gosling	Young goose.
Gaggle	Group of geese.

Turkey

Flock	Group of turkeys.
Hen	Intact female turkey.

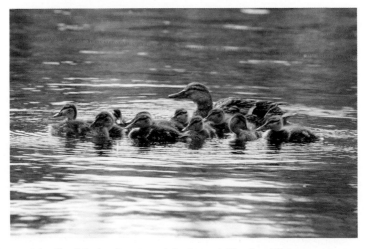

Figure 18.14A   A family of ducks. Courtesy of shutterstock/Kirychun Viktar.

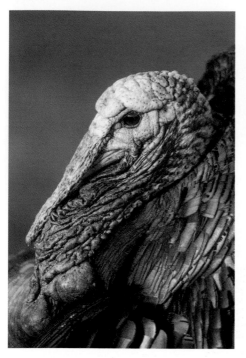

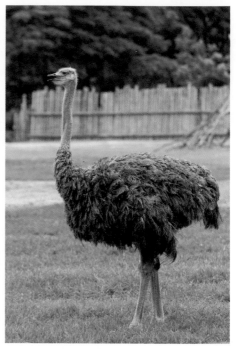

Figure 18.14B   Turkey close-up. Note the snood below the beak. Courtesy of shutterstock/Double Brow Imagery.

Figure 18.14C   Ostrich. Courtesy of shutterstock/Joy Brown.

Poult	Young turkey.
Tom	Intact male turkey.
Psittacine	Common name used for birds in the order Psittaciformes such as parrots, macaws, cockatoos, conures, lovebirds, parakeets, cockatiels, and budgies.
Chick	Young psittacine.
Cock	Intact male psittacine.
Flock	Group of psittacines.
Hen	Intact female psittacine.
Ratite	Group of running birds with a flat, raft-like sternum and strong muscular legs. These are flightless birds due to their lack of a keel bone. Examples include the ostrich, emu, rhea, and kiwi.
Chick	Young ratite.
Flock	Group of ratites.
Hen	Intact female ratite.
Rooster	Intact male ratite.

Pathology and Procedures

Care and management depends on the type of birds involved. The following terms are commonly used in avian husbandry.

Beak trim   In pet birds such as psitticines, this is a procedure using a dremel to trim the tip of the beak to ensure proper alignment. In poultry, special blades and cautery are used to trim beaks to prevent cannibalism.

Egg bound   Term used to describe the inability to pass an egg.

Feather picking Symptom that occurs due to disease or stress in which the bird removes its own feathers; also known as **feather plucking** or **depluming** (Figure 18.15).

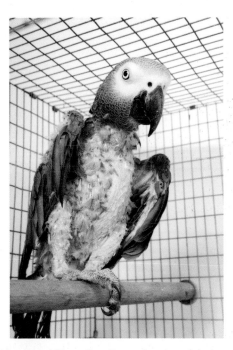

Figure 18.15   Feather picking in an African Grey Parrot. Courtesy of shutterstock/Michelle D. Milliman.

Flighted   Term used for birds with the ability to fly; often used to describe birds that need their wings trimmed.

Hand-raised   Commonly used term for pet birds raised by humans from birth.

Perch	This term can be used as a noun or a verb. A perch is a stick that can be placed in a cage for the bird to stand or rest upon. **Perching** is the act of the bird resting on the stick. An inability to perch can be an indication of sickness.
Preen	Term commonly used to describe a bird grooming itself, which includes cleaning its feathers.
Wing trim	Procedure in which wing feathers are clipped to prevent flight.

Reptiles

Reptiles are vertebrates that can be found living in water or on land. They have lungs in which to breathe air, a heart with three chambers—two atria and one ventricle—and their bodies are covered with horny scales. Animals in the class Reptilia are ectotherms, which means their body temperature varies with that of their environment. Depending on the species of reptile, they may or may not have legs. Those with legs have short legs which are strictly used for crawling. There are three notable subgroups of reptiles: Squamata, Chelonia, and Crocodilia.

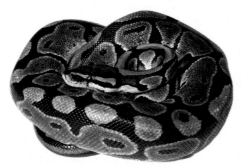

Figure 18.16A Ball python. Courtesy of shutterstock/Anita Patterson Peppers.

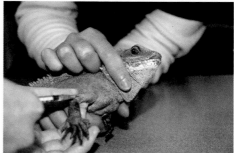

Figure 18.16B Bearded dragon. Courtesy of shutterstock/Julie Keen.

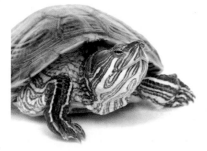

Figure 18.16C Pond terrapin turtle. Courtesy of shutterstock/Olga Popova.

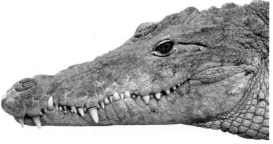

Figure 18.16D Alligator. Courtesy of shutterstock/AlexVirid.

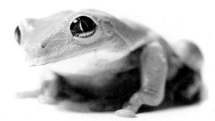

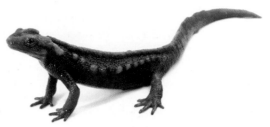

Figure 18.17A Frog. Courtesy of shutterstock/kornik.

Figure 18.17B Salamander. Courtesy of shutterstock/ Arun Roisri.

Animals in the order Squamata have scaly bodies and are capable of expanding their mouths to ingest large prey. Examples of animals in this order include snakes and lizards. Because of the varieties of snakes and lizards, this is one of the largest subgroups of reptiles.

Chelonia is an order of reptiles known for their tough, outer shell. Examples include turtles, sea turtles, tortoises, and terrapins.

Members of the order Crocodilia include the crocodile, alligator, and caiman.

Reproduction varies depending on the type of reptile. Some are oviparous, such as turtles, whereas others are ovoviviparous, such as some lizards.

Amphibians

Like reptiles, amphibians are ectotherms. Unlike reptiles, amphibians lack scales and instead have a smooth, moist body with which to absorb water, aid in breathing, and escape predators. In the earliest developmental stages, amphibians live in water and breathe through their gills. When the young mature, they undergo a developmental change in which they acquire lungs with which to breathe air on land. Once mature, amphibians may live on land or in water. Like reptiles, there are three orders of note: Anura, Caudata, and Gymnophiona.

Amphibians in the order Anura lack tails, have large eyes, and have long hindlimbs; for example, frogs and toads. The order Caudata consists of newts and salamanders, which have elongated bodies and tails. Finally, the order Gymnophiona contains worm-like amphibians called caecilians. These amphibians take on a snake-like appearance because they lack legs.

Amphibian and Reptile Terminology

Bask	To lie in the sun or under a heat lamp to absorb the heat.
Carapace	Dorsal aspect of the turtle's shell (Figure 18.18).

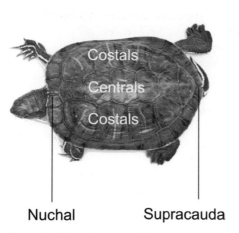

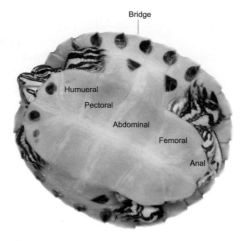

Figure 18.18A   Carapace of the turtle. Courtesy of shutterstock/kohy.

Figure 18.18B   Plastron of the turtle. Courtesy of shutterstock/Eric Isselée.

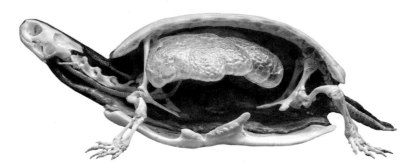

Figure 18.18C   Turtle skeleton. Courtesy of shutterstock/liubomir.

TECH TIP 18.4 Can Turtles Crawl Out of Their Shell?

The shell of the turtle is actually an extension of its ribs and vertebrae; therefore, it is impossible for a turtle to crawl out of its shell.

Clutch	Group of eggs.
Dysecdysis	Difficult shedding of skin (Figure 18.19B).
Ecdysis	Shedding of the external layer of skin (Figure 18.19A).
Ectotherm	Animal that is unable to regulate its own body temperature. Commonly called **cold-blooded animals,** ectotherms require the external environment to regulate their body temperature. Also called **poikilothermic.**
Envenomation	The introduction of venom from a venomous animal.

Impaction	Inability to pass waste from the intestines due to a buildup of foreign material, such as sand in herbivores.
Metabolic bone disease	Loss of bone tissue leading to malformations. Commonly seen in reptiles due to malnutrition.
Metamorphosis	Transition from one developmental stage to another such as a tadpole to a frog.
Mitotic parthenogenesis	The ability of a female to reproduce without a male for the survival of its species.
Pits	Organs found on some snakes to sense warm-blooded prey; also used for thermoregulation.
Plastron	The ventral aspect of the turtle's shell (Figure 18.18).
Scute	Thick epidermal plate found on the heads of snakes or shells of turtles.
Spectacle	Commonly called the eyecap, this is a transparent covering over the cornea of snakes. The spectacle is required for protection because snakes lack eyelids . The spectacle is shed during ecdysis.
Substrate	General term used to describe the material used on the bottom of a cage or tank.

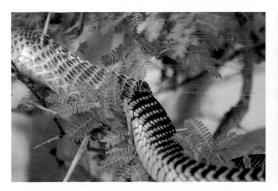

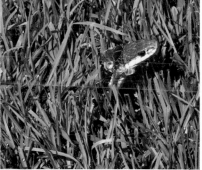

Figure 18.19A   Snake shedding its skin. Courtesy of shutterstock/Marietjie.

Figure 18.19B   Dysecdysis. Courtesy of shutterstock/JL Levy.

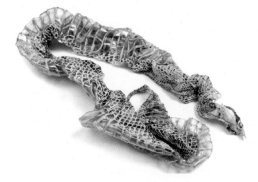

Figure 18.19C   Shed snake skin. Courtesy of shutterstock/Fribus Ekaterina.

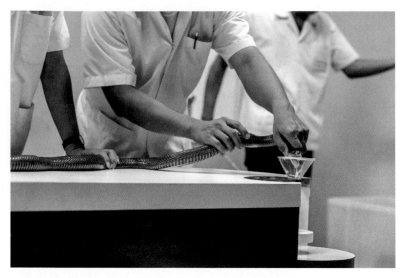

Figure 18.20 Collection of snake venom for production of antivenom. Courtesy of shutterstock/ LittleStocker.

Venom	Poison secreted by an animal or insect (Figure 18.20).
Venom gland	Salivary gland found in some snakes that produces venom.

Exercises

18-A: Give the term for the following definitions.

1. _____: Shedding and replacement of old feathers with new ones.
2. _____: External opening of the cloaca.
3. _____: Stomach of birds.
4. _____: Esophageal pouch near the throat of birds to temporarily store food.
5. _____: Intact male turkey.
6. _____: Order consisting of pigeons and doves.
7. _____: Developing feather with a blood supply.
8. _____: White portion of an egg.
9. _____: Fleshy part above the beak of birds.
10. _____: The breastbone of birds.

18-B: Define the following terms.

1. Clutch _____
2. Carapace _____
3. Ectotherm _____
4. Urodeum _____
5. Syrinx _____
6. Primary feathers _____
7. Cloaca _____

8. Yolk _____
9. Egg bound _____
10. Ecdysis _____

18-C: Circle the correct term in parentheses:

1. Small feathers that cover other feathers at the base. (barb, coverts, down)
2. Flight feathers of the wing. (rachis, rectrices, remiges)
3. Eyecap of a snake. (pit, scute, spectacle)
4. Material used on the bottom of a cage or tank. (scute, substrate, syrinx)
5. Bird cleaning its feathers. (bask, chalaza, preen)
6. A young bird whose wing feathers have just come in. (chick, fledgling, hatchling)
7. The wishbone of a bird. (coracoid, furcula, pygostyle)
8. Mid-portion of the oviduct known as the albumen-secreting zone. (isthmus, magnum, urodeum)
9. Group of birds including parrots and macaws. (aniserines, columbiformes, psittacines)
10. Tertiary bronchi that are tiny passages where gas exchange occurs. (apterium, choana, parabronchi)

18-D: List five functions of feathers.

1. _____
2. _____
3. _____
4. _____
5. _____

Answers can be found starting on page 571.

Go to www.wiley.com/go/taibo/terminology to find additional learning materials for this chapter:

• A crossword puzzle
• Flashcards
• Audio clips to show how to pronounce terms
• Case studies
• Review questions
• The figures from the chapter in PowerPoint

Chapter 19

Laboratory Animals

Laboratory animals are groups of animals used in laboratories for research. The category of laboratory animals is a broad one and can include anything from mice to nonhuman primates. This chapter focuses on the most commonly used laboratory animals. These animals are becoming more popular as pets and can be grouped into a category called pocket pets. Because these animals are not the typical dog and cat pets, they may also be considered exotic animals in some veterinary practices.

Rodents

Animals that fall in the order Rodentia include mice, rats, gerbils, hamsters, guinea pigs, and chinchillas. Rodents are a popular choice for research because they have short gestation periods and are therefore easy to observe for several generations.

Anatomically, all rodents share a similar dentition in that they generally lack canines and premolars. Rodents have a pair of upper and lower incisors which are used for gnawing and for defense. The number of molars varies depending on species.

Rats

Rats have pointed snouts and a long, almost hairless tail (Figure 19.1). They are nocturnal omnivores that originated in Asia. Throughout history these animals have been associated as disease-carrying pests causing such outbreaks as bubonic plague. The plague is actually caused by a flea, but because rats carried the fleas the outbreaks were associated with the rat population. Wild rats are carriers of many zoonotic diseases; however, pet rats are safe and typically disease free. While commonly used in research facilities, rats are also becoming popular as pets. The most common species today is the black rat, *Rattus rattus*, and the brown rat, *Rattus norvegicus*. Figure 19.2 shows the method of sexing rats using their anogenital distance—the distance between their anus and genitals.

Veterinary Medical Terminology Guide and Workbook, First Edition. Angela Taibo.
© 2014 John Wiley & Sons, Inc. Published 2014 by John Wiley & Sons, Inc.
Companion website: www.wiley.com/go/taibo/terminology

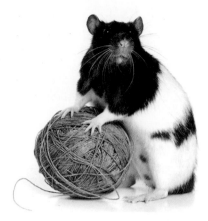

Figure 19.1A   Black and white rat. Courtesy of shutterstock.com/Utekhina Anna.

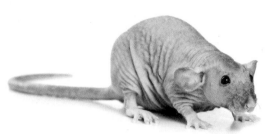

Figure 19.1B   Hairless rat. Courtesy of shutterstock.com/ Utekhina Anna.

(A)   (B)

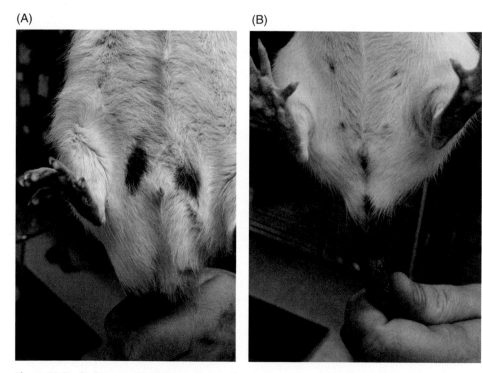

Figure 19.2   Sexing rats. (A) Male rat. (B) Female rat.

Mice

Like rats, mice are thought to have originated in Asia and have often been considered disease-carrying pests. However, like the rat, the mouse is a popular pet and is commonly used in research. Anatomically, the mouse and rat are similar with their pointed snouts and almost hairless tails. The internal anatomy is identical between the two species. The difference is that the mouse is much smaller. Mice have very poor eyesight and instead use their hearing and sense of smell to find food and detect predators. Mice are nocturnal omnivores that do best living in colonies of one male and multiple females. The most commonly seen species is *Mus musculus*, or house mouse. Figure 19.5 shows the anogenital difference between the male and female mouse.

Dam	Intact female rat or mouse (Figure 19.3).
Pup	Baby rat or mouse (Figure 19.3).
Pinkies	Newborn mice without fur (Figure 19.4).
Sire	Intact male rat or mouse (Figure 19.5).

(A)   (B)

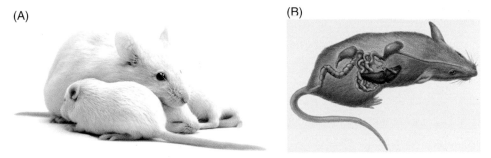

Figure 19.3   (A) Laboratory mice. A dam with her pups. Courtesy of shutterstock/anyaivanova. (B) Internal anatomy of a mouse. Courtesy of Getty Images/Dorling Kindersley.

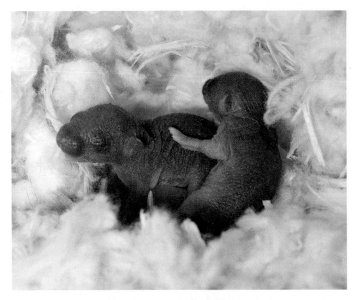

Figure 19.4   Pinkie mice. Courtesy of shutterstock.com/Jaroslav74.

(A)

(B)

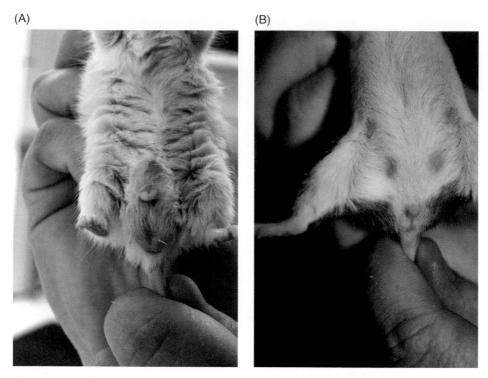

Figure 19.5   Sexing mice. (A) Male mouse. (B) Female mouse.

Gerbils

Gerbils are mouse-like animals with long, tufted tails which they use for balance while standing (Figure 19.6). Their movement and behavior are often described as kangaroo-like. Gerbils are diurnal omnivores thought to have originated in China. They are very social and easy to raise, which is why they are more popular than mice and rats as pets. A common problem with gerbils is tail sloughing, which

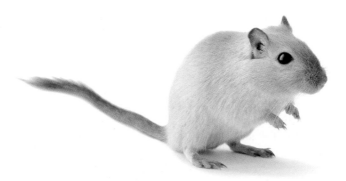

Figure 19.6   Gerbil. Courtesy of shutterstock.com/Anna Kucherova.

(A) (B)

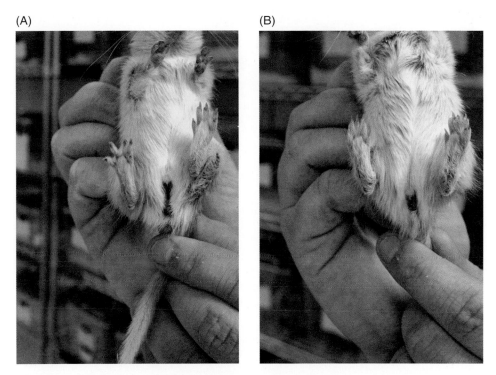

Figure 19.7 Sexing gerbils. (A) Male gerbil. (B) Female gerbil.

TECH TIP 19.1 Do You Know?

Gerbils and ferrets are illegal in the state of California. Several states and countries have restrictions on the ownership of ferrets. These laws were put in place due to concern about the animals escaping into the wild and altering the ecosystem.

---

results from improper restraint. Often new owners or children grab these animals by their tail and the tail breaks off when the gerbil tries to escape. The most common species of gerbil today is the Mongolian gerbil, which comes in a variety of colors. Sexing of gerbils is demonstrated in Figure 19.7.

Hamsters

Hamsters are popular as pets because of their cute teddy bear-like appearance (Figure 19.8). A variation of the hamster, the dwarf hamster, has risen in popularity because of its smaller size; however, it isn't as social as its larger counterparts. In general, hamsters are nocturnal omnivores with pronounced cheek pouches to temporarily store food. Unlike the previous rodents discussed, hamsters have a short, stubby tail and prefer to live alone. Figure 19.9 shows the differences between the male and female when sexing.

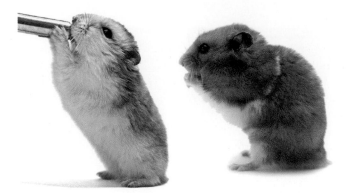

Figure 19.8   Hamsters. Courtesy of shutterstock/ADA_photo and shutterstock/AlexandreNunes.

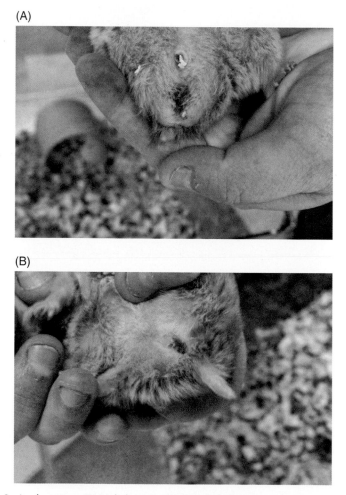

Figure 19.9   Sexing hamsters. (A) Male hamster. (B) Female hamster.

Guinea Pigs

Guinea pigs are popular as pets because of their easy-going nature (Figure 19.10). Commonly called **cavies**, guinea pigs have short, stout bodies and short, stubby legs. These animals originated in South America with the most common species being *Cavia porcellus*. Compared to the 20-day gestation period of mice, guinea pigs have a much longer gestation period of 63 days. Because of their longer gestation period, the newborns are much larger at birth which can create complications for the expectant female.

Guinea pigs are well known for their inability to synthesize vitamin C like other mammals. Owners must supplement their diets with food rich in Vitamin C to compensate for this.

Boar	Intact male guinea pig (Figure 19.11a).
Herd	Group of guinea pigs.
Pup	Young guinea pig (Figure 19.12).
Sow	Intact female guinea pig (Figure 19.11b).

(A)

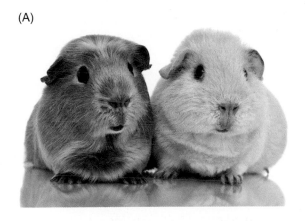

(B)

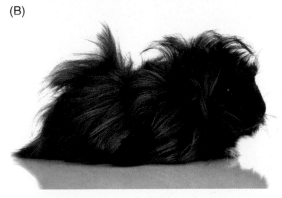

Figure 19.10   (A) American short-haired guinea pig. Courtesy of shutterstock/Photok.dk. (B) Peruvian guinea pig. Courtesy of shutterstock/Photok.dk.

(A)

(B)

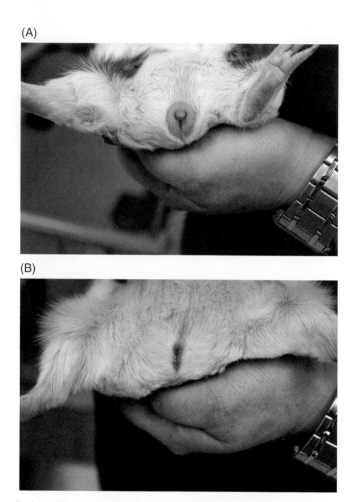

Figure 19.11   Sexing guinea pigs. (A) Male guinea pig. (B) Female guinea pig.

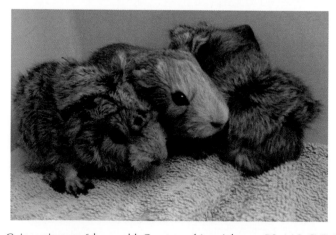

Figure 19.12   Guinea pig pups 6 hours old. Courtesy of Amy Johnson, BS, AAS, CVT, RLATG.

Chinchillas

Chinchillas are squirrel-like rodents well known for their thick, silver fur (Figure 19.13). Originating from South America, the most commonly seen species today is *Chinchilla laniger*. They are nocturnal omnivores with an unusual dentition compared to the previous rodents discussed. Chinchillas have premolars. Several species of Chinchilla have been extinct for years because they were hunted for their fur.

Chinchillas are known for their requirement of a dust bath. These animals can't get wet because their thick fur makes it impossible to get dry. If they get wet, the water can become trapped between their fur and skin, which can lead to fungal infections. To clean their fur, they are given a dust bath with dust from lava rocks or pumice. The dust absorbs the dirt and oils that accumulate on their fur and make it silky. It is also believed that the "dusting" is relaxing to the animal and helps to alleviate stress (Figure 19.14).

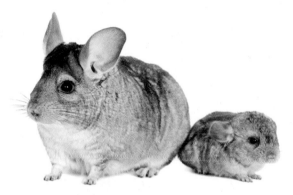

Figure 19.13   Chinchilla sow with her kit. Courtesy of shutterstock.com/Marina Jay.

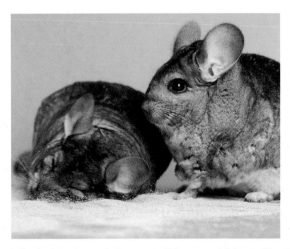

Figure 19.14   Chinchillas bathing in sand. Courtesy of shutterstock/Irina oxilixo Danilova.

Boar	Intact male chinchilla.
Herd	Group of chinchillas.
Kit	Young chinchilla.
Sow	Intact female chinchilla.

Ferrets

Ferrets are nocturnal carnivores with elongated, thin bodies that allow them to crawl into very small spaces (Figure 19.15). This is why ferrets were historically used for hunting small animals such as moles, rabbits, and rodents. Today, ferrets are used in research, as pets, and for hunting pests in certain countries. Like many rodents, ferrets have poor eyesight, especially in the daylight. Instead they use their keen senses of smell and hearing to find food and sense danger. Ferrets have all four types of teeth and scent glands similar to those of a skunk. When startled, ferrets can release their anal glands to detract enemies, so it is common for pet ferrets to be de-scented when purchased. De-scenting is the removal of the anal glands, which many believe to be inhumane. Even if de-scented, ferrets tend to have a musky smell. Common health issues in ferrets include insulinomas and canine distemper virus.

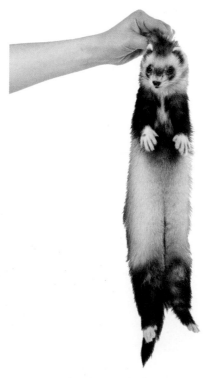

Figure 19.15 A ferret, shown with the scruff and hang technique used to restrain ferrets. Courtesy of shutterstock/IrinaK.

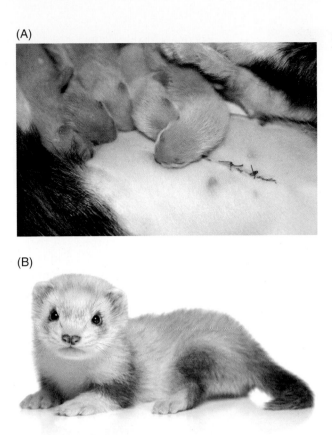

Figure 19.16 (A) Newborn ferrets from C-section. Courtesy of shutterstock/Radka Tesarova. (B) Kit. Courtesy of shutterstock/Jagodka.

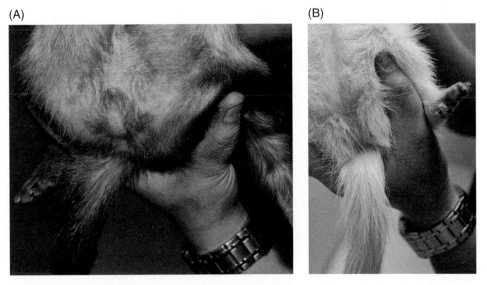

Figure 19.17 Sexing ferrets. (A) Male ferret. (B) Female ferret.

Gib	Neutered male ferret.
Hob	Intact male ferret.
Jill	Intact female ferret.
Kit	Young ferret (Figure 19.16).
Kindling	Giving birth to ferrets.
Sprite	Spayed female ferret.

Rabbits

Rabbits are animals that fall in the order Lagomorpha, so they are commonly called Lagomorphs (Figure 19.18). These animals are used in research, as pets, as food, and for their fur. While rabbits vary in size, their basic anatomy is the same (Figure 19.19). Their keen eyesight and hearing allow them to detect enemies and

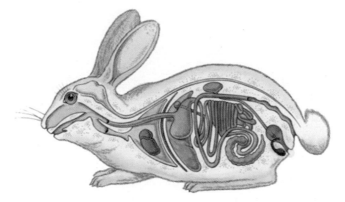

Figure 19.18   Internal anatomy of the rabbit. Courtesy of Getty Images/John Woodcock.

(A)   (B)

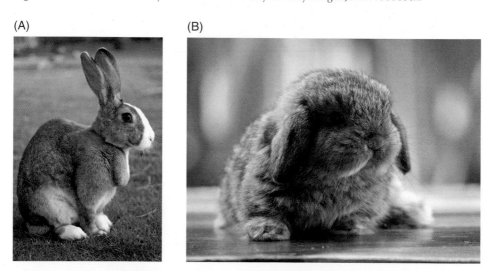

Figure 19.19   Breeds of rabbits. (A) Giant. Courtesy of shutterstock/Caroline Vancoillie. (B) Lop-eared. Courtesy of shutterstock/artemisphoto_. (C) Mini. Courtesy of shutterstock/Hayball. (D) Dwarf. Courtesy of shutterstock/oksana2010.

(C)

(D)

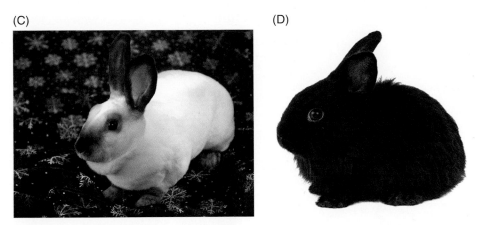

Figure 19.19 (Continued).

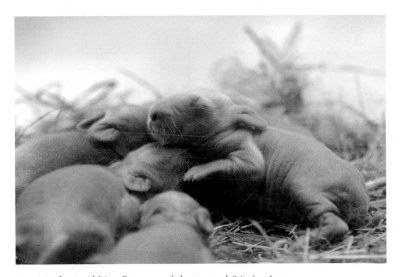

Figure 19.20 Newborn rabbits. Courtesy of shutterstock/Marina Jay.

their powerful hindlegs allow them to run fast or kick their predators. Care must be taken when restraining these animals because if done improperly, both the rabbit and restrainer can be hurt.

Rabbits are diurnal herbivores lacking canine teeth. Instead, they have two pairs of upper incisors. They are hindgut digesters with the bulk of digestion taking place in their large cecum. Therefore, nutrients may not be completely absorbed by the time the rabbit defecates. To compensate for this, rabbits are coprophagic so that they may re-ingest nutrients that had not been absorbed the first time. There are two types of feces from rabbits: feces still rich in nutrients and feces with processed roughage. Rabbits are unable to vomit, which can lead to serious health issues if foreign material such as fur is ingested.

(A)   (B)

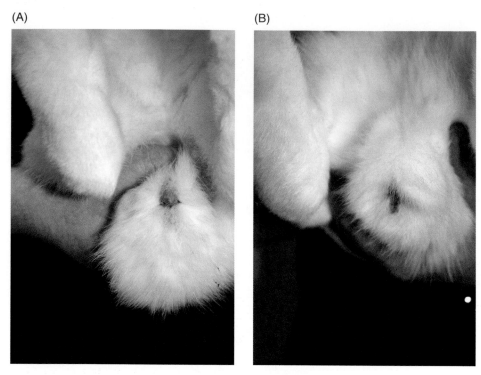

Figure 19.21   Sexing rabbits. (A) Male rabbit. (B) Female rabbit.

Buck	Intact male rabbit (Figure 19.21).
Doe	Intact female rabbit (Figure 19.21).
Herd	Group of rabbits.
Lapin	Neutered male rabbit.
Kit	Young rabbit.
Kindling	Giving birth to rabbits.

TECH TIP 19.2 Rabbits vs. Hares

Rabbits and hares are both lagomorphs; however, they are different species. Hares are much larger and considered wild, compared to species of rabbits that have been domesticated. Rabbits live in burrows and give birth to blind, hairless young. Hares live in nests above ground and give birth to young with hair and the ability to see. It is believed that because hares live above ground, it is necessary that their young can fend for themselves soon after birth.

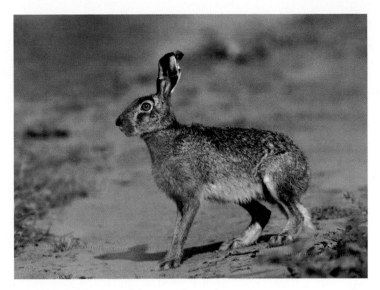

Figure 19.22   Wild hare. Courtesy of shutterstock/Borislav Borisov.

Professional Organizations and Laws

In 1966, the United States passed the Animal Welfare Act to ensure the humane treatment and care of animals used in research facilities. The United States Department of Agriculture inspects these facilities each year to ensure that the facilities meet or exceed the standards of these laws. The following are associations and laws that are in place to protect animals used in research facilities.

AAALAC	Association for Assessment and Accreditation of Laboratory Animal Care. This is a private, non-profit organization which facilities may voluntarily join to show that they treat animals humanely and exceed the standards set by laws. AAALAC inspects and accredits these organizations.
AALAS	American Association for Laboratory Animal Science. This organization is a membership program for laboratory professionals to communicate and find educational materials. AALAS certifies personnel in the laboratory animal field and provides materials for laboratory professionals.
ACLAM	American College of Laboratory Animal Medicine. This is a college that certifies licensed veterinarians in the laboratory animal field after they meet training requirements and take an exam. The college ensures the humane treatment of laboratory animals through their certification process.

APHIS   Animal and Plant Health Inspection Service. Agency of the
               United States Department of Agriculture which protects the
               health and wellbeing of plants and animals used in research.

AWA   Animal Welfare Act. Law passed by the United States to ensure
               the humane treatment and care of animals used in research
               facilities. APHIS and the USDA ensure that the laws are fol-
               lowed by research facilities.

FDA   Food and Drug Administration. Agency of the United States
               Department of Agriculture which protects the public through
               the inspection of food.

IACUC   Institutional Animal Care and Use Committee. Committee
               created by the research facility to ensure state requirements are
               followed.

NIH   National Institutes of Health. Agency of the United States
               Department of Agriculture to which the IACUC reports. NIH
               sets up the policies for the IACUC to follow.

PHS   Public Health Service. Division of the United States Department
               of Health which was created to protect, promote, and advance
               the health and safety of the American people.

USDA   United States Department of Agriculture. Government
               department that inspects research facilities each year to ensure
               that facilities meet or exceed the standards of the laws

Related Terms

The field of laboratory animal science is so broad that not all terms can be
discussed here. This section introduces basic laboratory animal terminology.

Axenic   Animal that is totally free of infection with
                        microorganisms.

Contact bedding   Bedding that an animal is in direct contact with
                        or will touch.

Crepuscular   Animal that is most active at dusk and/or
                        dawn.

Ecological typing   Classifies an animal based on microbiological
                        status. Examples include axenic, gnotobiotic,
                        or specific-pathogen free.

Genetic typing   Classifies an animal based on genetics.
                        Examples include inbred, outbred, or
                        transgenic.

Gnotobiotic   Animals whose microflora and microfauna are
                        known in complete detail.

Hybrid   Offspring from parents of different strains,
                        varieties, or species.

Hystricomorpha	Suborder of rodents consisting of guinea pigs, chinchillas, and porcupines.
Inbred	Strains resulting from the mating of closely related animals.
Lagomorpha	Taxonomic order of rabbits.
Murine	Pertaining to mice and rats.
Myomorpha	Suborder of rodents consisting of gerbils, hamsters, mice, and rats.
Noncontact bedding	Bedding that the animal will not touch; bedding in trays under the cage to help absorb waste.
Outbred	Stock from unrelated parents; also known as **random bred**.
Phenotype	Outward appearance of an animal including anatomical, physiological, and behavioral characteristics.
Progenitor	Ancestor or parent.
Progeny	Descendants or offspring.
Propagate	To reproduce.
Scuiromorpha	Suborder of rodents consisting of squirrels.
Scurvy	Disease caused by a deficiency of vitamin C.
Specific-pathogen free	An animal with normal flora bacteria. The bacterial agents may not be known, but the animal is free of specific bacterial agents. The animal is guaranteed to be free of specific pathogens.
Stock	Outbred animal lines and genetics.
Strain	Inbred animal lines and genetics.
Transgenic	An animal that has been genetically manipulated to contain DNA from another animal.

Exercises

19-A: Give the term for the following definitions.

1. _____: Intact male ferret.
2. _____: Young rabbit.
3. _____: Pertaining to mice and rats.
4. _____: Young guinea pig.
5. _____: Animal totally free of infection.
6. _____: To reproduce.
7. _____: Disease due to vitamin C deficiency.
8. _____: Animal most active at dusk or dawn.
9. _____: Offspring.
10. _____: Stock from unrelated parents.

19-B: Define the following terms.

1. Hybrid _____
2. Stock _____
3. Transgenic _____
4. Gnotobiotic _____
5. Lapin _____

19-C: Define the following abbreviations.

1. _____: IACUC   6. _____: AWA
2. _____: USDA   7. _____: FDA
3. _____: NIH   8. _____: PHS
4. _____: AALAS   9. _____: ACLAM
5. _____: APHIS 10. _____: AAALAC

16-E: Match the following animals with their taxonomic groups.

1. _____ Rabbits   A. Hystricomorpha
2. _____ Squirrels   B. Lagomorpha
3. _____ Guinea pigs, chinchillas, porcupines   C. Myomorpha
4. _____ Gerbils, hamsters, mice, rats   D. Sciuromorpha

Answers can be found starting on page 571.

Go to www.wiley.com/go/taibo/terminology to find additional learning materials for this chapter:

- A crossword puzzle
- Flashcards
- Audio clips to show how to pronounce terms
- Case studies
- Review questions
- The figures from the chapter in PowerPoint

Appendix A Pronunciation and Spelling of Terms Found in This Book

Similar Looks and Sounds of Terms

Spelling can be tricky with some of these medical terms. Just one letter can make a difference with certain words. For example, the terms hematoma and hepatoma look very similar on paper, but have very different meanings. Hematoma is a mass or collection of blood, whereas hepatoma is a tumor on the liver. Other terms may be pronounced exactly the same and have completely different meanings. For example, the ilium is a part of the pelvis and the ileum is the third part of the small intestine. Also be aware of terms with similar meanings. For example, the difference between a urethra and ureters. The urethra is a tube that transports urine from the urinary bladder to the outside of the body. The ureters are tubes that transport urine from the kidneys to the urinary bladder.

Spelling plays an important role in good record keeping. When hospitals are reviewed for accreditation, patient records are checked for detail and accuracy. Spelling is a part of that accuracy. In essence, you're writing in a legal document when you are writing in a patient file.

As a reminder, take advantage of the pronunciation section of the website that accompanies this book (www.wiley.com/go/taibo/terminology) which allows you to listen to how each term is pronounced.

Pronunciation of Certain Vowels

The symbols ˘ and ¯ above certain vowels help you sound out the vowels. For example, if the vowel has ¯ above it, the vowel sounds like the "capital form" or "long form" of itself. If the vowel has the ˘ above it, then it sounds like its "lowercase form" or "short form."

Veterinary Medical Terminology Guide and Workbook, First Edition. Angela Taibo.
© 2014 John Wiley & Sons, Inc. Published 2014 by John Wiley & Sons, Inc.
Companion website: www.wiley.com/go/taibo/terminology

ā	āte
ă	ăx
ē	ēleven
ĕ	ĕver
ī	pīe
ĭ	ĭnternal
ō	ōak
ŏ	lŏck
ū	ūnite
ŭ	ŭntie

Pronunciation of Certain Consonants

Consonants can have different sounds depending on what other letters they are attached to in a term. When viewing the pronunciation of terms pay attention to how the sounds of the consonants change in each term.

Rules for Plurals

There will always be exceptions to the following rules, but in general, these rules will apply:

Rule 1: If a word ends with "a," then add an "e" to make it plural. For example, the plural form of vertebra is vertebrae. The plural form of larva is larvae.

Rule 2: If a word ends with "um," then the plural form ends with an "a" instead of "um." For example, the plural form for bacterium is bacteria.

Rule 3: If a word ends with "is," then the plural form will end with "es." For example, the plural form of diagnosis is diagnoses. The plural form of metastasis is metastases.

Rule 4: If a word ends with "on," then the plural form will end with "a." For example, the plural form of ganglion is ganglia.

Rule 5: If a word ends with "ix" or "ex," then its plural form will end with "ices." For example, the plural form of index is indices.

Rule 6: If a word ends with "us," then its plural form will end with "i." For example, the plural form of nucleus is nuclei.

Pronunciation List of Medical Terms Found in This Book

Listen to an audio clip of bolded terms at www.wiley.com/go/taibo/terminology.

abdomen	Ăb-dō-mĕn	albino	ăl-BĪ-nō
abdominal	ăb-DŎM-ĭ-năl	albumin	ăl-BŪ-mĭn
abdominocentesis	ăb-dŏm-ĭ-nō-sĕn-TĒ-sĭs	albuminuria	ăl-bū-mĭ-NŪ-rē-ă
abducens	ăb-doo-sĕnz	aldosterone	ăl-DŎS-tĕ-rōn
abduction	ăb-DŬK-shŭn	alimentary	ăl-ĭ-MĔN-tăr-ē
ablation	ă-BLĀ-shŭn	alkaline phosphatase	ĂL-kă-lĭn FŎS-fă-tās
abomasum	ă-bō-MĀ-sŭm	allergen	Ăl-ĕr-jĕn
abortion	ă-BŎR-shŭn	allergy	Ăl-ĕr-jē
abscess	ĂB-sĕs	alopecia	ăl-ō-PĒ-shē-ă
absorption	ăb-SŌRP-shŭn	alveolar	ăl-VĒ-ō-lăr
accessory nerve	ăk-SĔS-ŏ-rē	alveoli; alveolus	ăl-VĒ-ō-lī; ăl-VĒ-ō-lŭs
accommodation	ă-kŏm-ō-DĀ-shŭn	amblyopia	ăm-blē-Ō-pē-ă
acetabular	ăs-ĕ-TĂB-ū-lăr	ambulatory	ĂM-bū-lă-tŏ-rē
acetabulum	ăs-ĕ-TĂB-ū-lŭm	amino acids	ă-MĒ-nō Ă-sĭdz
acetylcholine	ăs-ĕ-tĭl-KŌ-lēn	amniocentesis	ăm-nē-ō-sĕn-TĒ-sĭs
achalasia	ăk-ăh-LĀ-zē-ă	amnion	ĂM-nē-ŏn
achondroplasia	ā-kŏn-drō-PLĀ-zē-ă	amniotic fluid	ăm-nē-ŎT-ĭk FLOO-ĭd
acne	ĂK-nē	amniotic sac	ăm-nē-ŎT-ĭk SĂK
acoustic	ă-KOOS-tĭk	amphiarthroses	ăm-fē-ăr-THRŌ-sēs
acromegaly	ăk-rō-MĔG-ă-lē	amputation	ăm-pū-TĀ-shŭn
acromion	ă-KRŌ-mē-ŏn	amylase	ĂM-ĭ-las
acrophobia	ăk-rō-FŌ-bē-ă	anabolic	ăn-ă-BŎL-ĭc
acuity	ă-KŪ-ĭ-tē	anabolism	ă-NĂB-ō-lĭzm
acute	ă-KŪT	anal	Ā-năl
Addison's disease	ĂD ĭ-sŏn dĭ-ZĒZ	anal sac	Ā-nal săk
adduction	ă-DŬK-shŭn	anal sacculitis	Ā-năl săk-ū-LĪ-tĭs
adenectomy	ăd-ĕ-NĔK-tō-mē	analgesia	ăn-ăl-JĒ-zē-ă
adenitis	ăd-ĕ-NŎP-ă-thē	analysis	ă-NĂL-ĭ-sĭs
adenohypophysis	ăd-ĕ-nō-hī-PŎF-ĭ-sĭs	anaphylaxis	ăn-ă-fĭ-LĂK-sĭs
adenoidectomy	ăd-ĕ-noyd-ĔK-tō-mē	anastomosis	ă-năs-tō-MŌ-sĭs
adenoids	Ăd-ĕ-noydz	androgen	ĂN-drō-jĕn
adenoma	ăd-ĕ-NŌ-mă	anemia	ă-NĒ-mē-ă
adenopathy	ăd-ĕ-NĪ-tĭs	anencephaly	ăn-ĕn-SĔF-ă-lē
adhesion	ăd-HĒ-shŭn	anesthesia	ăn-ĕs-THĒ-zē-ă
adipose	Ă-dĭ-pōs	anestrus	ăn-ĔS-trŭs
adrenal	ă-DRĒ-năl	aneurysm	ĂN-ūr-ĭ-zĭm
adrenalectomy	ă-drē-năl-ĔK-tō-mē	angiogenesis	ăn-jē-ō-JĔN-ĕ-sĭs
adrenaline	ă-DRĔN-ă-lĭn	angiogram	ĂN-jē-ō-grăm
adrenectomy	ă-drē-ĔK-tō-mē	angiography	ăn-jē-ŎG-ră-fē
adrenocoricotropic hormone	ă-drē-nō-kŏr-tĭ-kō-TRŌP-ĭk HŌR-mŏn	angiopathy	ăn-jē-ŎP-ă-thē
		angioplasty	ăn-jē-ō-PLĂS-tē
adrenopathy	ă-drē-NŎP-ă-thē	angiorrhaphy	ăn-jē-ŎR-ă-fē
agalactia	ā-gă-LĂK-tē-ă	anisocoria	ăn-ē-sō-KŌ-rē-ă
agglutination	ă-gloo-tĭ-NĀ-shŭn	anisocytosis	ăn-ē-sō-sī-TŌ-sĭs
agonal	Ă-gŭ-nŭl	anisokaryosis	ăn-ē-sō-KĂR-ē-ō-sĭs
agranulocytes	ā-GRĂN-ū-lō-sīt	ankylosis	ăng-kĭ-LŌ-sĭs
akinetic	ā-kĭ-NĔT-ĭk	anomaly	ă-NŎM-ă-lē
alanine	ĂL-ă-nēn or ĂL-ă-nĭn	anophthalmos	ăn-ŏf-THĂL-mŏs
aminotransferase	ă-mē-nō-trănz-fĕr-ās	anoplasty	ā-nō-PLĂS-tē

anorchism	ăn-ŎR-kĭzm	arthrocentesis	ăr-THRŌ-sĕn-TĒ-sĭs
anorectal	ā-nō-RĔK-tăl	arthrodesis	ăr-thrō-DĒ-sĭs
anorexia	ăn-ō-RĔK-sē-ă	arthrodial joint	ăr-THRŌ-dē-ăl joynt
anovulation	ăn-ŎV-ū-lā-shŭn	arthrography	ăr-THRŎG-ră-fē
anoxia	ă-NŎK-sē-ă	arthrology	ăr-THRŌL-ō-jē
antagonist	ăn-TĂ-gō-nĭst	arthropathy	ăr-THRŎP-ă-thē
antecibum	ĂN-tē-SĒ-bŭm	arthroplasty	ăr-thrō-PLĂS-tē
antepartum	ĂN-tē-PĂR-tŭm	arthroscope	ăr-THRŌ-skōp
anterior	ăn-TĒ-rē-ŏr	arthroscopy	ăr-THRŌ-skō-pē
anterior chamber	ăn-TĒ-rē-ŏr CHĀM-bĕr	arthrosis	ăr-THRŌ-sĭs
anterior cruciate	ăn-TĒ-rē-ŏr KROO-shē-ĭt	arthrotomy	ăr-THRŌ-tō-mĕ
ligament	LĬG-ă-mĕnt	articular cartilage	ăr-TĬK-ū-lăr KĂR-tĭ-lăj
antibiotic	ăn-tĭ-tī-ŎT-ĭk	articulation	ăr-tĭk-ū-LĀ-shŭn
antibody	ĂN-tĭ-bŏd-ē	artifical insemination	ăr-tĭ-FĬSH-ăl
anticoagulant	ăn-tī-kō-ĂG-ū-lănt		ĭn-sĕm-ĭ-NĀ-shŭn
antidiarrheal	ăn-tī-dī-ū-RĒ-ăl	ascending colon	ă-SĔN-dĭng KŌ-lĕn
antidiuretic hormone	ăn-tī-dī-ū-RĒ-tĭk HŎR-mōn	ascites	ă-SĪ-tēz
antiemetic	ăn-tī-ĕ-MĔ-tĭk	aspermia	ā-SPĔR-mē-ă
antigen	ĂN-tĭ-jĕn	asphyxia	ăs-FĬK-sē-ă
antipyretic	ăn-tī-pī-RĔT-ĭk	aspiration	ăs-pĕ-RĀ-shŭn
antisepsis	ăn-tī-SĔP-sĭs	asthma	ĂZ-mă
antitoxin	ăn-tī-TŎK-sĭn	astroglial	ăs-trō-GLĒ-ăl sĕl
antitussives	ăn-tē-TŬ-sĭvz	asystole	ā-SĬS-tō-lē
antrum	ĂN-trŭm	ataxia	ā-TĂK-sē-ă
anuria	ăn-Ū-rē-ă	atelectasis	ă-tĕ-LĔK-tă-sĭs
anus	Ā-nŭs	atherosclerosis	ăth-ĕr-ō-sklĕ-RŌ-sĭs
aorta	ā-ŎR-tă	atlanto-axial	ăt-LĂN-tō-ĂX-ē-ăl joynt
aortic stenosis	ā-ŎR-tĭk stĕ-NŌ-sĭs	joint	
aortic valve	ā-ŎR-tĭk vălv	atlanto-occipital	ăt-LĂN-tō-ŏk-SĬP-ĭ-tăl
apex	Ā-pĕkz	joint	joynt
aplastic anemia	ā-PLĂS-tĭk ă-NĒ-mē-ă	atopy	ĂT-ō-pē
apnea	ĂP-nē-ă	atresia	ā-TRĔ-zē-ă
apocrine gland	ĂP-ō-krĭn glănd	atria; atrium	Ā-trē-ă; Ā-trē-ŭm
appendicular	ăp-ĭn-DĬK-ū-lăr	atrial	Ā-trē-ăl
appendicular	ăp-ĕn-DĬK-ū-lăr	atrioventricular	ā-trē-ō-vĕn-TRĬK-ū-lăr
skeleton	SKĔL-ĭ-tĭn	atrophy	ĂT-rō-fē
aqueous humor	Ā-kwē-ŭs or ĂK-wē-ŭs	audiometry	ăw-dē-ŎM-ĕ-trē
	HŪ-mĕr	auditory	ăw-dĭ-TŌ-rē
arachnoid membrane	ă-RĂK-noyd MĔM-brăn	auditory canal	ăw-dĭ-TŌ-rē kă-NĂL
arcade	ăr-KĀD	aural	ĂW-răl
arrector pili	ă-RĔK-tĕr PĒ-lē	auricle	ĂW-rĭ-kŭl
arrhythmia	ā-RĬTH-mē-ă	auricular	ăw-RĬK-ū-lăr
arterial	ăr-TĒ-rē-ăl	auscultation	ăw-skŭl-TĀ-shŭn
arteriectomy	ăr-tē-rē-ĔK-tō-mē	autoimmune	ăw-tō-ĭ-MŪN
arteriography	ăr-tē-rē-ŎG-ră-fē	autonomic nervous	ăw-tō-NŎM-ĭk
arteriole	ăr-TĔR-ē-ōl	system	NĔR-vŭs SĬS-tĕm
arteriosclerosis	ăr-tē-rē-ō-sklĕ-RŌ-sĭs	axial	ĂX-ē-ăl
arteriotomy	ăr-tē-rē-ŎT-ō-mē	axial skeleton	ĂX-ē-ăl SKĔL-ĭ-tĭn
artery	ĂR-tĕ-rē	axillary	ĂK-sĭ-lăr-ē
arthralgia	ăr-THRŎL-jă	axon	ĂK-sŏn
arthrectomy	ăr-THRĔK-tō-mē	azoospermia	ā-zō-ō-SPĔR-mē-ă
arthritis	ăr-THRĪ-tĭs	azotemia	ā-zō-TĒ-mē-ă

bacteriuria	băk-tē-rē-Ū-rē-ă	bronchoscopy	brŏng-KŎS-kō-pē
balanitis	băl-ă-NĪ-tĭs	bronchospasm	BRŎNG-kō-spăsm
barium study	BĂR-ē-ŭm STŬ-dē	bruxism	BRŬK-sĭ-zŭm
basal layer	BĀ-săl LĀ-ĕr	buccal	BŬK-ăl
basophil	BĀ-sō-fĭl	bulbourethral gland	bŭl-bō-ū-RĒ-thrăl glănd
benign	bē-NĪN	bulla; bullae	BŬL-ă; BŬL-ē
bicornuate	bī-KŎR-nāt	bundle of His	BŬN-dl of Hĭss
bicuspid valve	bī-KŬS-pĭd vălv	bursa; bursae	BĔR-să; BĔR-sē
bifurcation	bī-fŭr-KĀ-shŭn	bursitis	bĕr-SĪ-tĭs
bilateral	bī-LĂT-ĕr-ăl		
bile	BĪL	cachexia	kă-KĔK-sē-ă
biliary	BĬL-ē-ăr-ē	calcaneal	kăl-KĀ-nē-ăl
bilirubin	bĭl-ē-ROO-bĭn	calcaneus	kăl-KĀ-nē-ŭs
binocular	bī-NŎK-ū-lăr	calcification	kăl-sĭ-fĭ-KĀ-shŭn
biochemistries	bī-ō-KĔM-ĭs-trēz	calcitonin	kăl-sĭ-TŌ-nĭn
biological	bī-ō-LŎG-ĭk-ăl	calcium	KĂL-sē-ŭm
biologist	bī-ŎL-ō-jĭst	calculi	KĂL-kū-lī
biology	bī-ŎL-ō-jē	calici	kă-LĒ-sē
biopsy	BĪ-ŏp-sē	callus	KĂL-ŭs
blepharectomy	blĕf-ă-RĔK-tō-mē	calyces; calyx	KĀ-lĭ-sēz; KĀ-lĭks
blepharitis	blĕf-ă-RĪ-tĭs	cancellous bone	KĂN-sĕ-lŭs bōn
blepharoplasty	blĕ-fă-rō-PLĂS-tē	canine	KĀ-nīn
blepharoptosis	blĕ-fă-rŏp-TŌ-sĭs	canthectomy	kănth-ĔK-tō-mē
blepharorrhaphy	blĕ-fă-RŎR-ă fē	canthotomy	kănth-ŎT-ō-mē
blepharospasm	BLĔ-fă-rō-spăzm	canthus	KĂN-thŭs
blepharotomy	blĕ-fă-RŎT-ō-mē	capillary	KĂP-ĭ-lăr-ē
blood	blŭd	caprine	KĂP-rīn
bolus	BŌ-lŭs	carbon dioxide	kăr-bŏn dī-ŎK-sīd
bone marrow	bōn MĂ-rō	carcinogen	kăr-SĬN-ō-jĕn
borborygmus	bŏr-bō-RĬG-mŭs	carcinogenesis	kăr-sĭ-nō-JĔN-ĕ-sĭs
bovine	BŌ-vīn	carcinogenic	kăr-sĭ-nō-JĔN-ĭk
bovine respiratory	BŌ-vīn RĔS-pĭr-ă-tō-rē	carcinoma	kăr-sĭ-NŌ-mă
syncytial virus	sĭn-SĬSH-ăl VĪ-rŭs	cardiac	KĂR-dē-ăk
bovine spongiform	BŌ-vīn SPŬN-jĭ-fŏrm	cardiac muscle	KĂR-dē-ăk MŬS-ĕl
encephalopathy	ĕn-sĕf-ă-LŎP-ă-thē	cardiac tamponade	KĂR-dē-ăk tăm-pō-NŎD
bovine viral diarrhea	BŌ-vĭn VĪ-răl dī-ă-RĒ-ă	cardiology	kăr-dē-ŎL-ō-jē
bowel	BŎW-ĕl	cardiomegaly	kăr-dē-ō-MĔG-ă-lē
Bowman's capsule	BŌ-măn KĂP-sŭl	cardiomyopathy	kăr-dē-ō-mī-ŎP-ă-thē
brachial	BRĀ-kē-ăl	cardiopathy	kăr-dē-ŎP-ă-thē
brachycephalic	BRĀ-kē-sĕ-FĂL-ĭk	cardiopulmonary	kăr-dē-ō-PŬL-mō-nĕr-ē
brachygnathia	bră-kē-gNĀ-thē-ā	cerebral	sĕ-RĒ-brăl
bradycardia	brăd-ē-KĂR-dē-ă	resuscitation	rē-sŭ-sĭ-TĀ-shŭn
bradykinesia	bră-dē-kĭ-NĒ-zē-ă	cardiopulmonary	kăr-dē-ō-PŬL-mō-nĕr-ē
bradypnea	bră-DĬP-nē-ă	resuscitation	rē-sŭ-sĭ-TĀ-shŭn
brainstem	BRĀN-stĕm	carditis	kăr-DĪ-tĭs
bronchi; bronchus	BRŎNG-kī; BRŎNG-kŭs	carpals	KĂR-pălz
bronchial	BRŎNG-kē-ăl	carpus	KĂR-pŭs
bronchiectasis	brŏng-kē-ĔK-tă-sĭs	cartilage	KĂR-tĭ-lĭj
bronchiole	BRŎNG-kē-ōl	castration	kăs-TRĀ-shŭn
bronchiolitis	brŏng-kē-ō-LĪ-tĭs	catabolic	căt-ă-BŎL-ĭc
bronchitis	brŏng-KĪ-tĭs	catabolism	kă-TĂB-ō-lĭzm
bronchodilators	brŏng-kō-DĪ-lā-tĕr	cataplexy	KĂT-ŭ-plĕk-sē

cataract	KĂT-ă-răkt	chondral	KŎN-drăl
catecholamines	kăt-ě-KŌL-ă-mēnz	chondralgia	kŏn-DRĂL-jă
catheter	KĂ-thě-těr	chondrectomy	kŏn-DRĔK-tō-mē
catheterization	kăth-ě-těr-ĭ-ZĀ-shŭn	chondrocostal	kŏn-drō-KŎS-tăl
cauda equina	KĂW-dă ě-KWĪ-nă	chondroma	kŏn-DRŌ-mă
caudal	KAWD-ăl	chondromalacia	kŏn-DRŌ-mă-LĀ-shă
cauterization	kăw-těr-ĭ-ZĀ-shŭn	chondrosarcoma	kŏn-drō-săr-KŌ-mă
cecal	SĒ-kăl	chorion	KŌ-rē-ŏn
cecum	SĒ-kŭm	choroid	KŎR-oyd
celiac	SĒ-lē-ăk	choroid plexus	KŎR-oyd PLĔK-sŭs
cell membrane	sěl MĔM-brăn	chromosomes	KRŌ-mō-sōm
cellulitis	sěl-ū-LĪ-tĭs	chronic	KRŎN-ĭk
cementum	sē-MĔN-tŭm	cilia	SĬL-ē-ă
centrioles	SĔN-trē-ōl	ciliary body	SĬL-ē-ăr-ē BŎ-dē
cephalic	sě-FĂL-ĭk	circulation	sěr-kū-LĀ-shŭn
cerebellar	sěr-ě-BĔL-ăr	cirrhosis	sĭr-RŌ-sĭs
cerebellum	sěr-ě-BĔL-ŭm	clavicle	KLĂV-ĭ-kŭl
cerebral	sě-RĒ-brăl	clitoris	KLĬ-tō-rĭs
cerebrospinal fluid	sěr-ě-brō-SPĪ-năl FLŪ-ĭd	coagulation	kō-ăg-ū-LĀ-shŭn
cerebrovascular	sě-RĔ-brō-VĂS-kū-lăr	coagulopathy	kō-ăg-ū-LŎP-ă-thē
cerebrum	sě-RĒ-brŭm	coccygeal	kŏk-sĭ-JĒ-ăl
cerumen	sě-ROO-měn	cochlea	KŎK-lē-ă
cervical	SĔR-vĭ-kăl	cochlear	KŎK-lē-ăr
cervicitis	sěr-vĭ-SĪ-tĭs	coitus	KŌ-ĭ-tŭs
cervix	SĔR-vĭks	colectomy	kō-LĔK-tō-mě
cesarean section	sě-SĀ-rē-ăn SĔK-shŭn	colic	KŎL-ĭk
chalazion	kă-LĀ-zē-ŏn	colitis	kō-LĪ-tĭs
cheilosis	kī-LŌ-sĭs	collagen	KŎL-ă-jěn
chemonucleolysis	kē-mō-nū-klē-ŎL-ĭ-sĭs	colon	KŌ-lěn
chemotherapy	kē-mō-THĔR-ě-pē	colonectomy	kō-lěn-ĔK-tō-mē
cholangiectasia	kŏl-ăn-jē-ěk-TĀ-zē-ă	colonic	kō-LŎN-ĭk
cholangiocarcinoma	kŏl-ăn-jē-ō-kăr-sĭ-NŌ-mă	colonitis	kō-lŏn-Ī-tĭs

cholangio-
    enterostomy
	kŏl-ăn-jē-ō-ěn-tě-RŎS-
	    tō-mē
		colonopathy	kō-lŏn-Ŏ-pă-thē

cholangio-
    gastrostomy
	kŏl-ăn-jē-ō-găs-TRŎS-
	    tō-mē
		colonoscopy	kō-lŏn-ŎS-kō-pē

		colostomy	kō-LŎS-tō-mē
		colostrom	kō-LŎ-strŭm
cholangiohepatitis	kŏl-ăn-jē-ō-hěp-ă-TĪ-tĭs	colotomy	kō-LŎ-tō-mē
cholangiostomy	kŏl-ăn-jē-ŎS-tō-mē	colporrhaphy	kŏl-PŎR-ă-fē
cholecystectomy	kō-lē-sĭs-TĔK-tō-mē	colposcopy	kŏl-PŎS-kō-pē
cholecystic	kō-lē-SĬS-tĭk	coma	KŌ-mă
cholecystitis	kō-lē-sĭ-STĪ-tĭs	comatose	KŌ-mă-tōs

cholecystoje-
    junostomy
	kō-lē-sĭs-tō-jě-jū-NŎS-
	    tō-mē
		comedo; comedones	KŎM-ě-dō; kŏm-ě-DŌNZ

		common bile duct	KŎ-mŭn BĪL dŭkt
cholecystolithiasis	kō-lē-sĭs-tō-lĭ-THĪ-ă-sĭs	compact bone	KŎM-păkt bōn
choledochal	kō-lē-DŎK-ăl	conception	kŏn-SĔP-shŭn

choledochoje-
    junostomy
	kō-lēd-ō-kō-jĭ-jū-NŎS-
	    tō-mē
		concussion	kŏn-KŬS-shŭn

		condyle	KŎN-dĭl
choledocholithiasis	kō-lēd-ō-kō-lĭ-THĪ-ă-sĭs	congenital	kŏn-JĔN-ĭ-tăl

choledochotomy	kō-lēd-ō-KŎT-ō-mē	congestive heart
		    failure
			kŏn-GĔS-tĭv hărt
			    FĀL-ŭr

cholelithiasis	kō-lē-lĭ-THĪ-ă-sĭs		
cholestasis	kō-lē-STĀ-sĭs	conjunctiva	kŏn-jŭnk-TĪ-vă
cholesterol	kŭ-LĔS-těr-ŏl	conjunctival	kŏn-jŭnk-TĪ-văl

conjunctivits	kŏn-jŭnk-tĭ-VĪ-tĭs	cystostomy	sĭs-TŎS-tō-mē
conjunctivoplasty	kŏn-JŬNK-tĭ-vō-plăs-tē	cystotomy	sĭs-TŎ-tō-mē
conscious	KŎN-shŭs	cytological	sī-tŏ-LŎG-ĭc-ăl
constipation	cŏn-stĭ-PĀ-shŭn	cytologist	sī-TŎL-ō-jĭst
contract	kŭn-TRĂKT	cytology	sī-TŎL-ō-jē
contraction	kŭn-TRĂK-shŭn	cytoplasm	SĪ-tō-plăzm
contraindication	kŏn-tră-ĭn-dĭ-KĀ-shŭn		
contralateral	kŏn-tră-LĂT-ĕr-ăl	dacryoadenitis	dăk-rē-ō-ăd-ĕ-NĪ-tĭs
contusion	kŏn-TŪ-shŭn	dacryocystectomy	dăk-rē-ō-sĭs-TĚK-tō-mē
coprophagia	kŏ-prō-FĀ-jē-ă	dacryocystitis	dăk-rē-ō-sĭs-TĪ-tĭs
coprophagic	kŏ-prō-FĀ-jĭk	dacryocystotomy	dăk-rē-ō-sĭs-TŎ-tō-mē
copulation	kŏp-ū-LĀ-shŭn	debridement	dĭ-BRĒD-mĭnt
cornea	KŎR-nē-ă	decalcificataion	dē-kăl-sĭ-fĭ-KĀ-shŭn
corneal	KŎR-nē-ăl	deciduous teeth	dĭ-SĬ-dū-ŭs tēth
corneoscleral	kŏr-nē-ō-SKLĚ-răl	decubitus ulcers	dē-KŪ-bĭ-tŭs Ŭl-sĕrs
corona	kŭ-RŌ-nă	defecation	dĕf-ĕ-KĀ-shŭn
coronary arteries	KŎR-ō-năr-ē ĂR-tĕ-rēz	degloving	dē-GLŪ-vĭng
cortex	KŎR-tĕks	deglutition	dē-glū-TĬ-shŭn
cortical	KŎR-tĭ-kăl	dehydration	dē-hī-DRĀ-shŭn
corticosteroid	kŏr-tĭ-kō-STĚ-royd	dendrite	DĚN-drīt
cortisol	KŎR-tĭ-sŏl	dental calculus	DĚN-tăl KĂL-kū-lŭs
cortisone	KŎR-tĭ-zŏn	dental caries	DĚN-tăl KĂR-ēz
costal	KŎS-tăl	dentin	DĚN-tĭn
cough	KŎF	dentition	dĕn-TĬ-shŭn
coxofemoral	kŏk-sō-FĚM-ŏr-ăl	deoxygenated	dē-ŎK-sĭ-jĕ-NĀ-tĕd
cranial	KRĀ-nē-ăl	dermatitis	dĕr-mă-TĪ-tĭs
cranioplasty	KRĀ-nē-ō-plăs-tē	dermatologist	dĕr-mă-TŎL-ŏ-jĭst
craniosacral	KRĀ-nē-ō-SĀ-krăl	dermatology	dĕr-mă-TŎL-ŏ-jē
craniotome	KRĀ-nē-ō-tōm	dermatomycosis	dĕr-mă-tō-mī-KŌ-sĭs
craniotomy	krā-nē-ŎT-ō-me	dermis	DĚR-mĭs
creatinine	krē-ĂT-ĭ-nēn	descending colon	dē-SĚN-dĭng KŌ-lĕn
crepitation	krĕ-pĭ-TĀ-shŭn	dexamethasone	dĕk-sŭ-MĚTH-ŭ-sōn
crepitus	KRĚP-ĭ-tŭs	diabetes insipidus	dī-ă-BĒ-tēz ĭn-SĬP-ĭ-dŭs
crest	krĕst	diabetes mellitus	dī-ă-BĒ-tē MĚL-ĭ-tŭs
crown	krŏwn	diabetic ketoacidosis	dī-ă-BĚT-ĭk
cryosurgery	krī-ō-SŪR-jĕr-ē		kē-tō-ă-sĭ-DŌ-sĭs
cryptorchid	krĭp-TŎR-kĭd	diagnosis	dī-ăg-NŌ-sĭs
cryptorchism	krĭp-TŎR-kĭzm	dialysis	dī-ĂL-ĭ-sĭs
crystalluria	krī-stăl-Ū-rē-ă	diameter	dī-ĂM-ĭ-tĕr
culture	KŬL-chĕr	diapedesis	dī-ă-pĭ-DĒ-sĭs
Cushing syndrome	KŬSH-ĭng SĬN-drōm	diaphragm	DĪ-ă-frăm
cyanosis	sī-ă-NŌ-sĭs	diaphragmatic	dī-ă-frăg-MĂ-tĭk
cyanotic	sī-ă-NŌT-ĭk	hernia	HĚR-nē-ă
cyst	sĭst	diaphyses	dī-ĂF-ĭ-sēs
cystalgia	sĭs-TĂL-jă	diaphysis	dī-ĂF-ĭ-sĭs
cystectomy	sĭs-TĚK-tō-mē	diarrhea	dī-ă-RĒ-ă
cystitis	sĭs-TĪ-tĭs	diarthroses	dī-ăr-THRŌ-sēs
cystocele	SĬS-tō-sēl	diastole	dī-ĂS-tō-lē
cystocentesis	sĭs-TŌ-sĕn-TĒ-sĭs	diestrus	dī-ĚS-trŭs
cystogram	sĭs-TŌ-grăm	diethylstilbestrol	dī-ĕth-ĭl-stĭl-BĚ-strŏl
cystopexy	sī-tŏ-PĚK-sē	diffusion	dĭ-FŪ-zhŭn
cystoscopy	sĭs-TŎS-kō-pē	digestion	dĭ-JĚST-yŭn

dilation	dī-LĀ-shŭn	electromyogram	ē- lĕk-trō-MĪ-ō-grăm
disk (disc)	dĭsk	electromyography	ē- lĕk-trō-mī-ŎG-ră-fē
dislocation	dĭs-lō-KĀ-shŭn	electroretinography	ē-lĕk-trō-rĕ-tĭn-ŎG-ră-fē
disseminated	dĭs-SĔM-ĭ-nā-tĕd	elimination	ē-lĭm-ĭ-NĀ-shŭn
intravascular	ĭn-tră-VĂS-kū-lăr	emaciation	ē-mā-sē-Ā-shŭn
coagulation	kō-ăg-ū-LĀ-shŭn	emboli; embolus	ĔM-bō-lī; ĔM-bō-lŭs
distal	DĬS-tăl	embolism	ĔM-bō-lĭzm
distemper	dĭs-TĔM-pĕr	embryo	ĔM-brē-ō
distichiasis	dĭs-tĭ-KĪ-ă-sĭs	emesis	Ĕ-mĭ-sĭs
diuresis	dī-ŭr-RĒ-sĭs	emetic	ĕ-MĚ-tĭk
diverticulitis	dī-vĕr-tĭk-ū-LĪ-tĭs	emphysema	ĕm-fĭ-ZĒ-mă
diverticulum	dī-vĕr-TĬK-ū-lŭm	empyema	ĕm-pī-Ē-mă
dolichocephalic		emulsification	ē-mŭl-sĭ-fĭ-KĀ-shŭn
dopamine	DŌ-pă-mēn	enamel	ē-NĂM-ĕl
dorsal	DŎR-săl	enarthroses	ĕn-ăr-THRŌ-sēs
dorsiflexion	dŏr-sē-FLĔK-shŭn	encephalic	ĕn-sĕ-FĂL-ĭk
drench	drĕnch	encephalitis	ĕn-sĕf-ă-LĪ-tĭs
duodenal	dū-ŎD-dĕ-năl or	encephalocele	ĕn-SĔF-ă-lō-sēl
	dū-ō-DĒ-năl	encephalogram	ē-lĕk_trō-ĕn-SĔF-ă-lō-
duodenum	dū-ŎD-dĕ-nŭm or		grăm
	dū-ō-DĒ-nŭm	encephalography	ē-lĕk_trō-ĕn-SĔF-ă-
dura mater	DŬR-ă MĂT-tĕr		LŎG-ră-fē
dyschezia	dĭs-KĒ-zē-ă	encephalomyelitis	ĕn-sĕf-ă-lō-mī-ĕ-LĪ-tĭs
dyscrasia	dĭs-KRĀ-zē-ă	encephalopathy	ĕn-sĕf-ă-LŎP-ă-thē
dyspepsia	dĭs-PĔP-sē-ă	endarterectomy	ĕnd-ăr-tĕr-ĔK-tō-mē
dysphagia	dĭs-FĀ-jē-ă	endocarditis	ĕn-dō-kăr-DĪ-tĭs
dysplasia	dĭs-PLĀ-zē-ă	endocardium	ĕn-dō-KĂR-dē-ŭm
dyspnea	DĬSP-nē-ă	endocervicitis	ĕn-dō-sĕr-vĭs-SĪ-tĭs
dystocia	dĭs-TŌ-sē-ă	endocrine gland	ĔN-dō-krĭn glăndz
dysuria	dĭs-Ū-rē-ă	endocrinologist	ĕn-dō-krĭ-NŎL-ō-jĭst
		endocrinology	ĕn-dō-krĭ-NŎL-ō-jē
ecchymoses;	ĕk-ĭ-MŌ-sēz; ĕk-ĭ-	endolymph	ĔN-dō-lĭmf
ecchymosis	MŌ-sĭs	endometriosis	ĕn-dō-mē-trē-Ō-sĭs
eccrine gland	ĕk-rĭn glănd	endometritis	ĕn-dō-mē-TRĪ-tĭs
echocardiogram	ĕk-ō-KĂR-dē-ō-grăm	endometrium	ĕn-dō-MĒ-trē-ŭm
eclampsia	ĕ-KLĂMP-sē-ă	endoplasmic	ĕn-dō-PLĂZ-mĭk
ectopic	ĕk-TŎP-ĭk	reticulum	rĕ-TĬK-ū-lŭm
ectropion	ĕk-TRŎ-pē-ŏn	endorphins	ĕn-DŎR-fĭnz
eczema	ĔK-zē-mă	endoscope	ĔN-dō-skōp
edema	ĕ-DĒ-mă	endoscopy	ĕn-DŎS-kō-pē
effusion	ĕ-FŪ-zhŭn	endosteum	ĕn-DŎS-tē-ŭm
ejaculation	ē-jăk-ū-LĀ-shŭn	endothelial cells	ĕn-dō-THĒ-lē-ăl sĕlz
ejaculatory duct	ē-JĂK-ū-lă-tŏr-ē dŭkt	endothelium	ĕn-dō-THĒ-lē-ŭm
electrocardiogram	ē-lĕk-trō-KĂR-dē-ō-grăm	endotracheal	ĕn-dō-TRĀ-kē-ăl
electrocardiograph	ē-lĕk-trō-KĂR-dē-ō-grăf	endotracheal	ĕn-dō-TRĀ-kē-ăl
electrocardiography	ē-lĕk-trō-kăr-dē-ŎG-ră-fē	intubation	ĭn-tū-BĀ-shŭn
electroejaculation	ē-lĕk-trō-ē-jă-kū-LĀ-shŭn	enema	Ĕ-nĕ-mă
electroencephalogram	ē- lĕk-trō-ĕn-SĔF-ă-lō-grăm	enteric	ĕn-TĔR-ĭc
electroencephalograph	ē- lĕk-trō-ĕn-SĔF-ă-lō-grăf	enteritis	ĕn-tĕ-RĪ-tĭs
electroencephalo	ē- lĕk-trō-ĕn-sĕf-ă-LŎG-	enterocolitis	ĕn-tĕr-ō-kō-LĪ-tĭs
graphy	ră-fē	enterocolostomy	ĕn-tĕr-ō-kō-LŎS-tō-mē
electrolyte	ē-LĔK-trō-līt	enterology	ĕn-tĕ-RŎL-ō-jē

enteropathy	ĕn-tĕ-RŎP-ă-thē	evisceration	Ē-VĬS-ĕr-ā-shŭn
enterostomy	ĕn-tĕ-RŎS-tō-mē	excision	ĕk-SĬZH-ŭn
enterotomy	ĕn-tĕr-ŎT-ō-mē	excretion	ĕks-KRĒ-shŭn
entropion	ĕn-TRŌ-pē-ŏn	exhalation	ĕks-să-LĀ-shŭn
enucleation	ē-nū-klē-Ā-shŭn	exocrine gland	ĔK-sō-krĭn glăndz
enuresis	ĕn-ū-RĒ-sĭs	exophthalmos	ĕk-sŏf-THĂL-mŏs
enzyme	ĔN-zīm	exotropia	ĕk-sō-TRŌ-pē-ă
eosinophil	ē-ō-SĬN-ō-fĭl	expiration	ĕks-pĭr-RĀ-shŭn
eosinophilia	ē-ō-sĭn-ō-FĬL-ē-ă	exsanguination	ĕk-SĂNG-wĭ-nā-shŭn
ependymal	ĕp-ĔN-dĭ-măl	extension	ĕk-STĔN-shŭn
epidermis	ĕp-ĭ-DĔR-mĭs	external	ĕks-TĔR-năl
epidermolysis	ĕp-ĭ-dĕr-MŎL-ĭ-sĭs	extraction	ĕk-STRĂK-shŭn
epididymis	ĕp-ĭ-DĬD-ĭ-mĭs	extraocular	ĕks-tră-ŎK-ū-lăr
epididymitis	ĕp-ĭ-dĭd-ĭ-MĪ-tĭs	exudate	ĔK-sū-dāt
epidural	ĕp-ĕ-DŪ-răl		
epigastric	ĕp-ĭ-GĂS-trĭk	facial	FĀ-shŭl
epiglottis	ĕp-ĭ-GLŎT-ĭs	fascia	FĂSH-ē-ă
epiglottitis	ĕp-ĭ-glŏ-TĪ-tĭs	fasciectomy	făsh-ē-ĔK-tō-mē
epilepsy	ĔP-ĭ-lĕp-sē	fasciitis	făsh-ē-Ī-tĭs
epinephrine	ĕp-ĭ-NĔF-rĭn	fecal	FĒ-kŭl
epiphora	ē-PĬF-ŏ-ră	feces	FĒ-sēz
epiphyseal plate	ĕ-pĭ-FĬZ-ē-ăl	feline	FĒ-lĭn ĭm-ū-nō-dē-
epiphysis	ē-PĬF-ĭ-sĭs	immunodeficiency	FĬSH-ĕn-sē VĪ-rŭs
episiotomy	ĕ-pĭs-ē-ŎT-o-mē	virus	
epistaxis	ĕp-ĭ-STĂK-sĭs	femoral	FĔM-ŏr-ăl
epithelial	ĕp-ĭ-THĒ-lē-ăl	femorotibial	fĕ-mŏ-rō-TĬ-bē-ăl
epithelium	ĕp-ĭ THĒ-lē-ŭm	femur	FĒ-mŭr
epulis	ĕp-ŭl-ŭs	fertilization	fĕr-tăl-ĭ-ZĀ-shŭn
eructation	e-rŭk-TĂ-shŭn	fetotomy	fĕ-TŎT-ō-mē
erythema	ĕr-ĭ-THĒ-mă	fetus	FĒ-tŭs
erythroblast	ĕ-RĬTH-rō-blăst	fibrillation	fĭb-rĭ-LĀ-shŭn
erythrocyte	ĕ-RĬTH-rō-sīt	fibrin	FĪ-brĭn
erythrocytopenia	ĕ-rĭth-rō-sī-tō-PĒ-nē-ă	fibrinogen	fĭ-BRĬN-ō-jĕn
erythrocytosis	ĕ-RĬTH-rō-sī-TŌ-sĭs	fibroma	fĭ-BRŌ-mă
erythropenia	ĕ-rĭth-rō-PĒ-nē-ă	fibrosarcoma	fĭ-brō-săr-KŌ-mă
erythropoiesis	ĕ-rĭth-rō-pō-Ē-sĭs	fibrosis	fĭ-BRŌ-sĭs
erythropoietin	ĕ-rĭth-rō-PŌ-ĭ-tĭn	fibula	FĬB-ū-lă
esophageal	ĕ-sŏf-ă-JĒ-ăl	fibular	FĬB-ū-lăr
esophageal atresia	ĕ-sŏf-ă-JĒ-ăl ā-TRĒ-zē-ă	filtration	fĭl-TRĀ-shŭn
esophageal reflux	ĕ-sŏf-ă-JĒ-ăl RĒ-flŭks	fimbriae	FĬM-brē-ē
esophageal spasm	ĕ-sŏf-ă-JĒ-ăl spăsm	fissure	FĬSH-ŭr
esophagitis	ĕ-sŏf-ă-JĪ-tĭs	fistula	FĬS-tū-lă
esophagoplasty	ĕ-SŎF-ă-gō-plăs-tē	flagella	flă-JĔL-ă
esophagus	ĕ-SŎF-ă-gŭs	flagellum	flă-JĔL-ŭm
esotropia	ĕ-sō-TRŌP-ē-ă	flatulence	FLĂ-tū-lĕns
estrogen	ĔS-trō-jĕn	flexion	FLĔK-shŭn
estrus	ĕs-TRŬS	fluorescein	floo-ō-RĔS-ē-ĭn
ethmoid bone	ĔTH-moyd bōn	flutter	FLŬ-tĕr
etiology	ē-tē-ŎL-ō-jē	follicle-stimulating	FŎL-lĭ-kŭl STĬM-ū-lā-
euphoria	ū-FŎR-ē-ă	hormone	tĭng HŎR-mōn
Eustachian tube	ū-STĀ-shŭn	fontanelle	fŏn-tă-NĔL
euthyroid	ū-THĪ-royd	foramen	fōr-Ā-mĕn

fossa	FŎS-ă
fovea centralis	FŌ-vē-ă sĕn-TRĂ-lĭs
fracture	FRĂK-shŭr
frontal bone	FRŎN-tăl bōn
fundus	FŬN-dŭs
gait	GĀT
galactorrhea	gă-lăk-tō-RĒ-ă
gallbladder	găwl-BLĂ-dĕr
gamete	GĂM-ēt
ganglion	GĂNG-lē-ŏn
gangrene	găng-GRĒN
gastrectomy	găs-TRĔK-tō-mē
gastric	GĂS-trĭk
gastric dilatation	GĂS-trĭk dĭ-lă-TĀ-shŭn
gastric dilatation	GĂS-trĭk dĭ-lă-TĀ-shŭn
volvulus	VŎL-vū-lŭs
gastritis	găs-TRĪ-tĭs
gastroduo	găs-trō-dū-ŏd-dĕ-
denostomy	NŎS-tō-mē
gastroenteritis	găs-TRŎ-ĕn-tĕ-RĪ-tĭs
gastroenterology	găs-trō-ĕn-tĕr-ŎL-ō-jē
gastrointestinal	găs-trō-ĭn-TĔS-tĭn-ăl
gastrojejunstomy	găs-trō-jĭ-jū-NŎS-tō-mē
gastropexy	găs-trō-PĔK-sē
gastrostomy	găs-TRŎS-tō-mē
gastrotomy	găs-TRŎT-ō-mē
gavage	gă-VĂJ
genes	jēnz
genital lock	JĔN-ĭ-tă lŏk
genitalia	jĕn-ĭ-TĀ-lē-ă
genitourinary	jĕn-ĭ-tō-ŪR-ĭ-năr-ē
gestation	jĕs-TĀ-shŭn
gingiva	JĬN-jĭ-vă
gingival	JĬN-jĭ-văl
gingival sulcus	JĬN-jĭ-văl SŬL-kŭs
gingivectomy	jĭn-jĭ-VĔK-tō-mē
gingivitis	jĭn-jĭ-VĪ-tĭs
glans penis	glănz PĒ-nĭs
glaucoma	glăw-KŌ-mă
glial cell	GLĒ-ăl sĕl
gliding	GLĪ-dĭng
globin	GLŌ-bĭn
globulin	GLŎB-ū-lĭn
glomerular	glō-MĔR-ū-lăr
glomerulonephritis	glō-mĕr-ū-lō-nĕ-FRĪ-tĭs
glomerulus	glō-MĔR-ū-lŭs
glossal	GLŎ-săl
glossitis	glŏ-SĪ-tĭs
glossopharyngeal	glŏs-ō-fă-rĭn-JĒ-ăl
glottis	GLŎ-tĭs
glucagon	GLOO-kă-gŏn

glucocorticoids	gloo-kō-KŎR-tĭ-koyds
gluconeogenesis	gloo-kō-nē-ō-JĔN-ĕ-sĭs
glucose	GLOO-kōs
glucosuria	gloo-kōs-Ū-rē-ă
glycemia	glī-SĒ-mē-ă
glycemic	gli-SĒ-mĭk
glycogen	GLĪ-kō-jĕn
glycogenolysis	glī-kō-jĕ-NŎL-ĭ-sĭs
glycolysis	glī-KŎL-ĭ-sĭs
glycosuria	glī-kōs-Ū-rē-ă
golgi apparatus	GŌL-jē ăp-ŭ-RĂ-tŭs
gonad	GŌ-năd
gonadotropin	gō-năd-ō-TRŌ-pĭn
goniotomy	gō-nē-ŎT-ō-ē
gout	GŎWT
grain	GRĀN
granuloctye	GRĂN-ū-lō-sīt
granulocytopenia	GRĂN-ū-lō-sī-tō-PĒ-nē-ă
granulocytosis	grăn-ū-lō-sī-TŌ-sĭs
granuloma	gră-nū-LŌ-mă
gynecology	gī-nĕ-KŎL-ō-jē
gyri; gyrus	JĪ-rē; JĪ-rŭs
hair follicle	hār FŎL-ĭ-kŭl
hard palate	hărd PĂL-ăt
Haversian canals	hă-VĔR-shăn kă-NĂLZ
hemangioma	hē-MĂN-jē-ō-mă
hemarthrosis	hēm-ăr-THRŌ-sĭs
hematemesis	hĕ-mă-TĔM-ĭ-sĭs
hematochezia	hĕ-mă-tō-KĒ-zē-ă
hematocrit	hē-MĂT-ō-krĭt
hematology	hē-mă-TŎL-ō-jē
hematoma	hē-mă-TŌ-mă
hematopoiesis	hĕ-mă-tō-pō-Ē-sĭs
hematopoietic	hĕ-mă-tō-pō-Ĕ-tĭk
hematuria	hēm-ă-TŪ-rē-ă
heme	hēm
hemiglossectomy	hĕm-ē-glŏs-SĔK-tō-mē
hemiparesis	hĕm-ē-pă-RĒ-sĭs
hemiplegia	hĕm-ē-PLĒ-jă
hemisphere	hĕm-ē-sfēr
hemodialysis	hē-mō-dī-ĂL-ĭ-sĭs
hemoglobin	HĒ-mō-glō-bĭn
hemoglobinopathy	HĒ-mō-glō-bĭn-ŎP-ă-thē
hemolysis	hē-MŎL-ĭ-sĭs
hemolytic	hē-mō-LĪ-tĭk
hemoperitoneum	hē-mō-pĕ-rĭ-tō-NĒ-ŭm
hemophilia	hē-mō-FĬL-ē-ă
hemopytsis	hē-MŎP-tĭ-sĭs
hemorrhage	HĔM-ŏr-ĭj
hemorrhagic anemia	hĕ-mō-RĂ-jĭk
	ă-NĒ-mē-ă

hemorrhagic	hĕ-mō-RĂ-jĭk
gastroenteritis	găs-TRŌ-ĕn-tĕ-RĪ-tĭs
hemosiderin	hē-mō-SĬ-dĕr-ĭn
hemostasis	hē-mō-STĀ-sĭs
hemothorax	hē-mō-THŌ-răks
hemolytic anemia	hē-mō-LĬ-tĭk ă-NĒ-mē-ă
heparin	HĔP-ă-rĭn
hepatic	hĕ-PĂT-ĭk
hepatic lipidosis	hĕ-PĂT-ĭk lĭ-pĭ-DŌ-sĭs
hepatitis	hĕp-ă-TĪ-tĭs
hepatocyte	hĕ-PĂ-tō-sīt
hepatoma	hĕp-ă-TŌ-mă
hepatomegaly	hĕp-ă-tō-MĔG-ă-lē
hepatotomy	hĕp-ă-TŎ-tō-mē
hernia	HĔR-nē-ă
herniation	hĕr-nē-Ā-shŭn
herniorrhaphy	hĕr-nē-ŌR-ă fē
hiatal hernia	hī-Ā-tăl HĔR-nē-ă
hidrosis	hī-DRŌ-sĭs or hĭ-DRŌ-sĭs
hinge	hĭnj
hippocampus	hĭ-pō-KĂM-pŭs
histocyte	HĬS-tō-sīt
histological	hĭs-tō-LŎG-ĭk-ăl
histologist	hĭs-TŎL-ō-jĭst
histology	hĭs-TŎL-ō-jē
histopathologist	hĭs-tō-pă-THŎL-ō-jĭst
histopathology	hĭs-tō-pă-THŎL-ō-jē
homeostasis	hō-mē-ō-STĀ-sĭs
hordeolum	hŏr-DĒ-ō-lŭm
hormonal	hŏr-MŌN-ăl
hormone	HŎR-mōn
humeral	HŪ-mĕr-ăl
humeroradioulnar	hū-mĕr-ō-rā-dē-ō-ŬL-năr
humerus	HŪ-mĕr-ŭs
humoral immunity	HŪ-mŏr-ăl ĭ-MŪ-nĭ-tē
hydrarthrosis	hī-drăr-THRŌ-sĭs
hydrocephalus	hī-drō-SĔF-ă-lŭs
hydrochloric acid	hī-drō-KLŎR-ĭk Ă-sĭd
hydronephrosis	hī-drō-nĕ-FRŌ-sĭs
hydrotherapy	hī-drō-THĔR-ă-pē
hydrothorax	hī-drō-THŌ-răks
hymen	HĪ-mĕn
hyperadrenocorticism	hī-pĕr-ă-drē-nō-KŎR-tĭ-sĭ-zm
hyperbilirubinemia	hī-pĕr-bĭl-ē-roo-bĭ-NĒ-mē-ă
hypercalcemia	hī-pĕr-kăl-SĒ-mē-ă
hypercapnia	hī-pĕr-KĂP-nē-ă
hypercholesterolemia	hī-pĕr-kō-lĕs-tĕr-ŏl-Ē-mē-ă
hyperchromic	hī-pĕr-KRŌ-mĭk
hypercrinism	hī-pĕr-KRĬN-ĭzm
hyperesthesia	hī-pĕr-ĕs-THĒ-zē-ă
hyperglycemia	hī-pĕr-glī-SĒ-mē-ă
hypergonadism	hī-pĕr-GŌ-năd-ĭzm
hyperinsulinism	hī-pĕr-ĬN-sŭ-lĭn-ĭzm
hyperkalemia	hī-pĕr-kā-LĒ-mē-ă
hyperkeratosis	hī-pĕr-kĕr-ă-TŌ-sĭs
hyperkinesis	hī-pĕr-kĭ-NĒ-sĭs
hypernatremia	hī-pĕr-nā-TRĒ-mē-ă
hyperparathyroidism	hī-pĕr-pă-ră-THĪ-royd-ĭzm
hyperpituitarism	hī-pĕr-pĭ-TŪ-ĭ-tăr-ĭzm
hyperplasia	hī-pĕr-PLĀ-zē-ă
hyperpnea	hī-PĔRP-nē-ă
hypersensitivity	hī-pĕr-sĕn-sĭ-TĬV-ĭ-tē
hypersplenism	hī-pĕr-SPLĔN-ĭzm
hypertension	hī-pĕr-TĔN-shŭn
hyperthyroidism	hī-pĕr-THĪ-royd-ĭzm
hypertrophy	hī-PĔR-trō-fē
hypertropia	hī-pĕr-TRŌ-pē-ă
hyperventilation	hī-pĕr-vĕn-tĭ-LĀ-shŭn
hypoadrenocorticism	hī-pō-ă-drē-nō-KŎR-tĭ-sĭ-zm
hypoalbuminemia	hī-pō-ăl-bū-mĭ-NĒ-mē-ă
hypocalcemia	hī-pō-kăl-SĒ-mē-ă
hypocapnia	hī-pō-KĂP-nē-ă
hypochondriac	hī-pō-KŎN-drē-ăk
hypochromic	hī-pō-KRŌ-mĭk
hypocrinism	hī-pō-KRĬN-ĭzm
hypodermic	hī-pō DĔR-mĭk
hypogastric	hī-pō-GĂS-trĭk
hypoglossal	hī-pō-GLŎ-săl
hypoglycemia	hī-pō-glī-SĒ-mē-ă
hypogonadism	hī-pō-GŌ-năd-ĭzm
hypoinsulinism	hī-pō-ĬN-sŭ-lĭn-ĭzm
hypokalemia	hī-pō-kā-LĒ-mē-ă
hyoid bone	HĪ-oyd
hyponatremia	hī-pō-nā-TRĒ-mē-ă
hypoparathyroidism	hī-pō-pă-ră-THĪ-royd-ĭzm
hypophysis	hī-PŎF-ĭ-sĭs
hypopituitarism	hī-pō-pĭ-TŪ-ĭ-tăr-ĭzm
hypoplasia	hī-pō-PLĀ-zē-ă
hypopnea	hī-PŎP-nē-ă
hypopyon	hī-PŎP-ē-ŏn
hypotension	hī-pō-TĔN-shŭn
hypothalamus	hī-pō-THĂL-ă-mŭs
hypothyroidism	hī-pō-THĪ-royd-ĭzm
hypotropia	hī-pō-TRŌ-pē-ă
hypoxia	hī-PŎK-sē-ă
hypoxic	hī-PŎK-sĭk
hysterectomy	hĭs-tĕr-ĔK-tō-mē
hysteroscopy	hĭs-tĕr-ŎS-kō-pē

iatrogenic	ī-ăt-rō-JĚN-ĭk
icterus	ĬK-tĕr-ŭs
idiopathic	ĭd-ē-ō-PĂTH-ĭk
ileitis	ĭl-ē-Ī-tĭs
ileocecal	ĭl-ē-ō-SĒ-kăl
ileostomy	ĭl-ē-ŎS-tō-mē
ileum	ĬL-ē-ŭm
ileus	ĬL-ē-ŭs
iliac	ĬL-ē-ăk
ilium	ĬL-ē-ŭm
immobilization	ĭ-mō-bŭl-ĭ-ZĀ-shŭn
immune response	ĭ-MŪN rē-SPŎNS
immunity	ĭ-MŪ-nĭ-tē
immunodeficiency	ĭm-ū-nō-dē-FĬSH-ĕn-sē
immunofluorescent antibody test	ĭm-ū-nō-flŏ-RĔS-sĕnt ĂN-tĭ-bŏd-ē tĕst
immunoglobulin	ĭm-ū-nō-GLŎB-ū-lĭn
immunosorbent	ĭm-ū-nō-SŎR-bĕnt
immunosuppression	ĭm-ū-nō-sŭ-PRĔ-shŭn
implantation	ĭm-plăn-TĀ-shŭn
impulses	ĭm-PŬL-sĕs
inappetance	ĭn-ĂP-pĭ-tĕns
incision	ĭn-SĬZH-ŭn
incisive bone	ĭn-SĪ-sĭv
incisor	ĭn-SĪ-zŏr
incontinence	ĭn-KŎN-tĭ-nĕns
incus	ĬNG-kŭs
infarction	ĭn-FĂRK-shŭn
infection	ĭn-FĔK-shŭn
infectious	ĭn-FĔK-shŭs
infestation	ĭn-fĕ-STĀ-shŭn
inflammatory	ĭn-FLĂ-mă-tō-rē
infracostal	ĭn-fră-KŎS-tăl
infundibulum	ĭn-fŭn-DĬ-bū-lŭm
inguinal	ĬNG-gwĭ-năl
inhalation	ĭn-hă-LĀ-shŭn
injection	ĭn-JĔK-shŭn
innervation	ĭn-ĕr-VĀ-shŭn
inspiration	ĭn-spĭ-RĀ-shŭn
insulin	ĬN-sŭ-lĭn
insulinoma	ĭn-sŭ-lĭ-NŌ-mă
intact	ĭn-TĂKT
integumentary	ĭn-tĕg-ū-MĔN-tăr-ē
interatrial	ĭn-tĕr-Ā-trē-ăl
interbrain	ĭn-tĕr-BRĀN
intercostal	ĭn-tĕr-KŎS-tăl
internal	ĭn-TĔR-năl
interstitial	ĭn-tĕr-STĬ-shŭl
interventricular	ĭn-tĕr-vĕn-TRĬK-ū-lăr
intervertebral	ĭn-tĕr-VĔR-tē-brăl
intracardiac	ĬN-tră-KĂR-dē-ăk
intracranial	ĭn-tră-KRĀ-nē-ăl

intradermal	ĬN-tră-DĔR-mŏl
intrahepatic	ĬN-tră-hĕ-PĂT-ĭk
intramuscular	ĭn-tră-MŬS-kū-lăr
intraocular	ĭn-tră-ŎK-ū-lăr
intravenous	ĭn-tră-VĒ-nŭs
intravenous catheter	ĭn-tră-VĒ-nŭs KĂ-thĕ-tĕr
intussusception	ĭn-tŭs-sŭs-SĔP-shŭn
involution	ĭn-vō-LŪ-shŭn
iridectomy	ĭr-ĭ-DĔK-tō-mē
iridic	ĭ-RĬD-ĭk
iris	Ī-rĭs
iritis	ī-RĪ-tĭs
ischemia	ĭs-KĒ-mē-ă
ischemic	ĭs-KĒ-mĭk
ischial	ĬSH-ē-ăl
ischiatic	ĬSH-ē-ă-tĭk
ischium	ĬSH-ē-ŭm
jaundice	JĂWN-dĭs
jejunostomy	jĕ-joo-NŎS-tō-mē
jejunum	jĕ-JOO-nŭm
keloid	KĒ-loyd
keratectomy	kĕr-ă-TĔK-tō-mē
keratin	KĔR-ă-tĭn
keratitis	kĕr-ă-TĪ-tĭs
keratocentesis	kĕr-ă-tō-sĕn-TĒ-sĭs
keratoconjunctivitis	kĕr-ă-tō-kŏn-jŭnk-tĭ-VĪ-tĭs
keratoplasty	kĕr-ă-tō-PLĂS-tē
keratotomy	kĕr-ă-TŎT-ō-mē
ketones	KĒ-tōnz
ketonuria	kē-tōn-Ū-rē-ă
ketosis	kē-TŌ-sĭs
kidney	KĬD-nē
kinesiology	kĭ-nē-sē-ŎL-ō-jē
kyphosis	kī-FŌ-sĭs
labia	LĀ-bē-ă
labial	LĀ-bē-ăl
labium	LĀ-bē-ŭm
labyrinth	LĂB-ĭ-rĭnth
laceration	lă-sĕ-RĀ-shŭn
lacrimal	LĂ-krĭ-măl
lacrimal bone	LĂ-krĭ-măl bōn
lacrimation	lă-krĭ-MĀ-shŭn
lactation	lăk-TĀ-shŭn
lactogenesis	lăk-tō-JĔN-ĕ-sĭs
lame	lām
lameness	LĀM-nĕs
lamina	LĂM-ĭ-nă
laminectomy	lăm-ĭ-NĔK-tō-mē
lance	lăns

laparoscope	LĂP-ă-rō-skōp	lymphocyte	LĬM-fō-sīt
laparoscopy	lă-pă-RŎS-kō-pē	lymphocytopenia	lĭm-fō-sī-tō-PĒ-nē-ă
laparotomy	lăp-ă-RŎT-ō-mē	lymphocytosis	lĭm-fō-sī-TŌ-sĭs
laryngeal	lă-RĬN-jē-ăl	lymphoid	LĬM-foyd
laryngectomy	lăr-ĭn-JĔK-tō-mē	lymphoma	lĭm-FŌ-mă
laryngitis	lă-rĭn-JĪ-tĭs	lymphopoiesis	lĭm-fō-pō-Ē-sĭs
laryngopharynx	lă-RĬN-jō-făr-ĭnks	lysosome	LĪ-sō-sōm
laryngoscopy	lă-rĭn-GŎS-kō-pē		
laryngospasm	lă-RĬNG-jō-spăzm	macrocephaly	măk-rō-SĔF-ă-lē
larynx	LĂR-ĭnks	macrocytic	măk-rō-SĬ-tĭk
lateral	LĂT-ĕr-ăl	macrocytosis	măk-rō-sī-TŌ-sĭs
lavage	lă-VĂJ	macrophage	MĂK-rō-fāj
laxity	LĂK-sĭ-tē	macrophthalmia	măk-rŏf-THĂL-mē-ă
leiomyoma	lī-ō-mī-Ō-mă	macrotia	măk-RŌ-shē-ă
leiomyosarcoma	lī-ō-mī-ō-săr-KŌ-mă	macula	MĂK-ū-lă
lens	lĕnz	macular	MĂK-ū-lăr
lensectomy	lĕn-ZĔK-tō-mē	degeneration	dē-jĕn-ĕ-RĀ-shŭn
leptospirosis	lĕp-tō-SPĪ-rō-sĭs	macule	MĂK-ul
lesion	LĒ-zhŭn	malabsorption	măl-ăb-SŎRP-shŭn
lethargic	lĕ-THŎR-jĭk	malaise	măl-ĀZ
lethargy	LĔ-thĕr-jē	maldigestion	măl-dĭ-JĔST-yŭn
leukemia	lū-KĒ-mē-ă	malignant	Mă-LĬG-nănt
leukocyte	LŪ-kō-sīt	malleolar	mă-LĒ-ō-lŭs
leukocytopenia	lū-kō-sī-tō-PĒ-nē-ă	malleolus	mă-LĒ-ō-lăr
leukocytosis	lū-kō-sī-TŌ-sĭs	malleus	MĂL-ē-ŭs
leukorrhea	loo-kō-RĒ ă	malocclusion	măl-ŏ-KLOO-zhŭn
ligament	LĬG-ă-mĕnt	mammary	MĂM-ŏr-ē
ligamentous	lĭg-ă-MĔN-tŭs	mammoplasty	MĂM-ō-plăs-tē
lingual	LĬNG-wăl	mandible	MĂN-dĭ-hŭl
lipase	LĪ-pās	mandibular	măn-DĬB-ū-lăr
lipemia	lī-PĒ-mē-ă	mange	mānj
lipid	LĬ-pĭd	manubrium	mă-NŪ-brē-ŭm
lipocyte	LĬP-ō-sīt	mastectomy	măs-TĔK-tō-mē
lipoma	lī-PŌ-mă	mastication	măs-tĭ-KĀ-shŭn
lithotripsy	LĬTH-ō-trĭp-sē	mastitis	măs-TĪ-tĭs
litter	LĬ-tĕr	maxillary bone	MĂK-sĭ-lă-rē bōn
liver	LĬ-vĕr	mean corpuscular	mĕn kŏr-PŬS-kū-lăr
lobectomy	lō-BĔK-tō-mē	hemoglobin	HĒ-mō-glō-bĭn
lordosis	lŏr-DŌ-sĭs	mean corpuscular	mēn kŏr-PŬS-kū-lăr
lumbar	LŬM-băr	volume	VŎL-ūm
lumbosacral	lŭm-bō-SĀ-krăl	meatus	mē-Ā-tŭs
lupus erythematosus	LŪ-pŭs ĕ-rĭ-thē-mă-TŌ-sŭs	meconium	mĕ-KŌ-nē-ŭm
luteinizing hormone	LŪ-tĕ-nī-zĭng HŎR-mōn	medial	MĒ-dē-ăl
luxation	lŭk-SĀ-shŭn	median	MĒ-dē-ăn
Lyme disease	līm dĭ-ZĒZ	mediastinal	mē-dē-ă-STĪ-năl
lymph	lĭmf	mediastinum	mē-dē-ă-STĪ-nŭm
lymphadenitis	lĭmf-ă-dĕ-NĪ-tĭs	medulla	mĕ-DŪL-ă or mĕ-DŬL-ă
lymphadenopathy	lĭmf-ă-dĕ-NŎP-ă-thē	medulla oblongata	mĕ-DŪL-ă or mĕ-DŬL-ă
lymphangioma	lĭmf-ăn-jē-Ō-mă		ŏb-lŏn-GĂ-tă
lymphatic	lĭm-FĂ-tĭk	medullary	MĔD-ū-lăr-ē
lymphedema	lĭmf-ĕ-DĒ-mă	megacolon	mĕ-gă-KŌ-lĕn
lymphoblast	LĬM-fō-blăst	megaesophagus	mĕ-gă-ĕ-SŎF-ă-gŭs

megakaryocyte	mĕ-gă-KĂR-ē-ō-sīt	multipara	mŭl-TĬP-ă-ră
melanin	MĔL-ă-nĭn	murmur	MŬR-mĕr
melanocyte	mĕ-LĂN-ō-sīt	muscular	MŬS-kū-lăr
melanoma	mĕl-ă-NŌ-mă	myalgia	mī-ĂL-jă
melatonin	mĕl-ă-TŌ-nĭn	myasthenia	mī-ăs-THĒ-nē-ă
melena	MĔL-ĕ-nă or mĕ-LĒ-nă	myasthenia	mī-ăs-THĒ-nē-ă
membrane	MĔM-brān	gravis	GRĂ-vĭs
meningeal	mĕ-NĬN-jē-ăl or	mydriasis	mĭ-DRĪ-ă-sĭs
	mĕ-nĭn-JĒ-ăl	myectomy	mī-ĔK-tō-mē
meninges	mĕ-NĬN-jēz	myelin sheath	MĪ-ĕ-lĭn shēth
meningioma	mĕ-nĭn-jē-Ō-mă	myelitis	mī-ĕ-LĪ-tĭs
meningitis	mĕn-ĭn-JĪ-tĭs	myeloblast	MĪ-ĕ-lō-blăst
meningomyelocele	mĕ-nĭn-jō-MĪ-ĕ-lō-sēl	myelodysplasia	mī-ĕ-lō-dĭs-PLĀ-zē-ă
mesentery	MĔS-ĕn-tĕr-ē	myelogenous	mī-ĕ-LŎJ-ĕn-ŭs
metabolic	mĕ-tă-BŎL-ĭk	myelogram	MĪ-ĕ-lō-grăm
metabolism	mĕ-TĂB-ō-lĭzm	myeloid	MĪ-ĕ-loyd
metacarpal	mĕ-tă-KĂR-păl	myeloma	mī-ĕ-LŌ-mă
metacarpectomy	mĕ-tă-kăr-PĔK-tō-mē	myelopoiesis	mī-ĕ-lō-pō-Ē-sĭs
metamorphosis	mĕt-ă-MŎR-fŏ-sĭs	myocardial	mī-ō-KĂR-dē-ăl
metaphysis	mĕ-TĂ-fĭ-sĭs	myocardium	mī-ō-KĂR-dē-ŭm
metastasis	mĕ-TĂS-tă-sĭs	myoclonus	mī-ŎK-lŏ-nŭs
metatarsalgia	mĕ-tă-tăr-SĂL-jă	myoma	mī-Ō-mă
metatarsals	mĕ-tă-TĂR-sălz	myometrium	mī-ō-MĒ-trē-ŭm
metritis	mē-TRĪ-tĭs	myoneural	mī-ō-NŪ-răl
microcephaly	mĭ-krō-SĔF-ă-lē	myoparesis	mī-ō-pă-RĒ-sĭs
microcystosis	mī-krō-sī-TŌ-sĭs	myopathy	mī-ŎP-ă-thē
microcytic	mĭ-krō-SĬ-tĭk	myoplasty	mī-ō-PLĂS-tē
microglial	mĭ-krō-GLĒ-ăl sĕl	myosarcoma	mī-ō-săr-KŌ-mă
microphthalmia	mĭ-krōf-THĂL-mē-ă	myositis	mī-ō-SĪ-tĭs
microscope	MĪ-krō-skōp	myotomy	mī-ŎT-ō-mē
microtia	mī-KRŌ-shē-ă	myotonia	mī-ō-TŌ-nē-ă
micturition	mĭk-tū-RĬSH-ŭn	myringectomy	mēr-ĭn-JĔK-tō-mē
midbrain	mĭd-BRĀN	myringitis	mĭr-ĭn-JĪ-tĭs
mineralocorticoid	mĭn-ĕr-ăl-ō-KŎR-tĭ-koyd	myxoma	mĭk-SŌ-mă
miosis	mī-Ō-sĭs		
mitochondria	mī-tō-KŎN-drē-ă	narcolepsy	NĂR-kō-lĕp-sē
mitral valvulitis	MĪ-trăl văl-vū-LĪ-tĭs	nares	NĂ-rēz
molar	MŌ-lăr	nasal	NĀ-zăl
monoblast	mŏn-ō-blăst	nasal bone	NĀ-zăl bōn
monocyte	MŎN-ō-sīt	nasogastric	nā-zō-GĂS-trĭk
mononuclear	mŏn-ō-NŪ-klē-ăr	nasogastric	nā-zō-GĂS-trĭk
monoparesis	mŏn-ō-pă-RĒ-sĭs	intubation	ĭn-tū-BĀ-shŭn
monoplegia	mŏn-ō-PLĒ-jă	nasolacrimal	nā-zō-LĂ-krĭ-măl
monorchid	mŏn-ŎR-kĭd	nasopharynx	nā-zō-FĂR-ĭnks
morphology	mŏr-FŎL-ō-jē	nausea	NĂW-zē-ă
mount	mŏwnt	necropsy	NĒ-krŏp-sē
mucolytics	mū-kō-LĬ-tĭks	necrosis	nĕ-KRŌ-sĭs
mucosa	mū-KŌ-să	necrotic	nĕ-KRŌT-ĭk
mucous	MŪ-kŭs	neonatal	nē-ō-NĀ-tăl
mucous membranes	MŪ-kŭs MĔM-brāns	neonate	NĒ-ō-nāt
mucus	MŪ-kŭs	neonatology	nē-ō-nā-TŎL-ō-jē
multigravida	mŭl-tē-GRĂV-ĭ-dă	neoplasia	nē-ō-PLĀ-zē-ă

neoplasm	NĒ-ō-plăzm	nyctalopia	nĭk-tă-LŌ-pē-ă
nephralgia	nĕ-FRĂL-jă	obese	ō-BĒS
nephrectomy	nĕ-FRĔK-tō-mē	obstetrics	ŏb-STĔT-rĭks
nephritis	nĕ-FRĪ-tĭs	obstipation	ŏb-stĭ-PĀ-shŭn
nephrogram	nĕ-FRŎ-grăm	obstruction	ŏb-STRŬK-shŭn
nephrolithiasis	nĕ-frō-lĭ-THĪ-ă-sĭs	occipital bone	ŏk-SĬP-ĭ-tăl bōn
nephrolithotomy	nĕ-frō-lĭ-THŎT-ō-mē	occlusion	ō-KLū-jŭn
nephrologist	nĕ-FRŎL-ō-jĭst	ocular	ŎK-ū-lăr
nephrology	nĕ-FRŎL-ō-jē	ocular dermoid	ŎK-ū-lăr DĔR-moyd
nephroma	nĕ-FRŎ-mă	oculomotor	ŎK-ū-lō-mō-tĕr
nephromalacia	nĕ-frō-mă-LĀ-shă	olecranal	ō-LĔK-ră-năl
nephron	NĔF-rŏn	olecranon	ō-LĔK-ră-nŏn
nephropathy	nĕ-FRŎ-pă-thē	olfactory	ōl-FĂK-tĕ-rēē
nephroptosis	nĕ-FRŎP-Tō-sĭs	oligodendroglial	ōl-ē-gō-dĕn-drō-GLĒ-ăl
nephrosclerosis	nĕ-frō-sklĕ-RŌ-sĭs	oligospermia	ōl-ē-gō-SPĔR-mē-ă
nephrosis	nĕ-FRŎ-sĭs	oliguria	ōl-ē-GŪ-rē-ă
nephrostomy	nĕ-FRŎS-tō-mē	omasum	ō-MĀ-sŭm
nephrotic	nĕ-FRŎT-ĭk	omentum	ō-MĔN-tŭm
nerve	nĕrv	oncologist	ŏn-KŎL-ō-jĭst
neural	NŪ-răl	oncology	ŏn-KŎL-ō-jē
neuralgia	nū-RĂL-jă	onychectomy	ō-nĭ-KĔK-tō-mē
neurasthenia	nŭr-ăs-THĒ-nē-ă	onycholysis	ŏn-ĭ-KŎL-ĭ-sĭs
neurectomy	nū-RĔK-tō-mē	onychomycosis	ŏn-ĭ-kō-mī-KŌ-sĭs
neuritis	nū-RĪ-tĭs	oocyte	ō-ŭh-sīt
neurohypophysis	nū-rō-hī-PŎF-ĭ-sĭs	oogenesis	ō-ō-JĔN-ĕ-sĭs
neurological	nū-rō-LŎJ ĭk-ăl	oophorectomy	oo-fō-RĔK-tō-mē or
neurology	nū-RŎL-ō-jē		ō-ŏf-ō-RĔK-tō-mē
neuron	NŪ-rŏn	ophthalmic	ŏf-THĂL-mĭk
neuropathy	nū-RŎP-ă-thē	ophthalmologist	ŏf-thăl-MŎL-ō-jĭst
neuroplasty	nū-rō-PLĂS-tē	ophthalmology	ŏf-thăl-MŎL-ō-jē
neurorrhaphy	nū-RŎR-ă-fē	ophthalmoplegia	ŏf-thăl-mō-PLĒ-jă
neurotomy	nū-RŎT-ō-mē	ophthalmoscope	ŏf-THĂL-mō-skōp
neurotransmitter	nū-rō-trănz-MĬT-ĕr	ophthalmoscopy	ŏf-thăl-MŎS-kō-pē
neuter	NŪ-tĕr	opportunistic	ŏp-ĕr-too-NĬS-tĭk
neutropenia	nŭ-trō-PĒ-nē-ă	optic	ŎP-tĭk
neutrophil	nŭ-trō-FĬL-ē-ā	optic disc	ŎP-tĭk dĭsk
nictitating	NĬK-tĭ-tā-tĭng	optic nerve	ŎP-tĭk nĕrv
membrane	MĔM-brān	optical	ŎP-tĭk-ăl
nitrogen	NĪ-trō-jĕn	oral	ŎR-ăl
nitrogenous	nī-TRŎJ-ĕ-nŭs	orbit	ŎR-bĭt
nodule	NŎD-ūl	orchiectomy	ŏr-kē-ĔK-tō-mē
norepinephrine	nŏr-ĕp-ĭ-NĔF-rĭn	orchiopexy	ŏr-kē-ō-PĔK-sē
normochromic	nŏr-mō-KRŌ-mĭk	orchitis	ŏr-KĪ-tĭs
normocytic	nŏr-mō-SĪ-tĭk	orifice	ŎR-ĭ-fĭs
nostrils	NŎS-trŭlz	orogastric	ŏr-ō-GĂS-trĭk
nuclear	NŪ-klē-ăr	orogastric	ŏr-ō-GĂS-trĭk
nuclear sclerosis	NŪ-klē-ăr sklĕ-RŌ-sĭs	intubation	ĭn-tū-BĀ-shŭn
nucleic	nū-KLĔ-ĭk	oronasal	ŏr-ō-NĀ-zăl
nucleoplasm	NŪ-klē-ō-plăzm	oronasal fistula	ŏr-ō-NĀ-zăl FĬS-tū-lă
nucleus	NŪ-klē-ŭs	oropharynx	ŏr-ō-FĂR-ĭnks
nullipara	nŭl-LĬP-ă-ră	orthopedic	ŏr-thō-PĒ-dĭk
nutrients	NŪ-trē-ĕnts	os cordis	ŏs KŌR-dĭs

os penis	ŏs PĒ-nĭs	palatine bone	PĂL-ŭn-tīn bōn
os rostri	ŏs RŎS-trī	palatoplasty	PĂL-ă-tō-plăs-tē
osseus	ŎS-ē-ŭs	palatoschisis	păl-ă-TŎS-kĭ-sĭs
ossicle	ŎS-ĭ-kŭl	palliative	PĂ-lē-ă-tĭv
ossification	ŏs-ĭ-fĭ-KĀ-shŭn	pallor	PĂL-ĕr
ostealgia	ŏs-tē-ĂL-jă	palmar	PĂL-măr
ostectomy	ŏs-tē-ĔK-tō-mē	palpation	păl-PĀ-shŭn
osteitis	ŏs-tē-Ī-tĭs	palpebra	PĂL-pē-bră
osteoarthritis	ŏs-tē-ō-ăr-THRĪ-tĭs	palpebral	PĂL-pē-brăl
osteoblast	ŎS-tē-ō-blăst	palpitations	păl-pĭ-TĀ-shŭnz
osteocentesis	ŏs-tē-ō-sĕn-TĒ-sĭs	palsy	PĂL-zē
osteochondrosis	ŏs-tē-ō-kŏn-DRŌ-sĭs	pancreas	PĂN-krē-ăs
osteoclast	ŎS-tē-ō-klăst	pancreatectomy	păn-krē-ă-TĔK-tō-mē
osteocyte	ŎS-tē-ō-sīt	pancreatic	păn-krē-ĂH-tĭk
osteodystrophy	ŏs-tē-ō-DĬS-trō-fē	pancreatitis	PĂN-krē-ă-TĪ-tĭs
osteogenesis	ŏs-tē-ō-JĔN-ĕ-sĭs	pancreatotomy	păn-krē-ă-TŎ-tō-mē
osteogenic	ŏs-tē-ō-JĔN-ĭk	pancytopenia	păn-sī-tō-PĒ-nē-ă
osteology	ŏs-tē-ŎL-ŏ-jē	panhypopituitarism	păn-hī-pō-pĭ-TŪ-ĭ-tăr-ĭzm
osteomalacia	ŏs-tē-ō-mă-LĀ-shă	panleukopenia	păn-LŪ-kō-PĒ-nē-ă
osteomyelitis	ŏs-tē-ō-mī-ĕ-LĪ-tĭs	panophthalmitis	păn-ŏf-thăl-MĪ-tĭs
osteonecrosis	ŏs-tē-ō-nĕ-KRŌ-sĭs	panosteitis	păn-ŏs-tē-Ī-tĭs
osteopexy	ŎS-tē-ō-pĕk-sē	panotitis	păn-ō-TĪ-tĭs
osteoplasty	ŏs-tē-ō-PLĂS-tē	papillae	pă-PĬL-ē
osteoporosis	ŏs-tē-ō-pŏr-Ō-sĭs	papilledema	păp-ĕ-lĕ-DĒ-mă
osteosarcoma	ŏs-tē-ō-săr-KŌ-mă	papilloma	pă-pĭl-Ō-mă
osteosclerosis	ŏs-tē-ō-sklĕ-RŌ-sĭs	papule	PĂP-ūl
osteotome	ŎS-tē-ō-tōm	paracentesis	pă-ră-sĕn-TĒ-sĭs
osteotomy	ŏs-tē-ŎT-ō-mē	parainfluenza	pĕ-ră-ĬN-flū-ĕn-ză
otalgia	ō-TĂL-jă	paralysis	pă-RĂL-ĭ-sĭs
otic	Ō-tĭk	paranasal	pă-ră-NĀ-zăl
otitis	ō-TĪ-tĭs	paranephric	pă-ră-NĔF-rĭk
otitis externa	ō-TĪ-tĭs ĕx-TĔR-nă	paraparesis	pă-ră-pă-RĒ-sĭs
otitis interna	ō-TĪ-tĭs ĭn-TĔR-nă	paraphimosis	pă-ră-fī-MŌ-sĭs
otitis media	ō-TĪ-tĭs MĒ-dē-ă	paraplegia	păr-ă-PLĒ-jă
otolaryngology	ō-tō-lă-rĭn-GŎ-lō-jē	parasympathetic	păr-ă-sĭm-pă-THĔT-ĭk
otomycosis	ō-tō-mī-KŌ-sĭs	parathormone	pă-ră-THŎR-mōn
otopathy	ō-TŎ-păth-ē	parathyroid gland	păr-ă-THĪ-royd glănd
otopyorrhea	ō-tō-pī-ō-RĒ-ă	parathyroidectomy	păr-ă-thī-roy-DĔK-tō-mē
otorrhea	ō-tō-RĒ-ă	parenchyma	păr-ĔN-kĭ-mă
otoscope	Ō-tō-skōp	parenteral	pă-RĔN-tĕr-ăl
otoscopy	ō-TŎS-kō-pē	paresthesia	păr-ĕs-THĒ-zē-ă
ova	Ō-vă	parietal	pă-RĪ-ĕ-tăl
ovarian	ō-VĂ-rē-ăn	parietal bone	pă-RĪ-ĕ-tăl bōn
ovariohysterectomy	ō-VĂR-ē-ō-hĭs-tĕr-ĔK-tō-mē	paronychia	păr-ŏ-NĬK-ē-ă
		parotid gland	pă-RŎT-ĭd glănd
ovary	Ō-vă-rē	paroxysmal	păr-ŏk-SĬZ-măl
ovulation	ŏv-ū-LĀ-shŭn	parturition	păr-tū-RĬSH-ŭn
ovum	Ō-vŭm	parvo	PĂR-vō
oxygen	ŎK-sĭ-jĕn	patella	pă-TĔL-ă
oxytocia	ŏks-ē-TŌ-sē-ă	patellar	pă-TĔL-ăr
oxytocin	ŏks-ē-TŌ-sĭn	patent	PĀ-tĕnt
		patent ductus	PĀ-tĕnt DŬK-tŭs
palate	PĂL-ăt	arteriosus	ăr-tĕr-ē-Ō-sĭs

pathogenesis păth-ō-JĔN-ĕ-sĭs

pathogenic păth-ō-JĔN-ĭk

pathological păth-ō-LŎJ-ĭk-ăl

pathologist pă-THŎL-ŏ-jĭst

pathology pă-THŎL-ŏ-jē

pectoral pĕk-TŎR-ăl

pedunculated pĕ-DŬNG-kū-lāt-ĕd

pelvic PĔL-vĭk

pelvimetry pĕl-VĬM-ĭ-trē

pelvis PĔL-vĭs

percussion pĕr-KŬSH-ŭn

percutaneous pĕr-kū-TĀ-nē-ŭs

perfusion pĕr-FŪ-shŭn

perianal pĕ-rē-Ā-năl

pericardial pĕ-rē-KĂR-dē-ăl

pericardiocentesis pĕr-ĭ-KĂR-dē-ō-sĕn-TĒ-sĭs

pericarditis pĕr-ĭ-kăr-DĪ-tĭs

pericardium pĕr-ĭ-KĂR-dē-ŭm

perilymph PĔR-ĭ-lĭmf

perineal pĕ-rĭ-NĒ-ăl
  urethrostomy ū-rē-THRŎS-tō-mē

perineorrhaphy pĕ-rĭ-nē-ŎR-ră-fē

perineum pĕ-rĭ-NĒ-ŭm

periocular pĕ-rĭ-ŎK-ū-lăr

periodontal disease pĕr-ē-ō-DŎN-tăl dĭ-ZĒZ

periodontal ligament pĕr-ē-ō-DŎN-tăl
  LĬG-ă-mĕnt

periosteitis pĕr-ē-ŏs-tē-Ī-tĭs

periosteum pĕr-ē-ŎS-tē-ŭm

peripheral nervous pĕ-RĬF-ĕr-ăl NĔR-vŭs
  system SĬS-tĕm

peristalsis pĕr-ĭ-STĂL-sĭs

peritoneal pĕr-ĭ-tō-NĒ-ăl

peritoneum pĕ-rĭ-tō-NĒ-ŭm

peritonitis pĕ-rĭ-tō-NĪ-tĭs

peroneal pĕr-ō-NĒ-ăl

persistent frenulum pĕr-SĬS-tĕnt FRĔN-ū-lŭm

petechia; petechiae pĕ-TĒ-kē-ă; pĕ-TĒ-kē-ī

phagocyte FĂG-ō-sīt

phalangeal fă-lăn-JĒ-ăl

phalanges fă-LĂN-jēz

pharyngeal fă-RĬN-jē-ăl

pharyngitis fă-rĭn-JĪ-tĭs

pharyngoplasty fă-RĬN-gō-plăs-tē

pharyngostomy fă-rĭn-GŎS-tō-mē

pharyngotomy fă-rĭn-GŎT-ō-mē

pharynx FĂR-ĭnks

pheochromocytoma fē-ō-krō-mō-sī-TŌ-mă

phimosis fē-MŌ-sĭs

phlebotomy flĕ-BŎT-ō-mē

phlegm FLĔM

phosphorus FŎS-fō-rŭs

photophobia fō-tō-FŌ-bē-ă

phrenic FRĔN-ĭk

physiology fĭ-sē-ŎL-ō-jē

pia mater PĒ-ă MĂ-tĕr

pica PĪ-kă

piloerection PĪ-lō-ē-rĕk-shŭn

pilosebaceous pī-lō-sĕ-BĀ-shŭs

pineal gland pī-NĒ-ăl glănd

pinealopathy pĭn-ē-ăl-ŎP-ă-thē

pinna PĬN-ă

pituitarism pĭ-TŪ-ĭ-tăr-ĭzm

pituitary gland pĭ-TŪ-ĭ-tăr-ē glănd

pivot PĬ-vĭt

placenta plă-SĔN-tă

plane plān

plantar plăn-tĕr

plaque PLĂK

plasma PLĂZ-mă

platelet PLĀT-lĕt

pleomorphic plē-ō-MŎR-fĭk

pleura PLOO-ră

pleural PLOOR-ăl

pleurodynia Plŭr-ō-DĬN-ē-ă

plexus PLĔK-sŭs

pneumocolon nū-mō-KŌ-lĕn

pneumonectomy nū-mō NĔK-tō-mē

pneumonia nū-MŌN-ē-ă

pneumothorax nū-mō-THŌ-răks

pneumovagina nū-mō-vă-JĪ-nă

poikilocytosis poy kē-lō-sī-TŌ-sĭs

polioencepha- pō-lē-ō-ĕn-sĕf-ă-lō-mă-
  lomalacia LĀ-shă

polioencepha pō-lē-ō-ĕn-sĕf-ă-lō-mī-ĕ-
  lomyelitis LĪ-tĭs

pollakiuria PŎL-lă-kē-Ū-rē-ă

polyarthritis pŏl-ē-ăr-THRĪ-tĭs

polycystic pŏl-ē-SĬS-tĭk

polycythemia pŏl-ē-sī-THĒ-mē-ă

polydipsia pŏl-ē-DĬP-sē-ă

polymorphonuclear pŏl-ē-mŏr-fō-NŪ-klē-ăr

polymyalgia pŏl-ē-mī-ĂL-jă

polymyelitis pō-lē-ō-mī-ĕ-LĪ-tĭs

polymyositis pŏl-ē-mī-ō-SĪ-tĭs

polyneuritis pŏl-ē-nū-RĪ-tĭs

polyp PŎL-ĭp

polyphagia pŏl-ē-FĀ-jē-ă

polyuria pŏl-ē-Ū-rē-ă

pons pŏnz

portal vein PŎR-tăl Vān

portosystemic shunt pŏr-tō-sĭs-TĔM-ĭk SHŬNT

postauricular pŏst-ăw-RĬK-ū-lăr

postcibum pŏst-SĒ-bŭm

posterior pōs-TĒR-ē-ŏr

postmortem pŏst-MŎR-tĕm

postpartum	pōst-PĂR-tŭm	pyelolithotomy	pī-ĕ-lō-lĭ-THŎT-ō-mē
postprandial	pōst-PRĂN-dē-ăl	pyelonephritis	pī-ĕ-lō-nĕf-RĪ-tĭs
potassium	pō-TĂ-sē-ŭm	pyloric	pī-LŎR-ĭk
precancerous	prē-KĂN-sĕr-ŭs	pyloric stenosis	pī-LŎR-ĭk stĕ-NŌ-sĭs
pregnancy	PRĔG-nŭn-sē	pyloroplasty	pī-LŎR-ō-plăs-tē
premolar	prē-MŌ-lăr	pylorospasm	pī-LŎR-ō-spăsm
prenatal	prē-NĀ-tăl	pyoderma	pī-ō-DĔR-mă
preprandial	prē-PRĂN-dē-ăl	pyometra	pī-ō-MĒ-tră
prepuce	PRĒ-pūs	pyometritis	pī-ō-mē-TRĪ-tĭs
presentation	prĕ-sĕn-TĀ-shŭn	pyorrhea	pī-ō-RĒ-ă
priapism	PRĪ-ŭ-pĭ-zŭm	pyothorax	pī-ō-THŌ-răks
primigravida	prĭ-mĭ-GRĂV-ĭ-dă	pyuria	pī-Ū-rē-ă
primipara	prĭ-MĬ-pă-ră		
primiparous	prĭ-MĬP-ă-rŭs	quadriparesis	kwŏd-rĭ-pă-RĒ-sĭs
proctology	prŏk-TŎL-ō-jē	quadriplegia	kwŏd-rĭ-PLĒ-jă
prodrome	PRŌ-drōm		
proestrus	prō-ĔS-trŭs	rabies	RĀ-bēs
progesterone	prō-JĔS-tĕ-rōn	radial	RĀ-dē-ăl
prognathia	prō-gNĀ-thē-ā	radiculitis	ră-dĭk-ū-LĪ-tĭs
prognosis	prŏg-NŌ-sĭs	radiculopathy	ră-dĭk-ū-LŎP-ă-thē
prolactin	prō-LĂK-tĭn	radiograph	ră-dē-Ō-grăf
prolapse	PRŌ-lăps	radiographer	ră-dē-ŎG-ră-fĕr
pronation	prō-NĀ-shŭn	radiography	ră-dē-ŎG-ră-fē
prone	prōn	radiology	ră-dē-ŎL-ō-jē
proprioception	PRŌ-prē-ō-sĕp-shŭn	radiotherapy	ră-dē-ō-THĔ-ră-pē
proptosis	prŏp-TŌ-sĭs	radius	RĀ-dē-ŭs
prostate gland	PRŎS-tāt glănd	rales and crackles	răhlz and kră-kŭlz
prostatectomy	prŏs-tă-TĔK-tō-mē	reabsorption	rē-ăb-SŎRP-shŭn
prostatitis	prŏs-tă-TĪ-tĭs	rectal	RĔK-tăl
prostatomegaly	prŏs-tă-tō-MĔG-ă-lē	rectocele	RĔK-tō-sēl
protease	PRŌ-tē-āse	rectum	RĔK-tŭm
proteinuria	prō-tēn-Ū-rē-ă	recumbency	rē-KŬM-bĕn-sē
prothrombin	prō-THRŎM-bĭn	recumbent	rē-KŬM-bĕnt
protoplasm	PRŌ-tō-plăzm	reduction	rĕ-DŬK-shŭn
proximal	PRŎK-sĭ-măl	refraction	rē-FRĂK-shŭn
pruritus	prū-RĪ-tĭs	regurgitate	rē-GĔR-jĭ-tāt
pseudocyesis	sū-dō-sī-Ē-sĭs	relapse	RĒ-lăps
pubic	PŪ-bĭk	remission	rē-MĬ-shŭn
pubis	PŪ-bĭs	renal	RĒ-năl
pulmonary	PŬL-mō-nĕr-ē	renal pelvis	RĒ-năl PĔL-vĭs
pulp	pŭlp	renal tubule	RĒ-năl TŪ-būl
pulse	pŭls	renin	RĒ-nĭn
pulse oximeter	pŭls ŏk-SĬ-mĕ-tĕr	resection	Rē-SĔK-shŭn
pupil	PŪ-pĭl	respiration	rĕs-pĕ-RĀ-shŭn
pupillary	PŪ-pĭ-lăr-ē	respiratory	RĔS-pĭr-ă-tō-rē
Purkinje fibers	pĕr-KĬN-jē FĪ-bĕrz	reticulocyte	rĕ-TĬK-ū-lō-sīt
purpura	PŬR-pū-ră	reticulum	rĕ-TĬK-ū-lŭM
purulent	PŪR-ū-lĕnt	retina	RĔT-ĭ-nă
pus	PŬS	retinal	RĔT-ĭ-năl
pustule	PŬS-tūl	retinitis	rĕt-ĭ-NĪ-tĭs
pyelitis	pī-ĕ-LĪ-tĭs	retinopathy	rĕ-tĭ-NŎP-ă-thē
pyelogram	PĪ-ĕ-lō-grăm	retrocardiac	rĕ-trō-KĂR-dē-ăk

retroperitoneal	rĕ-trō-pĕr-ĭ-tō-NĒ-ăl	semicircular canal	sĕ-mē-SĔR-kū-lăr kă-NĂL
retrovirus	rĕ-trō-VĪ-rŭs	seminal vesicles	SĔM-ĭn-ăl VĔS-ĭ-kŭlz
rhabdomyoma	răb-dō-mī-Ō-mă	seminiferous tubules	sĕ-mĭ-NĬF-ĕr-ŭs TŪB-ūlz
rhabdomyosarcoma	răb-dō-mī-ō-săr-KŌ-mă	septa; septum	SĔP-tă; SĔP-tŭm
rheumatoid arthritis	ROO-mă-toyd ăr-THRĪ-tĭs	sequestrum	sĭ-KWĔS-trŭm
		serotonin	sĕr-ŭh-TŌ-nĭn
rhinitis	rī-NĪ-tĭs	serum	SĔ-rŭm
rhinoplasty	RĪ-nō-PLĂS-tē	sesamoid bone	SĔS-ă-moyd
rhinorrhea	rī-nō-RĒ-ăh	shock	SHŎK
rhinotracheitis	RĪ-nō-TRĀ-kē-ī-tĭs	shunt	SHŬNT
rhonchi	RŎNG-kī	sialadenitis	sī-ăl-ă-dĕ-NĪ-tĭs
ribosomes	RĪ-bō-sōm	sialadenosis	sī-ăl-ă-dĕ-NŌ-sĭs
ribs	rĭbz	sialocele	SĪ-ăl-ō-sēl
rod	rŏd	sinoatrial node	sī-nō-Ā-trē-ăl nōd
rostral	RŎS-trăl	sinus	SĪ-nŭs
rotation	rō-TĀ-shŭn	sinus rhythm	SĪ-nŭs RĬTH-ŭm
rouleaux	ROO-lō	sinusitis	sī-nū-SĪ-tĭs
rugae	ROO-gē	sinusotomy	sī-nū-SŎ-tō-mē
rumen	ROO-mĕn	skeletal muscle	SKĔL-ĕ-tăl MŬS-ĕl
ruminant	ROO-mĕ-nănt	skull	skŭl
		sodium	SŌ-dē-ŭm
sacral	SĀ-krăl	soft palate	sŏft PĂL-ăt
sacralgia	sā-KRĂL-jă	somatotropin	sō-mă-tō-TRŌ-pĭn
sacrocaudal	SĀ-krō-KAWD-ăl	spasm	SPĂ-zĭm
sacrococcygeal	SĀ-krō-kŏk-sĭ-JĒ-ăl	spasticity	spă-STĬ-sĭ tē
sacroiliac	SĀ-krō-ĬL-ē-ăk	spermatic cord	spĕr-MĂT-ĭk kŏrd
sacropelvic	SĀ-krō-PĔL-vĭk	spermatogenesis	spĕr-mă-tō-JĔN-ĕ-sĭs
sacrum	SĀ-krŭm	spermatozoa	spĕr-mă-tō-ZŌ-ă
saddle	SĂ-dŭl	spermatozoon	spĕr-mă-tō-ZŌ-ŏn
sagittal	SĂJ-ĭ-tăl	spermolytic	spĕr-mō-LĬT-ĭk
saliva	să-LĪ-vă	sphenoid bone	SFĔ-noyd bōn
salivary gland	SĂL-ĭ-vĕr-ē glănd	spherocytosis	sfēr-ō-sī-TŌ-sĭs
salivary mucocele	SĂL-ĭ-vĕr-ē MŪ-kō-sēl	spheroid joint	SFĔ-royd joynt
sarcoma	săr-KŌ-mă	sphincter	SFĬNGK-tĕr
scabies	SKĀ-bēz	sphygmomanometer	sfĭg-mō-mă-NŎM-ĕ-tĕr
scapula	SKĂP-ū-lă	spina bifida	SPĪ-nă BĬF-ĭ-dă
scapular	SKĂP-ū-lăr	spinal	SPĪ-năl
scapulohumeral	SKĂP-ū-lō-HŪ-mĕr-ăl	spinal cavity	SPĪ-năl KĂ-vĭ-tē
scar	skŏr	spinal column	SPĪ-năl KŎL-ŭm
schwann	shwŏn	spinal cord	SPĪ-năl kŏrd
sclera	SKLĔ-ră	spirometer	spī-RŎM-ĕ-tĕr
scleral	SKLĔ-răl	splanchnic skeleton	SPLĂNGK-nĭk SKĔL-ĭ-tĭn
scleritis	sklĕ-RĪ-tĭs	spleen	splēn
scours	SKOW-ĕrz	splenectomy	splĕ-NĔK-tō-mē
scrotal circumference	SKRŌ-tăl sĕr-KŬM-fĕr-ĕns	splenic rupture	SPLĔ-nĭk RŬP-shŭr
scrotal hydrocele	SKRŌ-tăl HĪ-drō-sēl	splenomegaly	splē-nō-MĔG-ă-lē
scrotum	SKRŌ-tŭm	spondylitis	spŏn-dĭ-LĪ-tĭs
sebaceous gland	sĕ-BĀ-shŭs glănd	spondylosis	spŏn-dĭ-LŌ-sĭs
seborrhea	sĕb-ō-RĒ-ă	sputum	SPŪ-tŭm
sebum	SĒ-bŭm	squamous	SKWĀ-mŭs
seizure	SĒ-zhŭr	stapes	STĀ-pēz
semen	SĒ-mĕn	staphylococcus	stăf-ĭ-lō-KŎK-ŭs

stasis	STĀ-sĭs	synarthroses	sĭn-ăr-THRŌ-sēs
steatitis	stē-ă-TĪ-tĭs	syncopal	SĬN-kō-păl
steatolysis	stē-ă-TŎL-ĭ-sĭs	syncope	SĬN-kō-pē
steatoma	stē-ă-TŌ-mă	syndactyly	sĭn-DĂK-tĭ-lē
steatorrhea	stē-ă-tō-RĒ-ă	syndrome	SĬN-drŏm
stem cell	stĕm sĕl	synergistic	sĭn-ĕr-JĬS-tĭk
stenosis	stĕ-NŌ-sĭs	synovial cavity	sĭ-NŌ-vē-ăl KĂ-vĭ-tē
stent	stĭnt	synovial fluid	sĭ-NŌ-vē-ăl FLOO-ĭd
sterility	stĕ-RĬL-ĭ-tē	synovial joint	sĭ-NŌ-vē-ăl joynt
sterilization	stĕr-ĭ-lĭ-ZĀ-shŭn	synovial membrane	sĭ-NŌ-vē-ăl MĔM-brān
sternal	STĔR-năl	synovitis	sĭn-ō-VĪ-tĭs
sternum	STĔR-nŭm	synthesis	SĬN-thĕ-sĭs
steroid	STĔR-oyd	systemic	sĭs-TĔM-ĭk
stethoscope	STĔTH-ō-skōp	systole	SĬS-tō-lē
stifle	STĪ-fŭl		
stimulus	STĬM-ū-lŭs	tachycardia	tăk-ē-KĂR-dē-ă
stoma	STŌ-mă	tachypnea	tă-KĬP-nē-ă
stomach	STŬ-măk	tactile	tăk-TĪL
stomatitis	stō-mă-TĪ-tĭs	tapetum lucidum	tă-PĒ-tŭm LOO-sĭ-dŭm
stomatogastric	stō-mă-tō-GĂS-trĭk	tarsals	TĂR-sălz
stomatology	stō-mă-TŎL-ō-jē	tarsectomy	tăr-SĔK-tō-mē
strabismus	stră-BĬZ-mŭs	tarsorrhaphy	tăr-SŌR-ă-fē
stranguria	străng-Ū-rē-ă	tarsus	TĂR-sŭs
stratum corneum	STRĂ-tŭm KŎR-nē-ŭm	temporal bone	TĔM-pĕr-ăl bōn
streptococci	strĕp-tō-KŎK-sī	tendinectomy	tĕn-dĭ-NĔK-tō-mē
striated	STRĪ-ā-tĕd	tendinitis	tĕn-dĭ-NĪ-tĭs
stricture	STRĬK-shŭr	tendon	TĔN-dŭn
stridor	STRĪ-dŏr	tenectomy	tĕn-ĔK-tō-mē
stroma	STRŌ-mă	tenesmus	tĕ-NĔZ-mŭs
stupor	STOO-pŏr	tenorrhaphy	tĕn-ŎR-ă-fē
subarachnoid	sŭb-ă-RĂK-noyd	tenosynovitis	tĕn-ō-sĭ-nō-VĪ-tĭs
subcostal	sŭb-KŎS-tăl	tenotomy	tĕn-Ŏ-tō-mē
subcutaneous	sŭb-kū-TĀ-nē-ŭs	testes	TĔS-tēs
subdural	sŭb-DŪ-răl	testicles	TĔS-tĭ-kŭlz
subhepatic	sŭb-hĕ-PĂT-ĭk	testicular	tĕs-TĬK-ū-lăr
sublingual	sŭb-LĬNG-wăl	testis	TĔS-tĭs
subluxation	sŭb-lŭk-SĀ-shŭn	testosterone	tĕs-TŎS-tĕ-rōn
submandibular	sŭb-măn-DĬB-ū-lăr	tetany	TĔT-ă-nē
subpatellar	sŭb-pă-TĔL-lăr	tetraiodothyronine	tĕ-tră-ī-ō-dō-THĪ-rō-nēn
subungual	sŭb-ŬNG-wăl	tetralogy of fallot	tĕ-TRĂL-ō-jē of fă-LŌ
sulci; sulcus	SŬL-sī; SŬL-kŭs	tetraparesis	tĕ-tră-pă-RĒ-sĭs
superficial	sū-pĕr-FĬSH-ăl	tetraplegia	tĕ-tră-PLĒ-jă
supination	sū-pĭ-NĀ-shŭn	thalamus	THĂL-ă-mŭs
supine	SŪ-pīn	theriogenology	thĕr-ē-ō-jĕ-NŎL-ō-jē
suppurative	SŬ-pĕr-ă-tĭv	thoracentesis	thō-ră-sĕn-TĒ-sĭs
supraclavicular	sū-pră-klă-VĬK-ū-lăr	thoracentesis	thō-ră-sĕn-TĒ-sĭs
suprascapular	sū-pră-SKĂP-ū-lăr	thoracic	thō-RĂS-ĭk
susceptible	sŭs-SĔP-tĭ-bŭl	thoracocentesis	thōr-ră-sĕn-TĒ-sĭs
suture	SŪ-tŭr	thoracoscopy	thōr-ră-KŎS-kō-pē
symmetry	SĬM-mĕ-trē	thoracotomy	thō-ră-KŎT-ō-mē
sympathetic	sĭm-pă-THĔT-ĭk	thorascopy	thō-RŎS-kō-pē
symphysis	SĬM-fĭ-sĭs	thorax	thō-RĂKS
synapse	SĬN-ăps	thrill	thrĭl

thrombin	THRŎM-bǐn	tricuspid valve	trī-KŬS-pǐd vălv
thrombocyte	THRŎM-bō-sīt	trigeminal	trī-JĔM-ǐ-nǎl
thrombocytopenia	thrŏm-bō-sī-tō-PĒ-nē-ă	trigone	TRĪ-gōn
thrombocytosis	THRŎM-bō-sī-TŌ-sǐs	triiodothyronine	trī-ī-ō-dō-THĪ-rō-nēn
thromboembolic	thrŏm-bō-ĕm-BŎL-ǐk	trochanter	trō-KĂN-tĕr
meningoence-	mĕ-NĬN-gō-ĕn-sĕf-ă-	trochlear	TRŌ-klē-ăr
phalitis	LĪ-tǐs	trypsin	TRĬP-sǐn
thrombolysis	thrŏm-BŎL-ǐ-sǐs	tubercle	TŪ-bĕr-kŭl
thrombolytic	thrŏm-bō-LĬ-tǐk	tuberosity	tū-bĕ-RŎS-ǐ-tē
thromboplastin	thrŏm-bō-PLĂS-tǐn	tympanic membrane	tǐm-PĂN-ǐk MĔM-brăn
thrombosis	thrŏm-BŌ-sǐs	tympanoplasty	tǐm-pă-nō-PLĂS-tē
thrombus	THRŎM-bŭs		
thymectomy	thī-MĔK-tō-mē	ulcer	ŬL-sĕr
thymoma	thī-MŌ-mă	ulna	ŬL-nă
thymosin	THĪ-mŭ-sǐn	ulnar	ŬL-năr
thymus gland	THĪ-mŭs glănd	ultrasound	ŬL-tră-sound
thyroid gland	THĪ-royd glănd	umbilical	ŭm-BĬL-ǐ-kăl
thyroiditis	thī-royd-Ī-tǐs	umbilical cord	ŭm-BĬL-ǐ-kăl kŏrd
thyromegaly	thī-ro-MĔG-ă-lē	umbilicus	ŭm-BĬL-ǐ-kŭs
thyrotoxicosis	thī-ro-tŏk-sǐ-KŌ-sǐs	ungulates	ŬN-gū-lŭt or ŬN-gū-lāts
thyrotropin	thī-rō-TRŌ-pǐn	unilateral	ū-nē-LĂT-ĕr-ăl
thyroxine	thī-RŎK-sǐn	urea	ū-RĒ-ă
tibia	TĬB-ē-ă	uremia	ū-RĒ-mē-ă
tibial	TĬB-ē-ăl	ureter	Ū-rĕ-tĕr
tidal volume	TĪ-dăl VŎL-ūm	ureteroileostomy	ū-rē-tĕr-ō-ĭl ē-ŎS-tō-mē
tissue	TĬSH-ū	ureterolithotomy	ū-rē-tĕr-ō-lǐ-THŎT-ō-mē
tomography	tō-MŎG-ră-fē	ureteroplasty	ū-rē-tĕr-ō-PLĂS-tē
tongue	TŬNG	urethra	ū-RĒ-thră
tonometer	tō-NŎ-mĕ-tĕr	urethral stricture	ū-RĒ-thrăl STRĬK-shŭr
tonometry	tō-NŎM-ĕ-trē	urethritis	ū-rē-THRĪ-tǐs
tonsil	TŎN-sǐl	urethroplasty	ū-rē-thrō-PLĂS-tē
tonsillectomy	tŏn-sǐ-LĔK-tō-mē	uric acid	Ū-rǐk ĂS-ǐd
tonsillitis	tŏn-sǐ-LĪ-tǐs	urinalysis	ū-rǐn-ĂL-ǐ-sǐs
tonus	TŌ-nŭs	urinary bladder	ŪR-ǐ-năr-ē BLĂ-dĕr
torsion	TŎR-shŭn	urinary retention	ŪR-ǐ-năr-ē rē-TĔN-shŭn
toxic	TŎK-sǐk	urination	ūr-ǐ-NĀ-shŭn
toxin	TŎK-sǐn	urine	ū-rǐn
trachea	TRĀ-kē-ă	urolithiasis	ūr-ō-lǐ-THĪ-ă-sǐs
tracheal	TRĀ-kē-ăl	urological	ūr-ō-LŎG-ǐk-ăl
tracheal stenosis	TRĀ-kē-ăl stĕ-NŌ-sǐs	urology	ū-RŎL-ō-jē
tracheoplasty	trā-kē-ō-PLĂS-tē	uropoiesis	ū-rō-pō-Ē-sǐs
tracheostomy	trā-kē-ŎS-tō-mē	urticaria	ŭr-tǐ-KĀ-rē-ă
tracheotomy	trā-kē-ŎT-ō-mē	uterine	Ū-tĕr-ǐn
transfusion	trăns-FŪ-zhŭn	uterus	Ū-tĕ-rŭs
transhepatic	trănz-hĕ-PĂT-ǐk	uvea	Ū-vē-ă
transtracheal	trănz-TRĀ-kē-ăl	uveitis	ū-vē-Ī-tǐs
transurethral	trăns-ū-RĒ-thrăl		
transverse	trănz-VĔRS	vaccination	văk-sǐ-NĀ-shŭn
transverse colon	trănz-VĔRS KŌ-lĕn	vaccine	văk-SĒN
tremor	TRĔ-mŏr	vacuole	VĂC-ū-ōl
triadan	TRĪ-ă-dăn	vagal	VĀ-găl
trichobezoar	trǐ-kō-BĒ-zŏr	vagina	vă-JĪ-nă
trichomycosis	trǐk-ō-mī-KŌ-sǐs	vaginal	VĂ-jǐ-năl

vaginitis	vă-jĭ-NĪ-tĭs
vagus	VĀ-gŭs
valvotomy	văl-VŎT-ō-mē
valvuloplasty	văl-vū-lō-PLĂS-tē
vas deferens	văs DĔF-ĕr-ĕnz
vascular	VĂS-kū-lăr
vasculitis	văs-kū-LĪ-tĭs
vasectomy	vă-SĔK-tō-mē
vasoconstriction	vă-zō-kŏn-STRĬK-shŭn
vasodilation	vă-zō-dī-LĀ-shŭn
vasopressin	văz-ō-PRĔS-ĭn
vasovasostomy	vă-zō-vă-ZŎS-tō-mē
vein	VĀN
vena cava; venae cavae	VĒ-nă KĀ-vă; VĒ-nē KĀ-vē
venipuncture	vĕ-nĭ-PŬNK-chŭr
venous	VĒ-nŭs
ventilation	vĕn-tĭ-LĀ-shŭn
ventral	VĔN-trăl
ventricle	VĔN-trĭ-kŭl
ventricular	vĕn-TRĬK-ū-lăr
ventricular septal defect	vĕn-TRĬK-ū-lăr SĔP-tăl DĔ-fĕkt
venule	VĔN-ūl
verruca; verrucae	vĕ-ROO-kă; vĕ-ROO-kē
vertebra	VĔR-tĕ-bră
vertebrae	VĔR-tĕ-brā
vertebral	VĔR-tĕ-brăl
vertigo	VĔR-tĭ-gō
vesicular	vĕ-SĬK-ū-lăr
vessel	VĔS-ĕl

vestibular disease	vĕs-TĬ-bū-lăr dĭ-ZĒZ
vestibule	VĔS-tĭ-būl
vestibulocochlear	vĕs-tĭb-ū-lō-KŎK-lē-ăr
viable	VĪ-ă-bŭl
villi	VĬL-ī
viral	VĪ-răl
viscera	VĬS-ĕr-ă
visceral	VĬS-ĕr-ăl
visceral muscle	VĬS-ĕr-ăl MŬS-ĕl
visceral skeleton	VĬS-ĕr-ăl SKĔL-ĭ-tĭn
visceralgia	VĬS-ĕr-ăl-jă
vitreous chamber	VĬT-rē-ŭs CHĀM-bĕr
vitreous humor	VĬT-rē-ŭs HŪ-mĕr
vocal cords	VŌ-kăl kŏrds
vocal folds	VŌ-kăl fōlds
voiding	VOY-dĭng
vomer	VŌ-mĕr
von Willebrand disease	fŏn VĬ-lĕ-brănts dĭ-ZĒZ
vovulus	VŎL-vū-lŭs
vulva	VŬL-vă
vulvovaginitis	vŭl-vō-vă-jĭ-NĪ-tĭs
warfarin	WĂR-fă-rĭn
wean	WĒN
wheal	wēl
xeroderma	zĕ-rō-DĔR-mă
xiphoid process	ZĬF-oyd PRŎS-ĕs
zygomatic bone	zī-gō-MĂ-tĭk bōnz

Go to www.wiley.com/go/taibo/terminology to find additional learning materials:

• Audio clips to show how to pronounce terms

Appendix B Commonly Used Veterinary Medical Abbreviations

%	Percent
A	Accommodation; ampere; anode; axial; anterior
A/P	Anterior/posterior
AAEVT	Academy of Equine Veterinary Nursing Technicians
AAFCO	American Association of Feed Control Officials
AAHA	American Animal Hospital Association
AALAS	American Association for Laboratory Animals
AB	Abortion
Ab	Antibody
ABC	Aspiration biopsy cytology
ABCDE	Airway, breathing, circulation, disability/dehydration, exposure
ABG	Arterial blood gas
ABVP	American Board of Veterinary Practitioners
ABVT	American Board of Veterinary Toxicology
ac	Before meals (ante cibum)
Ach	Acetylcholine
AChE	Acetylcholinestrase
ACL	Anterior cruciate ligament
ACLAM	American College of Laboratory Animal Medicine
ACPV	American College of Poultry Veterinarians
ACT	American College of Theriogenologists
ACTH	Adrenocorticotropic hormone
ACVA	American College of Veterinary Anesthesiologists
ACVB	American College of Veterinary Behaviorists
ACVCP	American College of Veterinary of Clinical Pharmacology
ACVD	American College of Veterinary Dermatology
ACVECC	American College of Veterinary Emergency and Critical Care
ACVIM	American College of Veterinary Internal Medicine
ACVM	American College of Veterinary Microbiologists
ACVN	American College of Veterinary Nutrition
ACVO	American College of Veterinary Ophthalmologists
ACVP	American College of Veterinary Pathologists
ACVPM	American College of Veterinary Preventative Medicine
ACVR	American College of Veterinary Radiology
ACVS	American College of Veterinary Surgeons
ACZM	American College of Zoological Medicine
AD	Right ear
ad. lib.	As desired
ADH	Antidiuretic hormone
ADR	Ain't doin right
AEMP	Animal emergency management program

AF	Atrial fibrillation	BAR	Bright, alert, responsive
Ag	Antigen	Baso	Basophils
AHT	Animal health technician	BBB	Blood brain barrier
AI	Artificial insemination	BCS	Body Condition Score
AIHA	Autoimmune hemolytic anemia	BD/LD	Big dog/little dog
AIMVT	Academy of Internal Medicine for Veterinary Technicians	BG	Blood gas
		BG	Blood glucose
AKC	American Kennel Club	BID	Twice daily; q12h
ALAT	Assistant laboratory animal technician	Bilat.	Bilateral
		Bili	Bilirubin
Alb	Albumin	BM	Bowel movement
Alk. phos.	Alkaline phosphatase (liver enzyme)	BMBT	Buccal mucosal bleeding time
		BP	Blood pressure
ALT	Alanine aminotransferase (liver enzyme)	BPM	Beats per minute/breaths per minute
		BRSV	Bovine respiratory syncytial virus
amp	ampule; ampere	BSA	Body surface area
amyl	Amylase	BSE	Bovine spongiform encephalopathy (mad cow disease)
ANS	Autonomic nervous system		
APHIS—VS	Animal and Plant—Health Inspection Services Veterinary Services	BUN	Blood urea nitrogen
		BVD	Bovine viral diarrhea
		bx	Biopsy
AS	Aortic stenosis		
AS	Left ear	$\bar{c}$	With
ASAP	As soon as possible	C	Castrated
ASM	Animal Shelter Management Certification	Ca	Calcium
		CA	Cancer
ASPCA	American Society for the Prevention of Cruelty to Animals	CAE	Caprine arthritis encephalitis virus
AST	Aspartate aminotransferase	cal	Calorie
ASVDT	American Society of Veterinary Dental Technicians	cap	Capsule
		CAPD	Continuous Abdominal Peritoneal Dialysis
AU	Both ears		
AVCPT	Academy of Veterinary Clinical Pathology Technicians	CAT scan	Computed tomography
		cath	Catheter
AVDC	American Veterinary Dental College	CAR	Congenital articular rigidity
		CBA	Cat bite abscess
AVDT	Academy of Veterinary Dental Technicians	CBC	Complete blood count
		cc	Cubic centimeter
AVECCT	Academy of Veterinary Emergency and Critical Care	CC	Chief complaint
		CCL	Cranial cruciate ligament
AVMA	American Veterinary Medical Association	CCU	Critical care unit
		CDC	Center for Disease Control
AVNT	Academy of Veterinary Nutrition Technicians	CFT	Complement fixation test
		CH	Certified herbalist
AVST	Academy of Veterinary Surgical Technicians	ChE	Cholinestrase
		CHD	Congenital Heart Disease
AVTA	Academy of Veterinary Technician Anesthetists	CHF	Congestive heart failure
		CHOL	Cholesterol
AVTCP	Academy of Veterinary Technicians in Clinical Practice	CK	Creatine kinase
		Cl	Chloride
AVTE	Association of Veterinary Technician Educators, Inc.	CM	Castrated male
		cm	centimeter
AVZMT	Association of Veterinary Zoological Medical Technicians	CMAR	Certified manager Animal Resources Program
AZVT	Association of Zoo Veterinary Technicians	CMT	California Mastitis Test
		CNS	Central nervous system

CO	Carbon monoxide	DMH	Domestic medium hair (a mixed breed cat with medium hair)
CO_2	Carbon dioxide		
conc	Concentration	DNA	Deoxyribonucleic acid
COPD	Chronic obstructive pulmonary disease	DOA	Dead on arrival
		DOB	Date of birth
CP	Conscious proprioception		
CPCR	Cardiopulmonary cerebral resuscitation	dr	Dram
		DSH	Domestic short hair
CPR	Cardiopulmonary resuscitation	DVM	Doctor of Veterinary Medicine
CREA	Creatinine	dx, ddx	Diagnosis; differential diagnosis
Creat	Creatinine		
CRF	Chronic renal failure	ECHO	Echocardiogram
CRT	Capillary refill time	ED	Effective dose
C-Sect	Cesarean section (c-section)	EDTA	Ethylenediaminetetraacetic acid
CSF	Cerebrospinal fluid	EEE	Eastern equine encephalitis
CSM	Cerebrospinal meningitis	EEG	Elecroencephalogram
CT	Computed tomography	EI	Equine influenza
CVA	Cerebrovascular accident (stroke)	EIA	Equine infectious anemia
CVA	Certified veterinary acupuncturist	EKG	Electrocardiogram; (ECG)
CVP	Central venous pressure	ELISA	Enzyme-linked Immunosorbent assay
CVPM	Certified veterinary practice manager		
		EMG	Electromyogram
CVS	Cardiovascular system	EOD	Every other day
CVT	Certified veterinary technician	Eos	Eosinophils
CVTEA	Committee on Veterinary Technician Education and Activities	EPM	Equine protozoal myeloencephalitis
		EPO	Erythropoietin
		ER	Emergency room
CVTS	Committee of Veterinary Technician Specialties	ESR	Erythrocyte sedimentation rate (sed rate)
		ET tube	Endotracheal tube
CWPM	Continue with previous medication	EVA	Equine viral arteritis
		EVR	Equine viral rhinopneumonitis
Cysto	Cystocentesis		
		F	Fahrenheit; female
D.Bili	Direct bilirubin	FA	Fatty acid
DA	Displaced abomasum	FAD	Flea allergy dermatitis
DC	Doctor of Chiropractic	FBS	Fasting blood sugar
DD	Differential diagnosis	FDA	Food and Drug Administration
DDN	Dull, depressed, nonresponsive	Fe	Iron
ddx	Differential diagnosis	FeLV	Feline leukemia virus
DEA	Drug Enforcement Administration	FIC	Feline idiopathic cystitis or Feline interstitial cystitis
Derm	Skin		
DES	Diethylstilbestrol	FIP	Feline infectious peritonitis
DHIA	Dairy Herd Improvement Association	FIV	Feline immunodeficiency virus
		fl oz	Fluid ounces
DHLPP-C	Distemper, hepatitis, leptospirosis, parvo virus, parainfluenza, coronavirus	FLUTD	Feline lower urinary tract disease
		FNA	Fine needle aspirate
		FSH	Follicle-stimulating hormone
DI	Diabetes insipidus	FSIS	Food Safety and Inspection Services
DIC	Disseminated intravascular coagulation		
		FUO	Fever of Unknown Origin
Diff	White blood cell differential	FUS	Feline urological syndrome
DKA	Diabetic ketoacidosis	FVRCP-C	Feline viral rhinotracheitis, calicivirus, panleukopenia, and chlamydia
DLE	Discoid lupus erythematosus		
DLH	Domestic long hair (a mixed breed cat with long hair)		
DM	Diabetes mellitus	fx	Fracture

g	Gram	ISO	Isolation unit
g/dl	Grams/deciliter	IT	Intrathecal
gal	Gallon	IU	International units
GDV	Gastric dilatation volvulus	IV	Intravenous
GFR	Glomerular filtration rate	IVAPM	International Veterinary Academy
GGT	Gamma glutamyltranspeptidase		of Pain Management
GH	Growth hormone	IVC	Intravenous catheter
GI	Gastrointestinal	IVD	Intervertebral disk (disc)
GLU	Glucose	IVDD	Intervertebral disc disease
g; gm	Gram	IVP	Intravenous pyelogram
gr	Grain		
GROS	Gross review of systems	K	Potassium
GSW	Gunshot wound	K+	Potassium
gt	Drop	K-9	Canine or Dog
gtt	Drops	KBH	Kicked by horse
GTT	Glucose tolerance test	KCl	Potassium chloride
Gyn	Gynecology	kg	Kilogram
		km	Kilometer
H	Hydrogen		
H&E	Hematoxylin and eosin stain	Ⓛ	Left
HGE	Hemorrhagic gastroenteritis	L (l)	Liter
H₂O	Water	LA	Large animal
H₂O₂	Hydrogen peroxide	LAT	Laboratory animal technician
Hb; Hgb	Hemoglobin	LATG	Laboratory animal technologist
HBC	Hit by car	lb or #	Pound
HCG	Human chorionic gonadotropin	LD	Lethal dose
HCl	Hydrochloric acid	LDA/RDA	Left displaced abomasum/right
HCT	Hematocrit		displaced abomasum
HDDS	High dose dexamethasone	LDDS	Low dose dexamethasone
	suppression test		suppression test
HDL	High-density lipoprotein	LDH	Lactic acid dehydrogenase
hpf	High power field	LDL	Low-density lipoprotein
HR	Heart rate	LE	Lupus erythematosus
hr	Hour	lg	Large
HW	Heartworm	LH	Luteinizing hormone
hx	History	LLQ/LL	Left lower quadrant
		LN	Lymph node
I	Iodine	LOC	Level of consciousness
I.Bili	Indirect bilirubin	LP	Lumbar puncture
IA	Intra-arterial	lpf	Low power field
IACUC	Institutional Animal Care and Use	LRS	Lactated Ringer's solution
	Committee	LUQ/LU	Left upper quadrant
IBR	Infectious bovine rhinotracheitis	LV	Left ventricle
IC	Intracardiac	LVT	Licensed veterinary technician
ICP	Intracranial pressure	Lymph	Lymphocytes
ICSH	Interstitial cell-stimulating hormone		
ICU	Intensive care unit	m	Meter
ID	Intradermal	M	Male
IFA	Immunofluorescent antibody test	mcg, μg	Microgram
	IgA, IgD, IgE, IgG, IgM	MCH	Mean corpuscular hemoglobin
	Immunoglobulins	MCHC	Mean corpuscular hemoglobin
IM	Intramuscular		concentration
IMHA	Immune-mediated hemolytic anemia	MCV	Mean corpuscular volume
inj	Injection	MDB	Minimum database
IOP	Intraocular pressure	ME	Myeloid-erythroid ratio
IP	Intraperitoneal	MED	Minimal effective dose

meq	Milliequivalents	OR	Operating room
mets	Metastasis	Ortho	Orthopedic or orthopedic procedure
mg	Milligram		
Mg	Magnesium	OS	Left eye
MG	Myasthenia gravis	OSHA	Occupational Safety and Health Administration
MI	Myocardial infarction		
MIC	Minimum inhibitory concentration	OT	Oxytocin
		OTC	Over the counter
MID	Minimum infective dose	OU	Both eyes
ml	Milliliter	oz	Ounce
MLD	Minimum lethal dose		
MLV	Modified live virus; modified live vaccine	$\bar{p}$	After
		p	Pulse
MM	Mucous membranes	P.T.	Physical therapy
mm	Millimeter	P/E	Physical examination
mmHG	Millimeters of mercury	PAC	Premature atrial contraction
Mono	Monocytes	pc	After meals (post cibum)
MRI	Magnetic resonance imaging	pCO_2	Partial pressure of carbon dioxide
MS	Mitral stenosis	PCR	Polymerase chain reaction
MSDS	Material data safety sheet	PCV	Packed cell volume
MSH	Melanocyte-stimulating hormone	PD	Polydipsia
MVP	Mitral valve prolapse	PDA	Patent ductus arteriosus
		PDR	Physicians' Desk Reference
N	Neutered; normal; nitrogen	PE	Pulmonary embolism
Na	Sodium	PEM	Polioencephalomalacia
NA (n/a)	Not applicable	PET	Positron emission tomography
Na	Sodium	PG	Pregnant
NADC	National Animal Disease Center	pH	Degree of acidity or alkalinity
NAF	No abnormalities found	PHF	Potomac horse fever
NAPCC	National Animal Poison Control Center	PHS	Public Health Service
		PI_3	Parainfluenzavirus 3
NAVTA	National Association of Veterinary Technicians of America	PKU	Phenylketonuria
		PLH	Pharyngeal lymphoid hyperplasia
neg or $\ominus$	Negative	PLR	Pupillary light reflex
NG tube	Nasogastric tube	Plt	Platelet
NH_3	Ammonia	PM	Postmortem; evening
NIH	National Institute of Health	PMI	Point of maximal intensity
NM (M/N)	Neutered male	PMN	Polymorphonuclear neutrophil
NPN	Nonprotein nitrogen; nonprotein nitrogenous waste	PMS	Pregnant mare's serum
		PMSG	Pregnant mare serum gonadotropin
NPO	Nothing by mouth (nil per os)	PNS	Peripheral nervous system
nRBC	Nucleated red blood cell	PO	By mouth (per os)
NS	Normal saline	pO_2	Partial Pressure of Oxygen
NSAID	Nonsteroidal anti-inflammatory drug	pos or $\oplus$	Positive
		POVMR	Problem-oriented veterinary medical records
NSF	No significant findings		
NVSL	National Veterinary Services Laboratories	PPH	Past pertinent history
		ppm	Parts per million
		PR	Per rectum
O_2	Oxygen	PRL	Prolactin
OB	Obstestrics	prn	As needed
OD	Right eye	PROM	Passive range of motion
OFA	Orthopedic Foundation for Animals	PRRS	Porcine respiratory and reproductive syndrome
OHE (OVH)	Spay	PSS	Physiological saline solution; porcine stress syndrome
OPP	Ovine progressive pneumonia		

PT	Prothrombin time; Physical therapy	SCC	Somatic cell count
pt	Pint	Seg	Neutrophils
pt.	Patient	SF (F/S)	Spayed female
PTH	Parathormone	SG	Specific gravity
PTT	Partial thromboplastin time	SGOT	Serum glutamic oxaloacetic transaminase
PU	Perineal urethrostomy; polyuria	SGPT	Serum glutamic pyruvic transaminase
PU/PD	Polyuria/polydipsia	SID	Once daily; q24h
Pulse Ox	Pulse oximeter; pulse oximetry	SLE	Systemic lupus erythematosus
PVC	Premature ventricular contraction	SMEDI	Stillborn, mummification, embryonic death, infertility
PZI	Protamine zinc insulin	SOAP	Subjective, objective, assessment, plan
q	Every	sol	Solution (sol'n, soln)
qd	Every day	sp. gr.	Specific gravity
qh	Every hour	SPF	Specific-pathogen free
QID	Four times daily; q6h	SQ	Subcutaneous (Sub Q)
qn	Every night	SR	Sedimentation rate (sed)
qns	Quantity not sufficient	Staph	*Staphylococcus spp.*
qp	As desired	stat	Immediately
qs	Quantity sufficient	Strep	*Streptococcus spp.*
qt	Quart	SVBT	Society of Veterinary Behavior Technicians
q24h	Once daily; every 24 hours	SVBT	Academy (formerly a Society) of Veterinary Behavior Technicians
q12h	Twice daily; every 12 hours		
q8h	Three times daily; every 8 hours		
q6h	Four times daily; every 6 hours	Sx	Surgery
		Sz	Seizure
®	Right		
®	Registered trademark	T	Tablespoon; tablet; temperature
R/O	Rule out	T_3	Triiodothyronine
RAI	Radioactive iodine; treatment for hyperthyroidism	T_4	Thyroxine; tetraiodothyronine
		tab	Tablet
RBC	Red blood cell	TB	Tuberculin
RLQ/RL	Right lower quadrant	Tbil T.Bili	Total bilirubin
RNA	Ribonucleic acid	Tbsp	Tablespoon; 1 Tbsp = 15 mls
ROM	Range of motion	TE	Tetanus
RP	Retained placenta	TEME, TME	Thromboembolic meningoencephalitis
rpm	Revolutions per Minute		
RR	Respiratory rate	TGE	Transmissible gastroenteritis
RTG	Ready to go (home)	THR	Total hip replacement
RUQ/RU	Right upper quadrant	TID	Three times daily; q8h
RV	Rabies vaccine	TLC	Tender loving care
RVT	Registered veterinary technician	TNTC	Too numerous to count
RVTG	Registered veterinary technologist	TP	Total protein
		TPLO	Tibial plateau leveling osteotomy
R_x	Prescription; medication	TPN	Total parenteral nutrition
		TPO	Triple pelvic osteotomy
s̄	Without	TPR(W)	Temperature, pulse, respiration, (weight)
S	Spayed		
SA	Small animal; sinoatrial	TR	Treatment
SAP	Serum alkaline phosphatase	TSH	Thyroid-stimulating hormone
SC	Scrotal circumference	tsp; t	Teaspoon; 1 tsp = 5 mls
SC, SQ, Sub Q	Subcutaneous	TTA	Tibial tuberosity advancement

TTW	Transtracheal wash	VPC	Ventricular premature contraction or ventricular premature complexes
Tx	Treatment		
U/A	Urinalysis	VS	Vesicular stomatitis
URI	Upper respiratory infection	VSD	Ventricular septal defect
USDA	United States Department of Agriculture	VT; V tach	Ventricular tachycardia
USG	Urine specific gravity	VTAS	Veterinary Technician Anesthetist Society
UTI	Urinary tract infection	VTS	Veterinary technician specialist
V fib	Ventricular Fibrillation	VWD	Von Willebrand's disease
V/D	Vomiting/diarrhea		
VA	Visual acuity	WBC	White blood cell
VEE	Venezuelan equine encephalitis	WEE	Western equine encephalitis
VESPA	Veterinary Emergency and Specialty Practice Associations	WMT	Wisconsin mastitis test
		WNL	Within normal limits
VMD	Veterinary medical doctor	WNV	West Nile virus
vol	Volume	wt	Weight
VPB	Veterinary pharmaceuticals and biologicals	µl	Microliters

Recommended Reading

American Association for Laboratory Animal Science. www.aalas.org/. Oct. 29, 2013.

Bassert, Joanna M., and Dennis M. McCurnin. *McCurnin's Clinical Textbook for Veterinary Technicians*, 7th ed. St. Louis: Elsevier Saunders, 2010.

Colville, Thomas P., and Joanna M. Bassert. *Clinical Anatomy and Physiology for Veterinary Technicians*, 2nd ed. St. Louis: Elsevier Health Sciences, 2008.

Dr. Greg Martinez on YouTube. www.youtube.com/drgregdvm. Oct. 29, 2013.

Harvey, John W. *Atlas of Veterinary Hematology: Blood and Bone Marrow of Domestic Animals*. Philadelphia: W.B. Saunders, 2001.

Hendrix, Charles M., and Ed Robinson. *Diagnostic Parasitology for Veterinary Technicians*, 4th ed. St. Louis: Elsevier Mosby, 2006.

Hendrix, Charles M., and Margi Sirois. *Laboratory Procedures for Veterinary Technicians*. St. Louis: Mosby Elsevier, 2007.

Holtgrew-Bohling, Kristin, and Elizabeth A. Hanie. *Large Animal Clinical Procedures for Veterinary Technicians*. St. Louis: Elsevier/Mosby, 2012.

Hrapkiewicz, Karen, Leticia Medina, and Donald D. Holmes. *Clinical Laboratory Animal Medicine: An Introduction*. Ames, Iowa: Blackwell, 2007.

Mader, Douglas R. *Reptile Medicine and Surgery*. Philadelphia: W.B. Saunders, 1996.

Mazzaferro, Elisa M. *Small Animal Emergency and Critical Care*. Oxford: Wiley-Blackwell, 2010.

Microscopy Learning Systems: https://lms.mlsedu.com/index.php. Oct. 29, 2013.

Pasquini, Chris, and Tom Spurgeon. *Anatomy of Domestic Animals*. Eureka, California: Sudz, 1987.

Reagan, William J., Teresa G. Sanders, and D.B. DeNicola. *Veterinary Hematology: Atlas of Common Domestic Species*. Ames: Iowa State University Press, 1998.

Samour, Jaime. *Avian Medicine*. Edinburgh: Mosby/Elsevier, 2008.

Sonsthagen, Teresa F. *Veterinary Instruments and Equipment: A Pocket Guide*. St. Louis: Elsevier Mosby, 2006.

Studdert, Virginia P., Clive C. Gay, and D.C. Blood. *Saunders Comprehensive Veterinary Dictionary*. Edinburgh: Saunders Elsevier, 2012.

Summers, Alleice. *Common Diseases of Companion Animals*, 2nd ed. St. Louis: Mosby, 2013.

Veterinary Medical Terminology Guide and Workbook, First Edition. Angela Taibo.
© 2014 John Wiley & Sons, Inc. Published 2014 by John Wiley & Sons, Inc.
Companion website: www.wiley.com/go/taibo/terminology

Thomas, John A., Phillip Lerche, and Diane McKelvey. *Anesthesia and Analgesia for Veterinary Technicians*. St. Louis: Mosby/Elsevier, 2011.

Thrall, Mary Anna. *Veterinary Hematology and Clinical Chemistry*. Philadelphia: Lippincott Williams & Wilkins, 2004.

Tracy, Diane L. *Small Animal Surgical Nursing*. St. Louis: Mosby, 2000.

USDA. www.usda.gov. Oct. 29, 2013.

Glossary

By Word Part

a-	no; not; without	acuit/o	sharp
ab-	away from	-acusia	hearing
abdomin/o	abdomen	-acusis	hearing
-able	capable of	acut/o	sharp
abort/o	premature expulsion of	ad-	toward
	fetus	-ad	in the direction of
abrad/o	scrape off		to; toward
abras/o	scrape off	aden/o	gland
abrupt/o	broken away from	adenoid/o	adenoids
abs-	away from	adhes/o	cling
absorpt/o	to suck up or in		stick
-ac	pertaining to	adip/o	fat
acanth/o	spiny	adnex/o	bound to
	thorny	adren/o	adrenal gland
acetabul/o	acetabulum	adrenal/o	adrenal gland
-acious	characterized by	aer/o	air
acne/o	point		gas
acous/o	hearing	aesthet/o	feeling
acoust/o	hearing		sensation
acr/o	extremities	af-	toward
	top	affect/o	exert influence on
acromi/o	acromion	ag-	toward
actin/o	light	agglutin/o	clumping
acu/o	severe		sticking together
	sharp	aggress/o	attack
	sudden		step forward

Veterinary Medical Terminology Guide and Workbook, First Edition. Angela Taibo.
© 2014 John Wiley & Sons, Inc. Published 2014 by John Wiley & Sons, Inc.
Companion website: www.wiley.com/go/taibo/terminology

-ago	attack		doubly
	disease condition		on both sides
-agon	to assemble	amput/o	cut off
	to gather		to cut away
agora-	marketplace	amputat/o	cut off
-agra	excessive pain		to cut away
	seizure	amyl/o	starch
-aise	comfort	an-	no
	ease		without
al-	similar	-an	pertaining to
-al	pertaining to	an/o	anus
alb/i	white		ring
alb/o	white		upward
albin/o	white	ana-	again
albumin/o	albumin		anew
alg/e	pain		apart
alg/o	pain		backward
alges/o	sensitivity to pain		up
algesi/o	sensitivity to pain	andr/o	male
-algesia	sensitivity to pain	aneurysm/o	aneurysm
-algesic	pertaining to sensitivity	angi-	vessel
	to pain	angi/o	blood vessel
algi-	sensitivity to pain		vessel
-algia	pain	angin/o	strangle
align/o	correct position	anis/o	unequal
	to bring in line	ankyl/o	stiff
aliment/o	to nourish	anomal/o	irregularity
all-	different	ante-	before
	other		forward
all/o	different	anter/o	front
	other	anthr/o	antrum of the stomach
alopec/o	baldness	anthrac/o	coal
alveol/o	air sac	anti-	against
	alveolus	anxi/o	anxious
amb-	both sides		uneasy
	double	anxiet/o	anxious
amb/i	both sides		uneasy
	double	aort/o	aorta
ambly/o	dim	-apheresis	removal
	dull	aphth/o	ulcer
ambul/o	to walk	apic/o	apex
ambulat/o	to walk		point
ametr/o	out of proportion	aplast/o	defective development
-amine	nitrogen		lack of strength
amni/o	amnion	apo-	away
amph-	around		off

aponeur/o	aponeurosis	auricul/o	ear
apth/o	ulcer	auscult/o	to listen
aqu/i	water	auto-	own
aqu/o	water		self
aque/o	water	ax/o	axis
-ar	pertaining to		main stem
arachn/o	arachnoid membrane	axill/o	armpit
	spider	azot/o	nitrogen
arc/o	arch		urea
	bow	bacill/o	bacillus
-arche	beginning	bacteri/o	bacteria
arrect/o	upright	balan/o	glans penis
arter/o	artery	bar/o	pressure
arteri/o	artery		weight
arteriol/o	arteriole	barthollin/o	Bartholin glands
arthr/o	joint	bas/o	base
articul/o	joint		opposite of acid
-ary	pertaining to	bi-	two
-ase	enzyme	bi/o	life
asphyxi/o	absence of a pulse	bifid/o	split into two
aspir/o	to breathe in		parts
aspirat/o	to breathe in	bifurcat/o	divide into two
asthen-	weakness		branches
-asthenia	lack of strength	bil/i	bile
	weakening		gall
asthmat/o	gasping	bilirubin/o	bilirubin
Astr/o	Star	-bin; bini-	double
at-	toward		twice
atel/o	incomplete		two
ather/o	plaque	bio-	life
athet/o	uncontrolled	bis-	twice
-ation	condition	-bis	double
	process		two
-atonic	lack of strength	-blast	embryonic
	tone		immature
atop/o	out of place	blast/i	embryonic
atres/i	closure		immature
	without an opening	-blastoma	immature tumor
atri/o	atrium	blephar/o	eyelid
attenuat/o	dilation	bol/o	to cast
	weak		to throw
aud-; aud/i	hearing	borborygm/o	rumbling sound
audi/o	hearing	brachi/o	arm
audit/o	hearing	brachy-	short
aur/i	ear	brady-	slow
aur/o	ear	brev/i	short

brev/o	short	cat-	down	
bronch/o	bronchial tube		downward	
bronchi/o	bronchial tube		lower	
bronchiol/o	bronchiole		under	
brux/o	to grind	cata-	down	
bucc/o	cheek	catabol/o	breaking down	
bucca-	cheek	cath-	down	
bulla-	blister		downward	
burs/o	bursa		lower	
	sac of fluid near a joint		under	
cac-	bad	cathart/o	cleansing	
	diseased		purging	
	weak	cathet/o	insert	
cac/o	bad		send down	
	diseased	caud/o	lower part of the	
	weak		body	
cadaver/o	dead body		tail	
calc/i	calcium	caus/o	burn	
calc/o	calcium		heat	
calcane/o	calcaneus	caust/o	burn	
calci/o	calyx		heat	
calic/o	calyx	caut/o	burn	
call/i	hard		heat	
callos/o	hard	cauter/o	burn	
calor/i	heart		heat	
canalicul/o	little duct	cav/i	hollow	
canth/o	corner of the eye	cav/o	hollow	
capillar/o	capillary	cavern/o	containing hollow	
capit/o	head		spaces	
capn/o	carbon dioxide	cec/o	cecum	
-capnia	carbon dioxide	-cele	hernia	
capsul/o	litter box	celi/o	abdomen	
	capsule		belly	
carb/o	carbon	cement/o	cementum	
carcin/o	cancer	cent-	hundred	
	cancerous	-centesis	surgical puncture to	
cardi/o	heart		remove fluid or gas	
cari/o	decay	cephal-	head	
carot/o	sleep	cephal/o	head	
	stupor	-ceps	head	
carp/o	carpals	cera-	wax	
	carpus	cerebell/o	cerebellum	
cartilag/o	cartilage	cerebr/o	cerebrum	
	gristle	cerumin/o	cerumen	
caruncul/o	bit of flesh	cervic/o	cervix	
	caruncles		neck	

chalas/o	relaxation	circumscrib/o	confined or limited to
-chalasia	relaxation	cirrh/o	orange-yellow
-chalasis	relaxation	cis/o	to cut
chalaz/o	hailstone	-clasis	to break
	small lump	-clast	to break
cheil/o	lip	clav/i	key
chem/i	chemical	clavicul/o	clavicle
	drug	clitor/o	clitoris
chem/o	chemical		female erectile tissue
	drug	clon/o	violent action
chemic/o	chemical	-clysis	irrigation
	drug		washing
-chezia	defecation	co-	together; with
	elimination of waste	coagul/o	clotting
chir/o	hand		clump
chlor/o	green		coagulation
chlorhydr/o	hydrochloric acid		congeal
chol/e	bile	coagulat/o	clump
cholangi/o	bile vessel		congeal
cholecyst/o	gallbladder	cocc/i	berry-shaped
choledoch/o	common bile duct		round
cholestrol/o	cholesterol	cocc/o	berry-shaped
chondr/o	cartilage		round
chondri/o	cartilage	-coccus; -cocci	berry-shaped
chord/o	cord		bacterium
	spinal cord	coccyg/o	coccyx
chore/o	dance		tailbone
chori/o	chorion	cochle/o	cochlea
chorion/o	chorion	-coel	hollow
choroid/o	choroid	coher/o	to stick together
chrom/o	color	cohes/o	to stick together
chromat/o	color	coit/o	coming together
chron/o	time	col/o	colon
chym/o	juice		large intestine
	to pour	coll/a	glue
cib/o	meal	coll/i	neck
-cidal	pertaining to killing	colon/o	colon
-cide	killing		large intestine
cili/o	insert	colp/o	vagina
	send down	column/o	pillar
cine/o	movement	com-	together
circi/o	circle	comat/o	deep sleep
	ring	comi/o	to care for
circulat/o	to go around in a	comminut/o	to break into pieces
	circle	communic/o	to share
circum-	around	compatibil/o	to sympathize with

con-	together	cord/o	heart
	with		spinal cord
concav/o	hollow	core-	pupil
concentr/o	remove excess water	core/o	pupil
	to condense	cori/o	leather
concept/o	to become pregnant	cori/o	skin
	to receive	corne/o	cornea
conch/o	shell	coron/o	crown
concuss/o	shaken together		heart
	violently	corp/u	body
condyl/o	knob	corpor/o	body
	knuckle	corpuscul/o	little body
confus/o	confusion	cort-	covering
	disorder	cortic/o	cortex
coni/o	dust		outer region
conjunctiv/o	conjunctiva	cost/o	rib
consci/o	aware	costal/o	rib
consolid/o	to become solid	cox/o	hip
constipat/o	pressed together	crani/o	skull
constrict/o	constrict	cras/o	mixture
	to draw together		temperament
	to narrow	-crasia	mixture
-constriction	narrowing	crepit/o	crackling
contact/o	touched	crepitat/o	crackling
contagi/o	infection	crin/o	to secrete
	touching of	-crine	separate
	something		to secrete
contaminat/o	to pollute	cris/o	turning point
contine/o	restrain	-crit	to separate
	to keep in	critic/o	turning point
continent/o	restrain	cruci-	cross
	to keep in	cry/o	cold
contra-	against	crypt/o	hidden
	opposite	crystall/o	crystals
contracept/o	prevention of	cubit/o	elbow
	fertilization	cuboid/o	cube-shaped
contus/o	bruise	culd/o	cul-de-sac
convalesc/o	to become strong	-cusis	hearing
convex/o	arched	cusp/i	pointed
convolut/o	coiled microorganism	cut-	skin
	twisted out	cutane/o	skin
convuls/o	to pull together	cyan/o	blue
copi/o	plentiful	cycl/o	ciliary body
copr/o	feces		circle
copulat/o	joining together		cycle
cor/o	pupil	-cyesis	pregnancy

cyst-	bag	dent-	teeth
	bladder	dent/i	tooth
cyst/o	cyst	dent/o	tooth
	sac of fluid	depilat/o	hair removal
	urinary bladder	depress/o	pressed
cyt/o	cell		sunken down
-cyte	cell	derm/o	skin
-cytic	pertaining to a cell	derma-	skin
-cytosis	condition of cells	-derma	skin
	increase in cell	dermat/o	skin
	numbers	desicc/o	drying
dacry-	tear	-desis	surgical fixation to
	tear duct		bind; to tie together
dacry/o	tear	deteriorat/o	worsening
dacryoaden/o	tear gland	deut-	second
dacryocyst/o	lacrimal sac	deuto-	second
	tear sac	dextr/o	right side
dactyl/o	digits	di-	twice
	fingers		two
	toes	dia-	complete
dart/o	skinned		through
de-	down	diaphor/o	sweat
	lack of strength	diaphragmat/o	diaphragm
	removal	diastol/o	expansion
dec/i	ten	didym/o	double
	tenth		testes
deca-	ten	diffus/o	spread out
	tenth	digest/o	divided
decem-	ten		to distribute
decidu/o	shedding	digit/o	digits
decubit/o	lying down	dilat/o	spread out
defec/o	free from waste	dilatat/o	spread out
defecat/o	free from waste	-dilation	expanding
defer/o	carrying down		stretching
degenerat/o	breakdown		widening
deglutit/o	swallow	dilut/o	separate
dehisc/o	to burst open		to dissolve
dek-	ten	diphther/o	membrane
deka-	ten	dipl/o	double
deliri/o	wandering of mind	dipla-	double
delta-	triangle	dips/o	thirst
dem/o	people	-dipsia	thirst
-dema	swelling	dis-	absence of; apart
demi-	half		duplicate
dendr/o	branching		negative
	resembling a tree		twice

dislocat/o	displacement	-ectasis	dilation
dissect/o	cutting apart		expansion
disseminat/o	widely scattered		stretching
dist/o	distant	ecto-	out
	far		outside
distend/o	to stretch apart	-ectomy	excision
distent/o	to stretch apart		removal
diur/o	increasing urine output		resection
diuret/o	increasing urine output	eczemat/o	eruption
divert/i	turning aside	-edema	swelling
dolich/o	long	edemat/o	fluid
domin/o	controlling		swelling
don/o	to give		tumor
dors/i	back	edentul/o	toothless
dors/o	back	ef-	out
-dote	to give	effect/o	to bring about a
drom/o	running		response
-drome	to run	effus/o	pouring out
du/o	two	ejactulat/o	to hurl out
-duct	opening		to throw out
duct/o	to carry	electr/o	electricity
	to lead	eliminat/o	to expel from the body
duoden/i	duodenum	em-	in
duoden/o	duodenum	-ema	condition
dur/o	dura mater	emaciat/o	lean
dy-	two		wasted away by disease
-dynia	pain	embol/o	something inserted
dyo-	two		thrown in
dys-	abnormal	embry/o	fertilized egg
	bad	-emesis	vomiting
	difficult	emet/o	vomit
	painful	-emia	blood condition
e-	out from	-emic	pertaining to a blood
	out of		condition
-eal	pertaining to	emmetr/o	in proper measure
ec-	out	emolli/o	to soften
	outside	en-	in
ecchym/o	pouring out of juice		within
echo-	reflected sound	encephal/o	brain
eclamps/o	flashing	endo-; end/o	in
	shining forth		within
eclampt/o	flashing	endocrin/o	to secrete within
	shining forth	enem/o	to inject
-ectasia	dilation	ennea-	nine
	expansion	enter/o	small intestine
	stretching	ento-	within

enzym/o	leaven	evacu/o	to empty out
eosin/o	dawn	evacuat/o	to empty out
	red	eviscer/o	disembowelment
	rosy	eviscerat/o	disembowelment
epi-	above	ex-	away from
	on		out
	upon		outside
epidemi/o	among the people	exacerbat/o	to aggravate
epididym/o	epididymis	exanthemat/o	rash
epiglott/o	epiglottis	excis/o	cutting out
episi/o	vulva	excori/o	to scratch
epithel/i	external surface covering	excoriat/o	to scratch
	outer layer of skin	excret/o	discharge
epitheli/o	epithelium		separate
	skin	excruciat/o	intense pain
equin/o	horse	exhal/o	to breathe out
-er	one who	exhalat/o	to breathe out
erect/o	upright	-exia	condition
erg/o	work	-exis	condition
eruct/o	to belch	exo-	away from
eructat/o	to belch		out
erupt/o	to burst forth		outside
erythem/o	flushed	exocrin/o	to secrete out of
	redness	expector/o	to cough up
crythemat/o	flushed	expir/o	die
	redness		to breathe out
erythr/o	red	expirat/o	die
es-	away from		to breathe out
	out of	exstroph/o	twisted out
-esis	abnormal condition	extern/o	outer
	condition		outside
eso-	inward	extra-	out
esophag/o	esophagus		outside
esthes/o	nervous sensation	extrem/o	extremities
esthesi/o	nervous sensation		outermost
-esthesia	nervous sensation	extremit/o	extremities
esthet/o	feeling		outermost
	sense of perception	extrins/o	contained outside
estr/o	female	exud/o	to sweat out
ethm/o	sieve	exudat/o	to sweat out
eti/o	cause	faci-	face
-etic	pertaining to a condition		form
eu-	good	faci/o	face
	normal	-facient	producing
	true	fasci/o; fasc/i	fascia
-eurysm	widening	fascicul/o	little bundle

fatal/o	death of tissue	follicul/o	follicle
	fate		small sac
fauc/i	narrow pass	foramin/o	opening
febr/i	fever	fore-	before
fec/i	upright		in front of
fec/o	sediment	-form	figure
femor/o	femur		form
fenestr/o	window		shape
fer/o	to bear	form/o	figure
	to carry		form
-ferent	carrying		shape
	to carry	fornic/o	arch
-ferous	carrying		vault
fertil/o	fruitful	foss/o	shallow depression
	productive	fove/o	pit
fet/i	fetus	fract/o	break
fet/o	fetus	fren/o	bridle
fibr/o	fiber		device to limit
fibrill/o	muscular twitching		movement
fibrin/o	fibrin	frigid/o	cold
	threads of a clot	front/o	forehead
fibros/o	fibrous connective tissue		front
fibul/o	fibula	-fuge	to drive away
-fic	forming	funct/o	to perform
	producing	function/o	to perform
fic/o	forming	fund/o	base
	producing		bottom
-fication	process of making		ground
-fida	split	fung/i	fungus
filtr/o	to strain through		mushroom
filtrat/o	to strain through	furc/o	branching
fimbri/o	fringe		forking
fiss/o	clear	furuncul/o	boil
	crack		infection
	split	-fusion	to come together
fissur/o	clear		to pour
	crack	galact/o	milk
	split	gamet/o	sex cell
fistul/o	pipe	gangli/o	ganglion
	tube	ganglion/o	ganglion
flamme/o	flame-colored	gangren/o	gangrene
flat/o	rectal gas	gastr/o	stomach
flex/o	to bend	gastrocnemi/o	calf muscle
fluor/o	luminous	gemin/o	double
foc/o	point		twin
foll/i	bag	-gen	forming
	sac		producing

gen/o	birth	gnath/o	jaw
	producing	gnos/o	knowledge
-gene	formation	goitr/o	enlargement of the
	origin		thyroid gland
	production	gon/i	angle
-genesis	forming		seed
	producing	gon/o	angle
-genic	produced by		seed
	produced in	gonad/o	sex glands
genit/o	birth	goni/o	angle
	producing		seed
-genous	producing	gracil/o	slender
ger/i	old age	grad/i	go
ger/o	old age		step
germin/o	bud		to move
	germ	-grade	to go
geront/o	old age	-gram	record
gest/o	pregnancy	granul/o	granules
gestat/o	pregnancy	-graph	instrument to record
gester/o	pregnancy	-graphy	process of recording
gigant/o	giant	gravid/o	pregnancy
	very large	-gravida	pregnancy
gingiv/o	gums	gutter/o	throat
glauc/o	gray	gynec/o	female
glen/o	pit		woman
	socket	gyr/o	folding
gli/o	glue		turning
	neuroglial tissue	hal/o	breath
-globin	protein	halit/o	breath
globin/o	protein	hallucin/o	hallucinate
globul/o	little ball	hecato-	hundred
-globulin	protein	hect-	hundred
glomerul/o	glomerulus	hector-	hundred
gloss/o	tongue	hem-	blood
glosso-	tongue	hem/e	deep red iron-
glott/i	tongue		containing pigment
glott/o	tongue	hem/o	blood
gluc/o	glucose	hemangi/o	blood vessel
	sugar	hemat/o	blood
glute/o	buttocks	hemi-	half
glyc/o	glucose	hemoglobin/o	hemoglobin
	sugar	hepa-	liver
glycer/o	sweet	hepat/o	liver
glycogen/o	animal starch	hepta-	liver
	glycogen	hered/o	inherited
glycos/o	glucose	heredit/o	inherited
	sugar	herni/o	hernia

herpet/o	creeping	iatr/o	doctor
heter/o	different		treatment
hex-	six	-ible	capable of being
hexa-	six	-ic	pertaining to
-hexia	habit	-ical	pertaining to
hiat/o	opening	ichthy/o	dry
hidr/o	sweat		scaly
hil/o	hilus	-icle	small
	opening from a body	icter/o	jaundice
	part	ictero-	jaundice
hirsut/o	hairy	idi/o	distinct
	rough		individual
hist/o	tissue		unknown
histi/o	tissue	-iferous	bearing
holo-	all		carrying
hom/o	same		producing
home/o	constant	-ific	producing
	sameness	-iform	resembling
	unchanging		shaped-like
hormon/o	hormone	-igo	disease condition
humer/o	humerus	-ile	capable of being
hyal/o	clear		pertaining to
	glassy	ile/o	ileum
hydr/o	fluid	ili/o	ilium
	water	illusi/o	deception
hydra-	water	immun/o	immune
hygien/o	healthful		safe
hymen/o	above	impuls/o	pressure
	hymen		urging on
	membrane	in-	in
hyper-	above		into
	excessive		not
	higher than	-in	pertaining to
	over	incis/o	cutting into
hypn/o	sleep	incubat/o	hatching
hypo-	below		incubation
	decrease	indurat/o	hardened
	deficient	-ine	a substance
	less than normal		pertaining to
	under	infarct/o	filled in
hypophys/o	pituitary gland		stuffed
hyster/o	uterus	infect/o	infected
-ia	condition		tainted
-iac	pertaining to	infer/o	below
-ial	pertaining to		beneath
-iasis	abnormal condition	infest/o	attack

inflammat/o	flame within	ipsi-	same
	set fire to	ir-	in
infra-	below	ir/i	iris
	beneath	ir/o	iris
	inferior to	irid/o	iris
infundibul/o	funnel	is/o	equal
ingest/o	pour in		same
	to carry	isch/o	back
inguin/o	groin		to hang
inhal/o	to breathe in	ischi/o	ischium
inhalat/o	to breathe in	-ism	condition
inject/o	throw in		process
	to force	-ist	specialist
innominat/o	nameless	-itis	inflammation
inocul/o	implant	-ium	structure
	to introduce		thing
insipid/o	tasteless		tissue
inspir/o	to breathe in	jaund/o	yellow
inspirat/o	to breathe in	jejun/o	jejunum
insul/o	island	jugul/o	jugular
insulin/o	insulin	juxta-	nearby
intact/o	whole	kal/i	potassium
inter-	between	kary/o	nucleus
intermitt/o	not continuous	karyo-	nucleus
intern/o	inner	kata-	down
	within	kath-	down
interstiti/o	space between things	kel/o	growth
intestin/o	intestine		tumor
intim/o	innermost	kera-	hardness
intoxic/o	to put poison in		horn
intra-	into	kerat/o	cornea
	within		hard
intrins/o	contained within		horny tissue
intro-	inside	kern-	nucleus
	into	ket/o	ketones
	within	keton/o	ketones
introit/o	entrance	kines/o	movement
	passage	kinesi/o	movement
intussuscept/o	to receive within	-kinesia	movement
involut/o	curled inward	-kinesis	movement
iod/o	iodine	-kinetic	pertaining to movement
-ion	process	koil/o	concave
ion/o	charged particle		hollow
	ion	kraur/o	dry
	to wander	kyph/o	bent
-ior	pertaining to		humpback

labi/o	lip	libidin/o	sexual drive
labyrinth/o	maze	ligament/o	ligament
lacer/o	torn	ligat/o	binding
lacerat/o	torn		tying off
lacrim/o	lacrimal duct	lingu/o	tongue
	tear	lip/o	fat
	tear duct		lipid
lact/i	milk	-listhesis	slipping
lact/o	milk	-lite	calculus
lactat/o	to secrete milk		stone
lacun/o	pit	-lith	calculus
lamin/o	lamina		stone
lapar/o	abdomen	lith/o	calculus
laps/o	fall		stone
	sag	-lithiasis	abnormal condition of
	slide		stones
-lapse	sag	-lithotomy	incision to remove a
	to fall		stone
	to slide	lob/i	lobe
laryng/o	larynx	lob/o	lobe
	voice box	loc/o	place
lat/i	broad	loch/i	birthing
lat/o	broad		confinement; birthing
later/o	side	log/o	study of
lax/o	loosen	-logy	study of
	relax	longev/o	long-lived
laxat/o	loosen	lord/o	bent backward
	relax		curve
leiomy/o	smooth muscle		swayback
	visceral muscle	-lucent	to shine
lemm/o	peel	lumb/o	loin
-lemma	covering		lower back
	sheath	lun/o	moon
lent/i	peel	lunul/o	crescent
lenticul/o	lens-shaped	lup/i	wolf
-lepsy	seizure	lup/o	wolf
lept/o	slender	lute/o	yellow
	thin	lux/o	to slide
-leptic	take hold of	lymph/o	lymph
	to seize	lymphaden/o	lymph gland
leth/o	death		lymph node
letharg/o	drowsiness	lymphangi/o	lymph vessel
leuco-	white	-lysis	breakdown
leuk/o	white		destruction
lev/o	to lift up		loosening
levat/o	to lift up		separation
libid/o	sexual drive	-lyst	agent that breaks down

-lytic	pertaining to the destruction or breakdown	medic/o	doctor healing medicine	
	to break down to destroy to reduce to separate	medicat/o	healing medication	
		medull/o	inner section marrow medulla middle soft	
macr/o	large			
macro-	large			
macul/o	spot			
magn/o	large	mega-	large	
major/o	larger	megal/o	large	
mal-	bad	-megaly	enlargement	
malac/o	softening	mei/o	less	
-malacia	softening	melan/o	black	
malign/o	bad evil	mellit/o	honey	
		membran/o	membrane thin skin	
malle/o	hammer			
malleol/o	little hammer malleolus	men/o	menstruation	
		mening/o	meninges	
mamm/o	breast mammary gland	meningi/o	meninges	
		menisc/o	crescent	
man/i	hand rage	mens-	menstruation	
		mens/o	menstruation	
man/o	hand	ment/o	middle mind	
mandibul/o	lower jaw mandible			
		mes-	middle	
-mania	obsessive preoccupation	mes/o	middle	
manipul/o	handful use of hands	mesenter/o	mesentery	
		mesi/o	median plane middle	
manubri/o	handle			
mast/o	breast mammary gland	meta-	beyond change	
		metabol/o	change	
mastic/o	chew	metacarp/o	metacarpals	
mastoid/o	mastoid process	metatars/o	metatarsals	
mastricat/o	chew	-meter	device for measurement to measure	
matern/o	of a mother			
matur/o	ripe	metr/i	uterus	
maxill/o	maxilla upper jaw	metr/o	measure uterus	
maxim/o	largest	metri/o	uterus	
meat/o	meatus opening	-metry	measurement	
		mi/o	less smaller	
med-	middle			
medi/o	middle	micr/o	small	
mediastin/o	in the middle mediastinum	micro-	small	

mictur/o	to urinate	myocardi/o	heart muscle
micturit/o	to urinate		myocardium
midsagitt/o	dividing into equal left	myom/o	muscle tumor
	and right halves	myos/o	muscle
milli-	one-thousandth	myring/o	ear drum
-mimetic	copy		tympanic membrane
	mimic	myx-	mucus
mineral/o	mineral	myx/o	mucus
	naturally occurring	myxa-	mucus
minim/o	smallest	myxo-	mucus
minor/o	smaller	nar/i	nostril
mio-	less	narc/o	numbness
-mission	to send		sleep
mit/o	thread		stupor
mobil/o	capable of moving	nas/i	nose
mon/o	one	nas/o	nose
	single	nat/i	birth
monil/o	string of beads	natr/o	sodium
mono-	one	nause/o	sick feeling in the
	single		stomach
morbid/o	disease	ne/o	new
moribund/o	dying	necr/o	death
morph/o	form	-necrosis	death of tissue
	shape	nect/o	to bind
mort/i	death		to connect
mort/o	death		to tie
mort/u	death	neo-	new
mortal/i	death	nephr/o	kidney
-mortem	death	nephra-	kidney
mot/o	movement	nerv/o	nerve
motil/o	movement	neu-	nerve
-motor	movement	neur/i	nerve
muc/o	mucus	neur/o	nerve
mucos/o	mucosa	neutr/o	neither
	mucous membranes		neutral
	mucus		neutrophil
multi-	many	nid/o	nest
muscul/o	muscle	nigr/o	black
mut/a	genetic change	niter-	nitrogen
mutagen/o	causing genetic	nitro-	nitrogen
	change	noct/i	night
my/o	muscle	nod/o	know
myc/e	fungus		swelling
myc/o	fungus	nodul/o	little knot
mydr/o	wide	nom/o	control
myel/o	bone marrow	non-	nine
	spinal cord		no

nona-	nine	olig/o	scanty
nonus-	nine	oligo-	scanty
nor-	normal	-oma	collection of fluid
	parent compound		mass
norm/o	normal		tumor
	order	oment/o	omentum
	rule	omphal/o	navel
nos/o	disease		umbilicus
not/o	back	onc/o	tumor
novem-	nine	-one	hormone
nuch/o	nape	onych/o	nail
nucle/o	nucleus	oo/o	egg
nulli-	none	oophor/o	ovary
numer/o	count	opac/o	dark
	number		shaded
nunci/o	messenger	opacit/o	dark
nutri/o	food		shaded
	nourishment	-opaque	obscure
nutrit/o	food	oper/o	perform
	nourishment		to work
nyct/o	night	operat/o	perform
nyctal/o	night		to work
o-	egg	opercul/o	cover
o/o	egg		lid
ob-	against	ophthalm/o	eye
obes/o	extremely fat	-opia	vision
obliqu/o	sideways	opisth/o	backward
	slanted	-opsia	vision
oblongat/o	elongated	-opsis	vision
	oblong	-opsy	to view
obstetr/o	one who receives		view of
occipit/o	back of the skull	opt/i	eye
occlud/o	to close up		vision
occlus/o	to close up	opt/o	eye
occult/o	hidden		vision
oct-	eight	opti/o	eye
octa-	eight		vision
octo-	eight	optic/o	eye
ocul/o	eye		vision
oculo-	eye	-or	one who
odont/o	tooth	or/o	mouth
odyn/o	pain	orbit/o	bony cavity
-oid	resembling		circle
-ole	little		socket
	small	orch/o	testes
olecran/o	olecranon	orchi/o	testes
olfact/o	smell	orchid/o	testes

orect/i	appetite	palpebr/o	eyelid
orex/i	appetite	palpit/o	throbbing
-orexia	appetite	pan-	all
organ/o	organ	pancreat/o	pancreas
orth/o	straight	papill/i	nipple-like
ortho-	straight		optic disc
-ory	pertaining to	papill/o	nipple-like
os-	bone		optic disc
	mouth	papul/o	pimple
-ose	full of; pertaining to	par-	abnormal
	sugar		other than
-osis	abnormal condition	par/o	abnormal
osm/o	pushing; smell		apart from
-osmia	smell		beside
oss/e	bone		near
oss/i	bone	para-	abnormal
ossicul/o	ossicle		along side of
oste/o	bone		apart from
-ostosis	condition of bone		beside
ot/o	ear		near
-otia	ear condition	-para	bring forth
-otic	pertaining to an		to bear
	abnormal condition	paralys/o	to disable
-ous	pertaining to	paralyt/o	to disable
ov/i	egg	parasit/o	near food
ov/o	egg	parathyroid/o	parathyroid glands
ovari/o	ovary	pares/i	to disable
ovul/o	egg	-paresis	slight paralysis
ox/i	oxygen		weakening
ox/o	oxygen	paret/o	to disable
ox/y	oxygen	-pareunia	sexual intercourse
-oxia	oxygen	pariet/o	wall
oxid/o	containing oxygen	parotid/o	parotid gland
oxy-	acid	-parous	bring forth
	oxygen		to bear
	rapid	paroxysm/o	sudden attack
	sharp	part/o	birth
oxysm/o	sudden		labor
pachy-	heavy	-partum	birth
	thick		labor
palat/o	palate	parturit/o	birth
pall/o	pale		labor
palliat/o	hidden	patell/a	patella
pallid/o	pale	patell/o	patella
palm/o	caudal surface of the	path/o	disease
	front foot (paw)	-pathic	pertaining to a disease
palpat/o	to touch		condition

-pathy	disease condition; emotion	phak/o	lens of the eye
paus/o	stopping	phalang/o	phalanges
pector/o	chest	phall/o	penis
ped/o	child; foot	pharmac/o	drug
pedi/a	child	pharmaceut/o	drug
pedicul/o	lice louse	pharyng/o	pharynx throat
pelv/i	hip hip bone pelvis	phe/o	dark dusky
		pher/o	to bear to carry
pelv/o	hip hip bone pelvis	-pheresis	removal
		-phil	attraction for
		phil/o	attraction to like
pen/i	penis		
pend/o	to hang	-philia	attraction for lincrease in cell number
-penia	decrease deficiency		
pent-	five	phim/o	muzzle
penta-	five	phleb/o	vein
peps/i	digestion	phlegm/o	phlegm thick mucus
-pepsia	digestion		
pept/o	digestion	phob/o	fear
per-	through	-phobia	fear
percept/o	to become aware	phon/o	sound voice
percussi/o	tap to beat	-phonia	sound voice
peri-	surrounding	phor/o	to bear
pericardi/o	pericardium	-phorcsis	carrying
perine/o	perineum	-phoria	feeling to bear to carry
peritone/o	peritoneum		
perme/o	to pass through		
pernici/o	destructive harmful	phot/o	light
		phren/o	diaphragm mind
perone/o	fibula		
pertuss/i	intense cough	-phthisis	wasting away
petechi/o	skin spot	-phylactic	prevention protective
-pexy	surgical fixation to put in place		
		-phylaxis	protection
phac/o	lens of the eye	physi/o	function; nature
phag/o	eat; swallow	physic/o	function nature
-phage	eat swallow		
		-physis	to grow
-phagia	eating swallowing	phys/o	growing; to grow
		phyt/o	plant

-phyte	plant	pneum/o	air
pigment/o	color		gas
	pigment		lung
pil/i	hair	pneumon/o	air
pil/o	hair		gas
pineal/o	pineal gland		lung
pinn/i	auricle	pod/o	foot
	external ear	-poiesis	formation
	pinna	-poietin	substance that forms
pituitar/o	pituitary gland	poikil/o	irregular
plac/o	flat patch		varied
placent/o	placenta	pol/o	extreme
-plakia	plaque	polio-	gray matter of the brain
plan/o	flat		and spinal cord
plant/i	caudal surface of the	poly-	many
	rear foot (paw)		much
plant/o	caudal surface of the	polyp/o	polyp
	rear foot (paw)		small growth
plas/i	development	pont/o	pons
	formation	poplit/o	caudal surface of the
plas/o	development		patella
	formation	por/o	pore
-plasia	development formation		small opening
	growth	-porosis	condition of pores
-plasm	formation	port/i	door
plasm/o	something formed		gate
-plast	primitive living cell	post-	after
plast/o	development		behind
	growth	poster/o	back
	mold		behind
-plastic	pertaining to formation	potent/o	powerful
-plasty	surgical repair	pract/i	practice
ple/o	many	practic/o	practice
	more	prandi/o	meal
-plegia	palsy	-prandial	meal
	paralysis	-praxia	action
-plegic	palsy	pre-	before
	paralysis		in front of
pleur/o	pleura	pregn/o	pregnancy
plex/o	network of nerves	prematur/o	too early
	plexus	preputi/o	prepuce
plic/o	fold	press/o	draw
	ridge		to press
-pnea	breathing	priap/o	penis
-pneic	pertaining to breathing	primi-	first
pneu-	air	pro-	before
	lung		forward

process/o	going forth	punct/o	puncture
procreat/o	to reproduce		sting
proct/o	rectum and anus	pupill/o	pupil
prodrom/o	precursor	pur/o	pus
product/o	to lead forward	purpur/o	purple
	to yield	purul/o	pus
prolaps/o	sag	pustul/o	blister
	slide	py/o	pus
	to fall	pyel/o	renal pelvis
prolifer/o	to reproduce	pylor/o	pyloric sphincter
pron/o	bent forward		pylorus
pront/o	bent forward	pyr/o	fever
pros-	before		fire
	forward	pyret/o	fever
prostat/o	prostate gland	pyrex/o	fever
prosth/o	addition	quadr/i	four
	appendage	quadr/o	four
prosthet/o	addition	quadri-	four
	appendage	quart-	fourth
prot-	first	quinqu-	five
prot/o	first	quint-	five
prote/o; protein/o	protein	rabi/o	madness
proto-	first		rage
proxim/o	near	rachi/o	spinal column
prurit/o	itching		vertebrae
pseud/o	false	radi/o	radioactivity
psor/i	itch		radius
psor/o	itch		x-ray
psych/o	mind	radiat/o	giving off radiation
ptomat/o	to fall	radicul/o	nerve root
-ptosis	droop	ram/o	branch
	fall	raph/o	seam
	prolapse		suture
	sag	-raphy	suture
-ptyalo	saliva	re-	again
	spit		backward
-ptysis	spitting	recept/o	receive
pub/o	pubis	recipi/o	receive
pubert/o	adult	rect/o	rectum
pudend/o	pudendum	recuperat/o	to recover
puerper/i	labor	reduct/o	to bring back together
pulm/o	lung	refract/o	to bend back
pulmon/o	air		turning aside
	gas	regurgit/o	gush back
	lung		to flood
pulpos/o	fleshy	remiss/o	give up
puls/o	beating		to let go

ren/o	kidney		sanguin/o	blood
restor/o	to rebuild		sanit/o	health
resuscit/o	to revive			soundness
retent/o	to hold back		saphen/o	apparent
reticul/o	network			clear
retin/o	retina		sapr/o	dead body
retract/o	to draw back			decaying
retro-	back		sarc/o	connective tissue
	backward			flesh
	behind		sarcomat/o	connective tissue
rhabd/o	rod			flesh
rhabdomy/o	skeletal muscle		scalp/o	scrape off
	striated muscle		scapul/o	scapula
-rhage	bursting forth		-schisis	to split
-rhagia	bursting forth		schiz/o	split
-rhaphy	suture		scint/i	spark
-rhea	discharge		scirrh/o	hard
	flow		scler/o	sclera
rheum/o	watery flow		-sclerosis	hardening
rheumat/o	watery flow		scoli/o	bent
-rhexis	rupture		-scope	instrument for visual
rhin/o	nose			examination
rhiz/o	root		-scopic	pertaining to visual
rhonc/o	to snore			examination
rhythm/o	rhythm		-scopy	process of visual
rhytid/o	wrinkle			examination
rigid/o	stiff		scot/o	darkness
roentgen/o	X-ray		scrot/o	bag
rostri	beak			pouch
rotat/o	to revolve			scrotum
-rrhage	bursting forth		seb/o	sebum
-rrhagia	bursting forth		sebace/o	sebum
-rrhaphy	suture		sect/o	to cut
-rrhea	discharge		secti/o	to cut
	flow		secundi-	second
rug/o	fold		segment/o	in pieces
	wrinkle			segmented
sacc/i	sac		sell/o	saddle
sacc/o	sac		semi-	half
sacr/o	sacrum		semin/i	secd
sagitta	arrow			semen
saliv/o	saliva		sen/i	old
	spit		sens/i	feeling
salping/o	uterine tube			sensation
-salpinx	uterine tube		sensitiv/o	sensitive to
sangu/i	blood		seps/o	infection

sept-	seven	sperm/o	sperm
sept/o	partition		spermatozoa
	septum	spermat/o	sperm
septi-	seven		spermatozoa
ser/o	clear	sphen/o	sphenoid bone
	serum		wedge
seros/o	serous	spher/o	globe-shaped
sesqui-	one and one-half		round
sex-	six	sphincter/o	sphincter
sial/o	saliva		tight band
sialaden/o	salivary gland	sphygm/o	pulse
sider/o	iron	-sphyxia	pulse
sigmoid/o	sigmoid colon	spin/o	backbones
silic/o	glass		spine
sin/o	sinus	spir/o	to breathe
sin/u	sinus	spirill/o	little coil
sinistr/o	left	spirochet/o	coiled microorganism
sinus/o	sinus	splanchn/o	internal organs
-sis	condition		viscera
	state of	splen/o	spleen
sit/u	place	spondyl/o	vertebrae
skelet/o	skeleton	spontane/o	unexplained
soci/o	companion		voluntary
-sol	solution	spor/o	seed
solut/o	dissolved	sput/o	spit
solv/o	dissolved	squam/o	scale
soma-	body	-stalsis	contraction
somat/o	body	staped/o	stapes
-some	body		stirrup
-somes	bodies	stapedi/o	stapes
somn/i	sleep		stirrup
somn/o	sleep	staphyl/o	clusters
-somnia	sleep		uvula
son/o	sound	stas/i	controlling
sopor/o	sleep		stopping
-spadia	to cut	-stasis	controlling
	to tear		stopping
-spasm	sudden, involuntary	stat/i	controlling
	contraction		stopping
spasm/o	sudden, involuntary	-static	controlling
	contraction		pertaining to stopping
spasmod/o	sudden, involuntary		stopping
	contraction	steat/o	fat
spec/i	a sort		sebum
	to look at	sten/o	contracted
specul/o	mirror		narrowing

-stenosis	narrowing	sulc/o	furrow
	stricture		groove
	tightening	super-	above
ster/o	solid structure		excessive
	steroid		higher than
stere/o	solid	super/o	above
	three dimensional		excessive
steril/i	barren		higher than
stern/o	sternum	superflu/o	excessive
stert/o	to snore		overflowing
steth/o	chest	supin/o	lying on the back
sthen/o	strength	supinat/o	bent forward
-sthenia	strength		to place on back
stigmat/o	point	suppress/o	to press down
	spot	-suppression	to stop
stimul/o	good	suppur/o	to form pus
	incite	suppurat/o	to form pus
-stitial	pertaining to standing	supra-	above
	to set		upper
stomat/o	mouth	sutur/o	to stitch
-stomia	condition of the mouth	sym-	together
-stomy	anastomosis		with
	new opening to the	symptomat/o	falling together
	outside of the body		symptom
strab/i	to squint	syn-	together
strat/i	layer		with
strept/o	twisted chains	synaps/o	point of contact
striat/o	groove		synapse
	stripe	synapt/o	point of contact
stric-	narrowing		synapse
strict/o	to draw tightly	syncop/o	cut off
	together		cut short
	to tie		faint
strid/o	harsh sound	syndesm/o	ligament
stup/e	stunned	syndrom/o	running together
styl/o	pen	synov/o	sheath around a tendon
	pointed instrument		synovial membrane
	pole	synovi/o	synovial fluid
	stake		synovial membrane
sub-	below	syring/o	tube
	under	system/o	entire body
subluxat/o	partial dislocation		system
sucr/o	sugar	systemat/o	entire body system
sudor/i	sweat	systol/o	contraction
suffoc/o	to choke	tachy-	fast
suffocat/o	to choke	tact/i	touch

tars/o	tarsals	tibi/o	tibia
	tarsus	-tic	pertaining to
tax/o	coordination	tine/o	ringworm
	order	tinnit/o	ringing
techn/o	skill	toc/o	birth
techni/o	skill		labor
tectori/o	covering	-tocia	birth
tel/o	complete		labor
tele/o	distant	-tocin	birth
tempor/o	temple		labor
ten/o	tendon	tom/o	to cut
tenac/i	sticky	-tome	instrument to cut
tendin/o	tendon	-tomy	incision
tens/o	extend		process of cutting into
	strain	ton/o	tension
	to stretch out	tone/o	to stretch
-tension	pressure	tonsill/o	tonsils
terat/o	malformed fetus	top/o	location
	monster		place
termin/o	end		position
tert-	third	tors/o	rotate
test/i	testes		to twist
test/o	testes	tort/i	twisted
tetan/o	rigid	tox/o	poison
tetra-	four	toxic/o	poison
thalam/o	thalamus	trabecul/o	beams
thalass/o	sea	trache/i	trachea
thanas/o	death		windpipe
thanat/o	death	trache/o	trachea
the/o	place		windpipe
	put	tract/o	bundle of nerve fibers
thec/o	sheath		path
thel/o	nipple		to draw back
therap/o	treatment		to pull
therapeut/o	treatment	tranquil/o	quiet
-therapy	treatment	trans-	across
therm/o	heat		through
thio-	sulfer	transfus/o	pour across
thorac/o	chest		to transfer
-thorax	chest	transit/o	changing
	pleural cavity	transvers/o	across
thromb/o	clot	traumat/o	injury
thym/o	thymus gland	trem/o	shaking
thyr/o	shield	tremul/o	shaking
	thyroid gland		tremor
thyroid/o	thyroid gland	treponem/o	coiled

-tresia	opening		umbilicus
tri-	three	un-	not
trich/o	hair	ungu/o	hoof
trigon/o	triangle		nail
	trigone	uni-	one
-tripsy	to crush	ur/o	urine
trit-	third	-uresis	urination
-trite	instrument	ureter/o	ureter
	for cutting	urethr/o	urethra
trito-	third	-uria	condition of urine
trochle/o	pulley		urination
trop/o	to change	urin/o	urine
	turn	urtic/o	hives
troph/o	development		rash
	nourishment	-us	structure
-trophy	development		thing
	nourishment		tissue
-tropia	to turn	uter/i	uterus
-tropic	turning	uter/o	uterus
-tropin	act on	uve/o	uvea
	stimulate		vascular layer of
tub/i	pipe		the eye
	tube	uvul/o	little grape
tub/o	pipe		uvula
	tube	vac/u	empty
tubercul/o	little knot	vaccin/i	vaccine
	swelling	vaccin/o	vaccine
tunic/o	covering	vag/o	vagus nerve
	sheath	vagin/o	vagina
turbinat/o	coiled	valg/o	bent
tuss/i	cough		twisted out
tympan/o	ear drum	valv/o	valve
	tympanic	valvul/o	valve
	membrane	varic/o	dilated vein
-type	classification		swollen vein
	picture	vas/o	duct
ulcer/o	core		vas deferens
	ulcer		vessel
-ule	little	vascul/o	blood vessel
	small		vessel
uln/o	ulna	vaso-	vessel
ultra-	beyond	vast/o	extensive
	excess		great
-um	structure	vect/o	convey
	thing		to carry
	tissue	ven/i	vein
umbilic/o	navel	ven/o	vein

vener/o	sexual intercourse	visc/o	sticky
	venereal	viscer/o	internal organs
venter-	abdomen		viscera
ventilat/o	to expose to air	viscos/o	sticky
ventr/o	belly side	vit/a	life
ventricul/o	ventricle	vit/o	life
venul/o	small vein	viti/o	blemish
	venule		defect
verg/o	incline	vitr/o	vitreous body
	to twist	vitre/o	glass
verm/i	worm	viv/i; vivi-	life
verruc/o	wart	viv/o	life
vers/o	turn	voc/i	vocal
-verse	to turn		voice
-version	to turn	vol/o	to roll
vert/o	turn	volv/o	roll
vertebr/o	backbones		to turn
	vertebrae	vulgar/i	common
vertig/o	revolution	vulv/o	vulva
	turning around	xanth/o	yellow
vertigin/o	revolution	xen/o	foreign
	turning around		strang
vesic/o	urinary bladder	xer/o	dry
vesicul/o	seminal vesicle	xiph/i	sword
vestibul/o	entrance	xiph/o	sword
	vestibule	-y	condition
vi/o	force		process
vill/i	villi	zo/o	animal life
vir/o	poison	zoo-	animal
	virus		life
viril/o	masculine	zygomat/o	cheekbone
vis/o	seeing		yoke
	sight	zygot/o	joined or yoked together

By Definition

a sort	spec/i	abnormal condition	-esis
a substance	-ine		-iasis
abdomen	abdomin/o		-osis
	celi/o	abnormal condition	
	lapar/o	of stones	-lithiasis
	venter-	above	epi-
abnormal	dys-		hyper-
	par-		super-
	par/o		super/o
	para-		supra-

absence of a pulse	asphyxi/o	anxious	anxi/o
absence of	dis-		anxiet/o
acetabulum	acetabul/o	aorta	aort/o
acid	oxy-	apart	ana-
acromion	acromi/o		dis-
across	trans-	apart from	par/o
	transvers/o		para-
act on	-tropin	apex	apic/o
action	-praxia	aponeurosis	aponeur/o
addition	prosth/o	apparent	saphen/o
	prosthet/o	appendage	prosth/o
adenoids	adenoid/o		prosthet/o
adrenal gland	adren/o	appetite	orect/i
	adrenal/o		orex/i
adult	pubert/o		-orexia
after	post-	arachnoid membrane	arachn/o
again	ana-	arch	arc/o
	re-		fornic/o
against	anti-	arched	convex/o
	contra-	arm	brachi/o
	ob-	armpit	axill/o
agent that breaks down	-lyst	around	amph-
air	aer/o		circum-
	pneu-	arrow	sagitta
	pneum/o	arteriole	arteriol/o
	pneumon/o	artery	arter/o
	pulmon/o		arteri/o
air sac	alveol/o	atrium	atri/o
albumin	albumin/o	attack	aggress/o
all	holo-		-ago
	pan-		infest/o
along side of	para-	attraction for	-phil
alveolus	alveol/o		-philia
amnion	amni/o	attraction to	phil/o
among the people	epidemi/o	auricle	pinn/i
anastomosis	-stomy	aware	consci/o
aneurysm	aneurysm/o	away	apo-
anew	ana-	away from	ab-
angle	gon/i		abs-
	gon/o		es-
	goni/o		ex-
animal	zoo-		exo-
animal life	zo/o	axis; main stem	ax/o
animal starch	glycogen/o	bacillus	bacill/o
antrum of the stomach	anthr/o	back	dors/i
anus	an/o		dors/o

	isch/o	beneath	infer/o
	not/o		infra-
	poster/o	bent	kyph/o
	retro-		scoli/o
back of the skull	occipit/o		valg/o
backbones	spin/o	bent backward	lord/o
	vertebr/o	bent forward	pron/o
backward	ana-		pront/o
	opisth/o		supinat/o
	re-	berry-shaped	cocc/i
	retro-		cocc/o
bacteria	bacteri/o	berry-shaped bacterium	-coccus;
bad	cac-		-cocci
	cac/o	beside	para-
	dys-		par/o
	mal-	between	inter-
	malign/o	beyond	meta-
bag	cyst-		ultra-
	-cyst	bile	bil/i
	foll/i		chol/e
	scrot/o	bile vessel	cholangi/o
baldness	alopec/o	bilirubin	bilirubin/o
barren	steril/i	binding	ligat/o
Bartholin glands	barthollin/o	birth	gen/o
base	bas/o		genit/o
	fund/o		nat/i
bit of flesh	caruncul/o		part/o
beak	rostri		-partum
beams	trabecul/o		parturit/o
bearing	-iferous		toc/o
beating	puls/o		-tocia
before	ante-		-tocin
	fore-	birthing	loch/i
	pre-	black	melan/o
	pro-		nigr/o
	pros-	bladder	cyst-
beginning	-arche		-cyst
behind	post-	blemish	viti/o
	poster/o	blister	bulla-
	retro-		pustul/o
belly	celi/o	blood	hem-
belly side	ventr/o		hem/o
below	hypo-		hemat/o
	infer/o		sangu/i
	infra-		sanguin/o
	sub-	blood condition	-emia

blood vessel	angi/o	bundle of nerve fibers	tract/o
	hemangi/o	burn	caus/o
	vascul/o		caust/o
blue	cyan/o		caut/o
bodies	-somes		cauter/o
body	corp/u	bursa	burs/o
	corpor/o	bursting forth	-rhage
	soma-		-rhagia
	somat/o		-rrhage
	-some		-rrhagia
boil	furuncul/o	buttocks	glute/o
bone	os-	calcaneus	calcane/o
	oss/e	calcium	calc/i
	oss/i		calc/o
	oste/o	calculus	-lite
bone marrow	myel/o		-lith
bony cavity	orbit/o		lith/o
both sides	amb-	calf muscle	gastrocnemi/o
	amb/i	calyx	calci/o
bottom	fund/o		calic/o
bound to	adnex/o	cancer	carcin/o
bow	arc/o	cancerous	carcin/o
brain	encephal/o	capable of	-able
branch	ram/o	capable of being	-ible
branching	dendr/o		-ile
	furc/o	capable of moving	mobil/o
break	fract/o	capillary	capillar/o
breakdown	degenerat/o	capsule	capsul/o
	-lysis	carbon	carb/o
breaking down	catabol/o	carbon dioxide	capn/o
breast	mamm/o		-capnia
	mast/o	carpals	carp/o
breath	hal/o	carpus	carp/o
	halit/o	carrying	-ferent
breathing	-pnea		-ferous
bridle	fren/o		-iferous
bring forth	-para		-phoresis
	-parous	carrying down	defer/o
broad	lat/i	cartilage	cartilag/o
	lat/o		chondr/o
broken away from	abrupt/o		chondri/o
bronchial tube	bronch/o	caruncles	caruncul/o
	bronchi/o	caudal surface of the	
bronchiole	bronchiol/o	front foot (paw)	palm/o
bruise	contus/o	caudal surface of the	
bud	germin/o	patella	poplit/o

caudal surface of the			saphen/o
rear foot (paw)	plant/i		ser/o
	plant/o	cling	adhes/o
cause	eti/o	clitoris	clitor/o
causing genetic change	mutagen/o	closure	atres/i
cecum	cec/o	clot	thromb/o
cell	cyt/o	clotting	coagul/o
	-cyte	clump	coagul/o
cementum	cement/o		coagulat/o
cerebellum	cerebell/o	clumping	agglutin/o
cerebrum	cerebr/o	clusters	staphyl/o
cerumen	cerumin/o	coagulation	coagul/o
cervix	cervic/o	coal	anthrac/o
change	meta-	coccyx	coccyg/o
	metabol/o	cochlea	cochle/o
changing	transit/o	coiled	treponem/o
characterized by	-acious		turbinat/o
charged particle	ion/o	coiled microorganism	convolut/o
cheek	bucc/o		spirochet/o
	bucca-	cold	cry/o
cheekbone	zygomat/o		frigid/o
chemical	chem/i	collection of fluid	-oma
	chem/o	colon	col/o
	chemic/o		colon/o
chest	pector/o	color	chrom/o
	steth/o		chromat/o
	thorac/o		pigment/o
	-thorax	comfort	-aise
chew	mastic/o	coming together	coit/o
	mastricat/o	common	vulgar/i
child	ped/o	common bile duct	choledoch/o
	pedi/a	companion	soci/o
cholesterol	cholestrol/o	complete	dia-
chorion	chori/o		tel/o
	chorion/o	concave	koil/o
choroid	choroid/o	condition	-ation
ciliary body	cycl/o		-ema
circle	circi/o		-esis
	cycl/o		-exia
	orbit/o		-exis
classification	-type		-ia
clavicle	clavicul/o		-ism
cleansing	cathart/o		-sis
clear	fiss/o		-y
	fissur/o	condition of bone	-ostosis
	hyal/o	condition of cells	-cytosis

condition of pores	-porosis	crackling	crepit/o
condition of the			crepitat/o
mouth	-stomia	creeping	herpet/o
condition of urine	-uria	crescent	lunul/o
confined or limited to	circumscrib/o		menisc/o
confinement	loch/i	cross	cruci-
confusion	confus/o	crown	coron/o
congeal	coagul/o	cube-shaped	cuboid/o
	coagulat/o	cul-de-sac	culd/o
conjunctiva	conjunctiv/o	curled inward	involut/o
connective tissue	sarc/o	curve	lord/o
	sarco-	cut off	amput/o
	sarcomat/o		amputat/o
constant	home/o		syncop/o
constrict	constrict/o	cut short	syncop/o
contained outside	extrins/o	cutting apart	dissect/o
contained within	intrins/o	cutting into	incis/o
containing hollow		cutting out	excis/o
spaces	cavern/o	cycle	cycl/o
containing oxygen	oxid/o	cyst	cyst/o
contracted	sten/o	dance	chore/o
contraction	-stalsis	dark	opac/o
	systol/o		opacit/o
control	nom/o		phe/o
controlling	domin/o	darkness	scot/o
	stas/i	dawn	eosin/o
	-stasis	dead body	cadaver/o
	stat/i		sapr/o
	-static	death	leth/o
convey	vect/o		mort/i
coordination	tax/o		mort/o
copy	-mimetic		mort/u
cord	chord/o		mortal/i
core	ulcer/o		-mortem
cornea	corne/o		necr/o
	kerat/o		thanas/o
correct position	align/o		thanat/o
cortex	cortic/o	death of tissue	fatal/o
cough	tuss/i		-necrosis
count	numer/o	decay	cari/o
cover	cort-	decaying	sapr/o
covering	-lemma	deception	illusi/o
	opercul/o	decrease	hypo-
	tectori/o		-penia
	tunic/o	deep red iron-containing	
crack	fiss/o	pigment	hem/e
	fissur/o	deep sleep	comat/o

defecation	-chezia	dissolved	solut/o
defect	viti/o		solv/o
defective development	aplast/o	distant	dist/o
deficient	hypo-		tele/o
deficiency	-penia	distinct	idi/o
destruction	-lysis	divide into two	
destructive	pernici/o	branches	bifurcat/o
development	plas/i	divided	digest/o
	plas/o	dividing into equal	
	-plasia	left and right halves	midsagitt/o
	plast/o	doctor	iatr/o
	troph/o		medic/o
	-trophy	door	port/i
device for measurement	-meter	double	amb-
device to limit movement	fren/o		amb/i
diaphragm	phren/o		-bin
die	expir/o		-bis
	expirat/o		didym/o
different	all-		dipl/o
	all/o		dipla-
	heter/o		gemin/o
difficult	dys-	doubly	amph-
digestion	peps/i	down	cat-
	-pepsia		cata-
	pept/o		cath-
digits	dactyl/o		de-
	digit/o		kata-
dilated vein	varic/o		kath-
dilation	attenuat/o	downward	cat-
	-ectasia		cath-
	-ectasis	draw	press/o
dim	ambly/o	droop	-ptosis
discharge	excret/o	drowsiness	letharg/o
	-rhea	drug	chem/i
	-rrhea		chem/o
disease	morbid/o		chemic/o
	nos/o		pharmac/o
	path/o		pharmaceut/o
disease condition	-ago	dry	ichthy/o
	-igo		kraur/o
	-pathy		xer/o
diseased	cac-	drying	desicc/o
	cac/o	duct	vas/o
disembowelment	eviscer/o	dull	ambly/o
	eviscerat/o	duodenum	duoden/i
disorder	confus/o		duoden/o
displacement	dislocat/o	duplicate	dis-

dura mater	dur/o	evil	malign/o
dusky	phe/o	excess	ultra-
dust	coni/o	excessive	hyper-
dying	moribund/o		hyper-
ear	aur/i		super-
	aur/o		super/o
	auricul/o		superflu/o
	ot/o	excessive pain	-agra
ear condition	-otia	excision	-ectomy
ear drum	myring/o	exert influence on	affect/o
	tympan/o	expanding	-dilation
ease	-aise	expansion	diastol/o
eat	phag/o		-ectasia
	-phage		-ectasis
eating	-phagia	extend	tens/o
egg	o-	extensive	vast/o
	o/o	external ear	pinn/i
	oo/o	external surface	
	ov/i	covering	epithel/i
	ov/o	extreme	pol/o
	ovul/o	extremely fat	obes/o
eight	oct-	extremities	acr/o
	octa-		extrem/o
	octo-		extremit/o
elbow	cubit/o	eye	ocul/o
electricity	electr/o		oculo-
elimination of waste	-chezia		ophthalm/o
elongated	oblongat/o		opt/i
embryonic	-blast		opt/o
	blast/i		opti/o
empty	vac/u		optic/o
end	termin/o	eyelid	blephar/o
enlargement	-megaly		palpebr/o
enlargement of the		face	faci-
thyroid gland	goitr/o		faci/o
entire body	system/o	faint	syncop/o
	systemat/o	fall	laps/o
entrance	introit/o		-ptosis
	vestibul/o	falling together	symptomat/o
enzyme	-ase	false	pseud/o
epididymis	epididym/o	far	dist/o
epiglottis	epiglott/o	fascia	fasci/o
epithelium	epitheli/o	fast	tachy-
equal	is/o	fat	adip/o
eruption	eczemat/o		lip/o
esophagus	esophag/o		steat/o

fate	fatal/o	flow	-rhea
fear	phob/o		-rrhea
	-phobia	fluid	edemat/o
feeling	aesthet/o		hydr/o
	esthet/o	flushed	erythem/o
	-phoria		erythem/o
	sens/i		erythemat/o
female	estr/o	fold	plic/o
	gynec/o		rug/o
female erectile tissue	clitor/o	folding	gyr/o
femur	femor/o	follicle	follicul/o
fertilized egg	embry/o	food	nutri/o
fetus	fet/i		nutrit/o
	fet/o	foot	ped/o
fever	febr/i		pod/o
	pyrex/o	force	vi/o
	pyret/o	forehead	front/o
	pyr/o	foreign	xen/o
fiber	fibr/o	forking	furc/o
fibrin	fibrin/o	form	faci-
fibrous connective tissue	fibros/o		-form
fibula	fibul/o		form/o
	perone/o		morph/o
figure	-form	formation	-gene
	form/o		plas/i
filled in	infarct/o		plas/o
fingers	dactyl/o		-plasia
fire	pyr/o		-plasm
first	primi-		-poiesis
	prot-	forming	-fic
	prot/o		fic/o
	proto-		-gen
five	pent-		-genesis
	penta-	forward	ante-
	quinqu-		pro-
	quint-		pros-
flame within	inflammat/o	four	quadr/i
flame-colored	flamme/o		quadri-
flashing	eclamps/o		quadr/o
	eclampt/o		tetra-
flat	plan/o	fourth	quart-
flat patch	plac/o	free from waste	defec/o
flesh	sarc/o		defecat/o
	sarco-	fringe	fimbri/o
	sarcomat/o	front	anter/o
fleshy	pulpos/o	front	front/o

fruitful	fertil/o	great	vast/o
full of	-ose	green	chlor/o
function	physi/o	gristle	cartilag/o
	physic/o	groin	inguin/o
fungus	fung/i	groove	sulc/o
	myc/e		striat/o
	myc/o	ground	fund/o
funnel	infundibul/o	growth	kel/o
furrow	sulc/o		-plasia
gall	bil/i		plast/o
gallbladder	cholecyst/o	gums	gingiv/o
ganglion	gangli/o	gush back	regurgit/o
	ganglion/o	habit	-hexia
gangrene	gangren/o	hailstone	chalaz/o
gas	aer/o	hair	pil/i
	pneum/o		pil/o
	pneumon/o		trich/o
	pulmon/o	hair removal	depilat/o
gasping	asthmat/o	hairy	hirsut/o
gate	port/i	half	demi-
genetic change	mut/a		hemi-
germ	germin/o		semi-
giant	gigant/o	hallucinate	hallucin/o
give up	remiss/o	hammer	malle/o
giving off radiation	radiat/o	hand	chir/o
gland	aden/o		man/i
glans penis	balan/o		man/o
glass	silic/o	handful	manipul/o
	vitre/o	handle	manubri/o
glassy	hyal/o	hard	call/i
globe-shaped	spher/o		callos/o
glomerulus	glomerul/o		kerat/o
glucose	gluc/o		scirrh/o
	glyc/o	hardened	indurat/o
	glycos/o	hardening	-sclerosis
glue	coll/a	hardness	kera-
	gli/o	harmful	pernici/o
glycogen	glycogen/o	harsh sound	strid/o
go	grad/i	hatching	incubat/o
going forth	process/o	head	capit/o
good	eu-		cephal-
	stimul/o		cephal/o
granules	granul/o		-ceps
gray	glauc/o	healing	medic/o
gray matter of			medicat/o
the brain and		health	sanit/o
spinal cord	polio-	healthful	hygien/o

hearing	acous/o	humpback	kyph/o
	-acusia	hundred	cent-
	-acusis		hecato-
	aud-		hect-
	audi/o		hector-
	audit/o	hydrochloric acid	chlorhydr/o
	-cusis	hymen	hymen/o
heart	calor/i	ileum	ile/o
	cardi/o	ilium	ili/o
	cordi/o	immature	-blast
	coron/o		blast/i
heart muscle	myocardi/o	immature tumor	-blastoma
heat	caus/o	immune	immun/o
	caust/o	implant	inocul/o
	caut/o	in	en-
	cauter/o		end/o
	therm/o		endo-
heavy	pachy-		in-
hemoglobin	hemoglobin/o		ir-
hernia	-cele	in front of	fore-
	herni/o		pre-
hidden	crypt/o	in pieces	segment/o
	occult/o	in proper measure	emmetr/o
	palliat/o	in the direction of	-ad
higher than	hyper-	in the middle	mediastin/o
	super-	incision	-tomy
	super/o	incision to remove	
hilus	hil/o	a stone	-lithotomy
hip	cox/o	incite	stimul/o
	pelv/i	incline	verg/o
	pelv/o	incomplete	atel/o
hip bone	pelv/i	increase in cell number	-cytosis
	pelv/o		-philia
hives	urtic/o	increasing urine output	diur/o
hollow	cav/i		diuret/o
	cav/o	incubation	incubat/o
	-coel	individual	idi/o
	concav/o	infected	infect/o
	koil/o	infection	contagi/o
honey	mellit/o		furuncul/o
hoof	ungu/o		seps/o
hormone	hormon/o	inferior to	infra-
	-one	inflammation	-itis
horn	kera-	inherited	hered/o
horny tissue	kerat/o		heredit/o
horse	equin/o	injury	traumat/o
humerus	humer/o	inner	intern/o

inner section	medull/o	key	clav/i
innermost	intim/o	kidney	nephr/o
insert	cathet/o		nephra-
	cili/o		ren/o
inside	intro-	killing	-cide
instrument for cutting	-trite	knob	condyl/o
instrument for visual		know	nod/o
examination	-scope	knowledge	gnos/o
instrument to cut	-tome	knuckle	condyl/o
instrument to record	-graph	labor	part/o
insulin	insulin/o		-partum
intense cough	pertuss/i		parturit/o
intense pain	excruciat/o		puerper/i
internal organs	splanchn/o		toc/o
	viscer/o		-tocia
intestine	intestin/o		-tocin
into	in-	lack of strength	aplast/o
	intra-		-asthenia
	intro-		-atonic
inward	eso-		de-
iodine	iod/o	lacrimal duct	lacrim/o
ion	ion/o	lacrimal sac	dacryocyst/o
iris	ir/i	lamina	lamin/o
	ir/o	large	macr/o
	irid/o		macro-
iron	sider/o		magn/o
irregular	poikil/o		mega-
irregularity	anomal/o		megal/o
irrigation	-clysis	large intestine	col/o
ischium	ischi/o		colon/o
island	insul/o	larger	major/o
itch	psor/i	largest	maxim/o
	psor/o	larynx	laryng/o
itching	prurit/o	layer	strat/i
jaundice	icter/o	lean	emaciat/o
	ictero-	leather	cori/o
jaw	gnath/o	leaven	enzym/o
jejunum	jejun/o	left	sinistr/o
joined or yoked together	zygot/o	lens of the eye	phac/o
joining together	copulat/o		phak/o
joint	arthr/o	lens-shaped	lenticul/o
	articul/o	less	mei/o
jugular	jugul/o		mi/o
juice	chym/o		mio-
ketones	ket/o	less than normal	hypo-
	keton/o	lice	pedicul/o

lid	opercul/o	luminous	fluor/o
life	bi/o	lung	pneu-
	bio-		pneum/o
	vit/a		pneumon/o
	vit/o		pulm/o
	viv/i		pulmon/o
	viv/o	lying down	decubit/o
	zoo-	lying on the back	supin/o
ligament	ligament/o	lymph	lymph/o
	syndesm/o	lymph gland	lymphaden/o
light	actin/o	lymph node	lymphaden/o
	phot/o	lymph vessel	lymphangi/o
like	phil/o	madness	rabi/o
lip	cheil/o	main stem	ax/o
	labi/o	male	andr/o
lipid	lip/o	malformed fetus	terat/o
litter box	capsul/o	malleolus	malleol/o
little	-ole	mammary gland	mamm/o
	-ule		mast/o
little ball	globul/o	mandible	mandibul/o
little body	corpuscul/o	many	multi-
little bundle	fascicul/o		ple/o
little coil	spirill/o		poly-
little duct	canalicul/o	marketplace	agora-
little grape	uvul/o	marrow	medull/o
little hammer	malleol/o	masculine	viril/o
little knot	nodul/o	mass	-oma
	tubercul/o	mastoid process	mastoid/o
liver	hepa-	maxilla	maxill/o
	hepat/o	maze	labyrinth/o
	hepta-	meal	cib/o
lobe	lob/i		prandi/o
	lob/o		-prandial
location	top/o	measure	metr/o
loin	lumb/o	measurement	-metry
long-lived	longev/o	meatus	meat/o
loosen	lax/o	median plane	mesi/o
	laxat/o	mediastinum	mediastin/o
loosening	-lysis	medication	medicat/o
louse	pedicul/o	medicine	medic/o
lower	cat-	medulla	medull/o
	cath-	membrane	diphther/o
lower back	lumb/o		hymen/o
lower jaw	mandibul/o		membran/o
lower part of		meninges	mening/o
the body	caud/o		meningi/o

menstruation	men/o		myxa-
	mens-		myxo-
	mens/o	muscle	muscul/o
mesentery	mesenter/o		my/o
messenger	nunci/o		myos/o
metacarpals	metacarp/o	muscle tumor	myom/o
metatarsals	metatars/o	muscular twitching	fibrill/o
middle	med-	mushroom	fung/i
	medi/o	muzzle	phim/o
	medull/o	myocardium	myocardi/o
	ment/o	nail	onych/o
	mes-		ungu/o
	mes/o	nameless	innominat/o
	mesi/o	nape	nuch/o
milk	galact/o	narrow pass	fauc/i
	lact/i	narrowing	-constriction
	lact/o		em-
mimic	-mimetic		sten/o
mind	ment/o		-stenosis
	phren/o		stric-
	psych/o	naturally occurring	mineral/o
mineral	mineral/o	nature	physi/o
mirror	specul/o		physic/o
mixture	cras/o	navel	omphal/o
	-crasia		umbilic/o
mold	plast/o	near	par/o
monster	terat/o		para-
moon	lun/o		proxim/o
more	ple/o	near food	parasit/o
mouth	or/o; stomat/o	nearby	juxta-
mouth; bone	os-	neck	cervic/o
movement	cine/o		coll/i
	kines/o	negative	dis-
	kinesi/o	neither	neutr/o
	-kinesia	nerve	nerv/o
	-kinesis		neu-
	mot/o		neur/i
	motil/o		neur/o
	-motor	nerve root	radicul/o
much	poly-	nervous sensation	esthes/o
mucosa	mucos/o		esthesi/o
mucous membranes	mucos/o		-esthesia
mucus	muc/o	nest	nid/o
	mucos/o	network	reticul/o
	myx-	network of nerves	plex/o
	myx/o	neuroglial tissue	gli/o

neutral	neutr/o	oblong	oblongat/o
neutrophil	neutr/o	obscure	-opaque
new	ne/o	obsessive preoccupation	-mania
	neo-	of a mother	matern/o
new opening to the		off	apo-
outside of the body	-stomy	old	sen/i
night	noct/i	old age	ger/i
	nyct/o		ger/o
	nyctal/o		geront/o
nine	ennea-	olecranon	olecran/o
	non-	omentum	oment/o
	nona-	on	epi-
	nonus-	on both sides	amph-
	novem-	one	mon/o
nipple	thel/o		mono-
nipple-like	papill/i		uni-
	papill/o	one and one-half	sesqui-
nitrogen	-amine	one who	-er
	azot/o		-or
	niter-	one who receives	obstetr/o
	nitro-	one-thousandth	milli-
no	a-	opening	-duct
	an-		foramin/o
	non-		hiat/o
none	nulli-		meat/o
normal	eu-		-tresia
	nor-	opening from a	
	norm/o	body part	hil/o
nose	nas/i	opposite	contra-
	nas/o	opposite of acid	bas/o
nose	rhin/o	optic disc	papill/i
nostril	nar/i		papill/o
not	a-	orange-yellow	cirrh/o
	in-	order	norm/o
	un-		tax/o
not continuous	intermitt/o	organ	organ/o
nourishment	nutri/o	origin	-gene
	nutrit/o	ossicle	ossicul/o
	troph/o	other	all-
	-trophy		all/o
nucleus	kary/o	other than	par-
	karyo-	out	ec-
	kern-		ecto-
	nucle/o		ef-lex-
number	numer/o		exo-
numbness	narc/o		extra-

out from	e-	passage	introit/o
out of	e-	patella	patell/a
	es-		patell/o
out of place	atop/o	path	tract/o
out of proportion	ametr/o	peel	lemm/o
outer	extern/o		lent/i
outer layer of skin	epithel/i	pelvis	pelv/i
outer region	cortic/o		pelv/o
outermost	extrem/o	pen	styl/o
	extremit/o	penis	pen/i
outside	ec-		phall/o
	ecto-		priap/o
	ex-	people	dem/o
	exo-	perform	oper/o
	extern/o		operat/o
	extra-	perineum	perine/o
ovary	oophor/o	peritoneum	peritone/o
	ovari/o	pertaining to	-ac
over	hyper-		-al
overflowing	superflu/o		-an
own	auto-		-ar
oxygen	ox/i		-ary
	ox/o		-eal
	ox/y		-iac
	-oxia		-ial
	oxy-		-ic
pain	alg/e		-ical
	alg/o		-ile
	-algia		-in
	-dynia		-ine
	odyn/o		-ior
painful	dys-		-ose
palate	palat/o		-ous
pale	pall/o		-tic
	pallid/o	pertaining to a blood	
palsy	-plegia	condition	-emic
	-plegic	pertaining to a cell	-cytic
pancreas	pancreat/o	pertaining to a disease	
paralysis	-plegia	condition	-pathic
	-plegic	pertaining to breathing	-pneic
parathyroid		pertaining to formation	-plastic
glands	parathyroid/o	pertaining to killing	-cidal
parent compound	nor-	pertaining to movement	-kinetics
parotid gland	parotid/o	pertaining to sensitivity	
partial dislocation	subluxat/o	to pain	-algesic
partition	sept/o	pertaining to standing	-stitial

pertaining to stopping	-static		vir/o
pertaining to the		pole	styl/o
destruction or		polyp	polyp/o
breakdown	-lytic	pons	pont/o
pertaining to visual		pore	por/o
examination	-scopic	position	top/o
phalanges	phalang/o	potassium	kal/i
pharynx	pharyng/o	pouch	scrot/o
phlegm	phlegm/o	pour across	transfus/o
picture	-type	pour in	ingest/o
pigment	pigment/o	pouring out	effus/o
pillar	column/o	pouring out of juice	ecchym/o
pimple	papul/o	powerful	potent/o
pineal gland	pineal/o	practice	pract/i
pinna	pinn/i		practic/o
pipe	tub/i	precursor	prodrom/o
	tub/o	pregnancy	-cyesis
	fistul/o		gest/o
pit	fove/o		gestat/o
	glen/o		gester/o
	lacun/o		gravid/o
pituitary gland	hypophys/o		-gravida
	pituitar/o		pregn/o
place	loc/o	premature expulsion	
	sit/u	of fetus	abort/o
	the/o	prepuce	preputi/o
	top/o	pressed	depress/o
placenta	placent/o	pressed together	constipat/o
plant	phyt/o	pressure	bar/o
	-phyte		impuls/o
plaque	ather/o		-tension
	-plakia	prevention	-phylactic
plentiful	copi/o	prevention of	
pleura	pleur/o	fertilization	contracept/o
pleural cavity	-thorax	primitive living cell	-plast
plexus	plex/o	process	-ation
point	acne/o		-ion
	apic/o		-ism
	foc/o		-y
	stigmat/o	process of cutting into	-tomy
point of contact	synaps/o	process of making	-fication
	synapt/o	process of recording	-graphy
pointed	cusp/i	process of visual	
pointed instrument	styl/o	examination	-scopy
poison	tox/o	produced by	-genic
	toxic/o	produced in	-genic

producing	-facient		urtic/o
	-fic	receive	recept/o
	fic/o		recipi/o
	-gen	record	-gram
	gen/o	rectal gas	flat/o
	-genesis	rectum	rect/o
	genit/o	rectum and anus	proct/o
	-genous	red	eosin/o
	-iferous		erythr/o
	-ific	redness	erythem/o
production	-gene		erythemat/o
productive	fertil/o	reflected sound	echo-
prolapse	-ptosis	relax	lax/o
prostate gland	prostat/o		laxat/o
protection	-phylaxis	relaxation	chalas/o
protective	-phylactic		-chalasia
protein	-globin		-chalasis
	globin/o	removal	-apheresis
	-globulin		de-
	prote/o		-ectomy
pubis	pub/o		-pheresis
pudendum	pudend/o	remove excess water	concentr/o
pulley	trochle/o	renal pelvis	pyel/o
pulse	sphygm/o	resection	-ectomy
	-sphyxia	resembling	-iform
puncture	punct/o		-oid
pupil	cor/o	resembling a tree	dendr/o
	core-	restrain	contine/o
	core/o		continent/o
	pupill/o	retina	retin/o
purging	cathart/o	revolution	vertig/o
purple	purpur/o		vertigin/o
pus	pur/o	rhythm	rhythm/o
	purul/o	rib	cost/o
	py/o		costal/o
pushing	osm/o	ridge	plic/o
put	the/o	right side	dextr/o
pyloric sphincter	pylor/o	rigid	tetan/o
pylorus	pylor/o	ring	an/o
quiet	tranquil/o		circi/o
radioactivity	radi/o	ringing	tinnit/o
radius	radi/o	ringworm	tine/o
rage	man/i	ripe	matur/o
	rabi/o	rod	rhabd/o
rapid	oxy-	roll	volv/o
rash	exanthemat/o	root	rhiz/o

rosy	eosin/o		steat/o
rotate	tors/o	second	deut-
rough	hirsut/o		deuto-
round	cocc/i		secundi-
	cocc/o	sediment	fec/o
	spher/o	seed	gon/i
rule	norm/o		gon/o
rumbling sound	borborygm/o		goni/o
running	drom/o		semin/i
running together	syndrom/o		spor/o
rupture	-rhexis	seeing	vis/o
sac	foll/i	segmented	segment/o
	sacc/i	seizure	-agra
	sacc/o		-lepsy
sac of fluid	cyst/o	self	auto-
sac of fluid near		semen	semin/i
a joint	burs/o	seminal vesicle	vesicul/o
sacrum	sacr/o	send down	cathet/o
saddle	sell/o		cili/o
safe	immun/o	sensation	aesthet/o
sag	laps/o		sens/i
	-lapse	sense of perception	esthet/o
	prolaps/o	sensitive to	sensitiv/o
	-ptosis	sensitivity to pain	alges/o
saliva	-ptyalo		algesi/o
	saliv/o		-algesia
	sial/o		algi
salivary gland	sialaden/o	separate	-crine
same	hom/o		dilut/o
	ipsi-		excret/o
	is/o	separation	-lysis
sameness	home/o	septum	sept/o
scale	squam/o	serous	seros/o
scaly	ichthy/o	serum	ser/o
scanty	olig/o	set fire to	inflammat/o
	oligo-	seven	sept-
scapula	scapul/o		septi-
sclera	scler/o	severe	acu/o
scrape off	abrad/o	sex cell	gamet/o
	abras/o	sex glands	gonad/o
	scalp/o	sexual drive	libid/o
scrotum	scrot/o		libidin/o
sea	thalass/o	sexual intercourse	-pareunia
seam	raph/o		vener/o
sebum	seb/o	shaded	opac/o
	sebace/o		opacit/o

shaken together violently concuss/o

shaking trem/o
 tremul/o

shallow depression foss/o

shape -form
 form/o
 morph/o

shaped-like -iform

sharp acu/o
 acuit/o
 acut/o
 oxy-

sheath -lemma
 thec/o
 tunic/o

sheath around a tendon synov/o

shedding decidu/o

shell conch/o

shield thyr/o

shining forth eclamps/o
 eclampt/o

short brachy-
 brev/i
 brev/o

sick feeling in the
 stomach nause/o

side later/o

sideways obliqu/o

sieve ethm/o

sight vis/o

sigmoid colon sigmoid/o

similar al-

single mon/o
 mono-

sinus sin/o
 sin/u
 sinus/o

six hex-
 hexa-
 sex-

skeletal muscle rhabdomy/o

skeleton skelet/o

skill techn/o
 techni/o

skin cori/o
 cut-

skin spot petechi/o

skinned dart/o

skull crani/o

slanted obliqu/o

sleep carot/o
 hypn/o
 narc/o
 somn/i
 somn/o
 -somnia
 sopor/o

slender gracil/o
 lept/o

slide laps/o
 prolaps/o

slight paralysis -paresis

slipping -listhesis

slow brady-

small -icle
 micr/o
 micro-
 -ole
 -ule

small growth polyp/o

small intestine enter/o

small lump chalaz/o

small opening por/o

small sac follicul/o

small vein venul/o

smaller mi/o
 minor/o

smallest minim/o

smell olfact/o
 osm/o
 -osmia

smooth muscle leiomy/o

socket glen/o
 orbit/o

sodium natr/o

soft medull/o

cutane/o
derm/o
derma-
-derma
dermat/o
epitheli/o

softening	malac/o		stapedi/o
	-malacia	starch	amyl/o
solid	stere/o	state of	-sis
solid structure	ster/o	step	grad/i
solution	-sol	step forward	aggress/o
something formed	plasm/o	sternum	stern/o
something inserted	embol/o	steroid	ster/o
sound	phon/o	stick	adhes/o
	-phonia	sticking together	agglutin/o
	son/o	sticky	tenac/i
soundness	sanit/o		visc/o
space between things	interstiti/o		viscos/o
spark	scint/i	stiff	ankyl/o
specialist	-ist		rigid/o
sperm	sperm/o	stimulate	-tropin
	spermat/o	sting	punct/o
spermatozoa	sperm/o	stirrup	staped/o
	spermat/o		stapedi/o
sphenoid bone	sphen/o	stomach	gastr/o
sphincter	pylor/o	stone	-lite
	sphincter/o		-lith
spider	arachn/o		lith/o
spinal column	rachi/o	stopping	paus/o
spinal cord	chord/o		stas/i
	cord/o		stasis
	myel/o		stat/i
	oste/o		-static
spine	spin/o	straight	orth/o
spiny	acanth/o		ortho-
spit	-ptyalo	strain	tens/o
	saliv/o	strang	xen/o
	sput/o	strangle	angin/o
spitting	-ptysis	strength	sthen/o
spleen	splen/o		-sthenia
split	-fida	stretching	-dilation
	fiss/o		-ectasia
	fissur/o		-ectasis
	schiz/o	striated muscle	rhabdomy/o
split into two parts	bifid/o	stricture	-stenosis
spot	macul/o	string of beads	monil/o
	stigmat/o	stripe	striat/o
spread out	diffus/o	structure	-ium
	dilat/o		-um
	dilatat/o		-us
stake	styl/o	study of	log/o
stapes	staped/o		-logy

stuffed	infarct/o	symptom	symptomat/o
stunned	stup/e	synapse	synaps/o
stupor	carot/o		synapt/o
	narc/o	synovial fluid	synovi/o
substance that forms	-poietin	synovial membrane	synov/o
sudden	acu/o		synovi/o
	oxysm/o	system	system/o
sudden attack	paroxysm/o		systemat/o
sudden, involuntary		tail	caud/o
contraction	-spasm	tailbone	coccyg/o
	spasm/o	tainted	infect/o
	spasmod/o	take hold of	-leptic
sugar	gluc/o	tap	percussi/o
	glyc/o	tarsals	tars/o
	glycos/o	tarsus	tars/o
	-ose; sucr/o	tasteless	insipid/o
sulfer	thio-	tear	dacry-
sunken down	depress/o		dacry/o
surgical fixation	-desis		lacrim/o
	-pexy	tear duct	dacry-
surgical puncture to			lacrim/o
remove fluid or gas	-centesis	tear gland	dacryoaden/o
surgical repair	-plasty	tear sac	dacryocyst/o
surrounding	peri-	teeth	dent-
suture	raph/o	temperament	cras/o
	-raphy	temple	tempor/o
	-rhaphy	ten	dec/i
	-rrhaphy		deca-
swallow	deglutit/o		decem-
	phag/o		dek-
	-phage		deka-
swallow	-phagia	tendon	ten/o
swayback	lord/o		tendin/o
sweat	diaphor/o	tension	ton/o
	hidr/o	tenth	dec/i
	sudor/i		deca-
sweet	glycer/o	testes	didym/o
swelling	-dema		orch/o
	-edema		orchi/o
	edemat/o		orchid/o
	nod/o		test/i
	tubercul/o		test/o
swollen vein	varic/o	thalamus	thalam/o
sword	xiph/i	thick	pachy-
	xiph/o	thick mucus	phlegm/o

thin	lept/o	to become aware	percept/o
thin skin	membran/o	to become pregnant	concept/o
thing	-ium	to become solid	consolid/o
	-um	to become strong	convalesc/o
	-us	to belch	eruct/o
third	tert-		eructat/o
	trit-	to bend	flex/o
	trito-	to bend back	refract/o
thirst	dips/o	to bind	-desis
	-dipsia		nect/o
thorny	acanth/o	to break	-clasis
thread	mit/o		-clast
threads of a clot	fibrin/o	to break into pieces	comminut/o
three	tri-	to breakdown	-lytic
three dimensional	stere/o	to breathe	spir/o
throat	gutter/o	to breathe in	aspir/o
	pharyng/o		aspirat/o
throbbing	palpit/o		inhal/o
through	dia-		inhalat/o
	per-		inspir/o
	trans-		inspirat/o
throw in	inject/o	to breathe out	exhal/o
thrown in	embol/o		exhalat/o
thymus gland	thym/o		expir/o
	thyr/o		expirat/o
	thyroid/o	to bring about a response	effect/o
tibia	tibi/o	to bring back together	reduct/o
tight band	sphincter/o	to bring in line	align/o
tightening	-stenosis	to burst forth	erupt/o
time	chron/o	to burst open	dehisc/o
tissue	hist/o	to care for	comi/o
	histi/o	to carry	duct/o
	-ium		fer/o
	-um		ferent
	-us		ingest/o
to	-ad		pher/o
to aggravate	exacerbat/o		-phoria
to assemble	-agon		vect/o
to bear	fer/o	to cast	bol/o
	-para	to change	trop/o
	-parous	to choke	suffoc/o
	pher/o		suffocat/o
	phor/o	to close up	occlud/o
	-phoria		occlus/o
to beat	percussi/o	to come together	-fusion

to condense	concentr/o	to hold back	retent/o
to connect	nect/o	to hurl out	ejaculat/o
to cough up	expector/o	to inject	enem/o
to crush	-tripsy	to introduce	inocul/o
to cut	cis/o	to keep in	contine/o
	sect/o		continent/o
	secti/o	to lead	duct/o
	-spadia	to lead forward	product/o
	tom/o	to let go	remiss/o
to cut away	amput/o	to lift up	lev/o
	amputat/o		levat/o
to cut off	syncop/o	to listen	auscult/o
to cut short	syncop/o	to look at	spec/i
to destroy	-lytic	to measure	-meter
to disable	paralys/o	to move	grad/i
	paralyt/o	to narrow	constrict/o
	pares/i	to nourish	aliment/o
	paret/o	to pass through	perme/o
to dissolve	dilut/o	to perform	funct/o
to distribute	digest/o		function/o
to draw back	retract/o	to place on back	supinat/o
	tract/o	to pollute	contaminat/o
to draw tightly together	strict/o	to pour	chym/o
to draw together	constrict/o		-fusion
to drive away	-fuge	to press down	suppress/o
to empty out	evacu/o	to press	press/o
	evacuat/o	to pull	tract/o
to expel from the body	eliminat/o	to pull together	convuls/o
to expose to air	ventilat/o	to put in place	-pexy
to faint	syncop/o	to put poison in	intoxic/o
to fall	-lapse	to rebuild	restor/o
	prolaps/o	to receive	concept/o
	ptomat/o	to receive within	intussuscept/o
to flood	regurgit/o	to recover	recuperat/o
to force	inject/o	to reduce	-lytic
to form pus	suppur/o	to reproduce	procreat/o
	suppurat/o		prolifer/o
to gather	-agon	to revive	resuscit/o
to give	don/o	to revolve	rotat/o
	-dote	to roll	vol/o
to go	-grade	to run	-drome
to go around in a circle	circulat/o	to scratch	excori/o
to grind	brux/o		excoriat/o
to grow	-physis	to secrete	crin/o; -crine
to hang	isch/o	to secrete milk	lactat/o
	pend/o	to secrete out of	exocrin/o

to secrete within	endocrin/o	to walk	ambul/o
to seize	-leptic		ambulat/o
to send	-mission	to wander	ion/o
to separate	-crit	to work	oper/o
	-lytic		operat/o
to set	-stitial	to yield	product/o
to share	communic/o	toes	dactyl/o
to shine	-lucent	together	co-
to slide	-lapse		com-
	lux/o		con-
to snore	rhonc/o		sym-
	stert/o		syn-
to soften	emolli/o	tone	-atonic
to split	-schisis	tongue	gloss/o
to squint	strab/i		glosso-
to stick together	coher/o		glott/i
	cohes/o		glott/o
to stitch	sutur/o		lingu/o
to stop	-suppression	tonsils	tonsill/o
to strain through	filtr/o	too early	prematur/o
	filtrat/o	tooth	dent/i
to stretch	tone/o		dent/o
to stretch apart	distend/o		odont/o
	distent/o	toothless	edentul/o
to stretch out	tens/o	top	acr/o
to suck up or in	absorpt/o	torn	lacer/o
to sweat out	exud/o		lacerat/o
	exudat/o	touch	tact/i
to sympathize with	compatibil/o	touched	contact/o
to tear	-spadia	touching of something	contagi/o
to throw	bol/o	toward	ad-
to throw out	ejaculat/o		-ad
to tie	nect/o		af-
	strict/o		ag-
to tie together	-desis		at-
to touch	palpat/o	trachea	trache/i
to transfer	transfus/o		trache/o
to turn	-tropia	treatment	iatr/o
	-verse		therap/o
	-version		therapeut/o
	volv/o		-therapy
to twist	verg/o	tremor	tremul/o
	tors/o	triangle	delta-
to urinate	mictur/o		trigon/o
	micturit/o	trigone	trigon/o
to view	-opsy	true	eu-

tube	fistul/o	unchanging	home/o
	syring/o	uncontrolled	athet/o
	tub/i	under	cat-
	tub/o		cath-
tumor	edemat/o		hypo-
	kel/o		sub-
	-oma	uneasy	anxi/o
	onc/o		anxiet/o
turn	trop/o	unequal	anis/o
	vers/o	unexplained	spontane/o
	vert/o	unknown	idi/o
turning	gyr/o	up	ana-
	-tropic	upon	epi-
turning around	vertig/o	upper	supra-
	vertigin/o	upper jaw	maxill/o
turning aside	divert/i	upright	arrect/o
	refract/o		erect/o
turning point	cris/o		fec/i
	critic/o	upward	an/o
twice	-bin	urea	azot/o
	bis-	ureter	ureter/o
	di-	urethra	urethr/o
	dis-	urging on	impuls/o
twin	gemin/o	urinary bladder	cyst/o
twisted	tort/i		vesic/o
twisted chains	strept/o	urination	-uresis
twisted out	convolut/o		-uria
	exstroph/o	urine	ur/o
	valg/o		urin/o
two	bi-	use of hands	manipul/o
	-bin	uterine tube	salping/o
	-bis		-salpinx
	di-	uterus	hyster/o
	du/o		metr/i
	dy-		metr/o
	dyo-		metri/o
tying off	ligat/o		uter/i
tympanic membrane	myring/o		uter/o
	tympan/o	uvea	uve/o
ulcer	aphth/o	uvula	staphyl/o
	apth/o		uvul/o
	ulcer/o	vaccine	vaccin/i
ulna	uln/o		vaccin/o
umbilicus	omphal/o	vagina	colp/o
	umbilic/o		vagin/o

vagus nerve	vag/o	vomiting	-emesis
valve	valv/o	vulva	episi/o
	valvul/o		vulv/o
varied	poikil/o	wall	pariet/o
vas deferens	vas/o	wandering of mind	deliri/o
vascular layer of the eye	uve/o	wart	verruc/o
vault	fornic/o	washing	-clysis
vein	phleb/o	wasted away by disease	emaciat/o
	ven/i	wasting away	-phthisis
	ven/o	water	aqu/i
venereal	vener/o		aqu/o
ventricle	ventricul/o		aque/o
venule	venul/o		hydr/o
vertebrae	rachi/o		hydra-
	spondyl/o	watery flow	rheum/o
	vertebr/o		rheumat/o
very large	gigant/o	wax	cera-
vessel	angi-	weak	attenuat/o
	angi/o		cac-; cac/o
	vas/o	weakening	-asthenia
	vascul/o		-paresis
	vaso-	weakness	asthen-
vestibule	vestibul/o	wedge	sphen/o
view of	-opsy	weight	bar/o
villi	vill/i	white	alb/i
violent action	clon/o		alb/o
virus	vir/o		albin/o
viscera	splanchn/o		leuco-
	viscer/o		leuk/o
visceral muscle	leiomy/o	whole	intact/o
vision	-opia	wide	mydr/o
	-opsia	widely scattered	disseminat/o
	-opsis	widening	-dilation
	opt/i		-eurysm
	opt/o	window	fenestr/o
	opti/o	windpipe	trache/i
	optic/o		trache/o
vitreous body	vitr/o	with	co-
vocal	voc/i		con-
voice	phon/o		sym-
	-phonia		syn-
	voc/i	within	en-
voice box	laryng/o		end/o
voluntary	spontane/o		endo-
vomit	emet/o		ento-

	intern/o	worm	verm/i
	intra-	worsening	deteriorat/o
	intro-	wrinkle	rhytid/o
without	a-		rug/o
	an-	X-ray	radi/o
without an opening	atres/i		roentgen/o
wolf	lup/i	yellow	jaund/o
	lup/o		lute/o
woman	gynec/o		xanth/o
work	erg/o	yoke	zygomat/o

Answers

Chapter 1   Case Study and Exercises

K-9:	Canine or Dog	Biopsy:	Removal of tissue for microscopic exam
TPR(W):	Temperature, pulse, respiration, weight	Hematology:	Study of blood
BAR:	Bright, alert, responsive	Erythrocyte:	Red blood cell
DOB:	Date of birth	Leukocyte:	White blood cell
PPH:	Past pertinent history	Thrombocyte:	Clotting cell or platelet
Radiograph:	Instrument for recording X-rays	WNL:	Within normal limits
Diagnose:	Estimation of the cause of disease	Hepatic:	Pertaining to the liver
Cardiopathy:	Disease condition of the heart	Electrocardiogram:	Record of electricity in the heart
Arthritis:	Inflammation of joints	OR:	Operating room
Hepatitis:	Inflammation of the liver	Incision:	Process of cutting into
P/E:	Physical examination	Excised:	Process of cutting out
Dermatitis:	Inflammation of skin	ICU:	Intensive care unit
Cytology:	Study of cells	Sarcoma:	Malignant tumor arising from connective tissue
NSF:	No significant findings	Prognosis:	Estimation of disease outcome
Hypogastric:	Pertaining to below the stomach		
Gastric:	Pertaining to the stomach		

1-A:

1.	B	7.	I
2.	H	8.	J
3.	G	9.	A
4.	L	10.	K
5.	F	11.	E
6.	D	12.	C

Veterinary Medical Terminology Guide and Workbook, First Edition. Angela Taibo.
© 2014 John Wiley & Sons, Inc. Published 2014 by John Wiley & Sons, Inc.
Companion website: www.wiley.com/go/taibo/terminology

1-B:

1. Histology
2. Hematoma
3. Encephalitis
4. Cardiopathy
5. Hepatoma
6. Hepatitis
7. Osteotomy
8. Thrombocytosis
9. Pathologist
10. Nephrosis
11. Ophthalmoscope
12. Electrocardiogram
13. Neural
14. Erythrocyte
15. Hypodermic
16. Subhepatic
17. Hyperglycemia
18. Diagnosis
19. Dermatitis
20. Extrahepatic

1-C:

1. Joint
2. Inflammation
3. Surgical puncture to remove fluid
4. Nose
5. Head
6. Red blood cells, Hemoglobin
7. Eye
8. Large Intestine (Colon)
9. Cutting into
10. Kidney

1-D:

1. Inflammation
2. Removal or excision
3. Incision or cutting into
4. Record
5. Process of visual examination
6. Abnormal condition
7. Specialist
8. Instrument for recording
9. Disease condition
10. Pain
11. Surgical puncture to remove fluid or gas
12. Blood condition

1-E:

1. D
2. B
3. B
4. D
5. B

1-F:

1. Bright, alert, responsive
2. Operating room
3. Domestic short hair
4. Intensive care unit
5. Temperature, pulse, respiration, weight
6. Date of birth
7. Physical examination
8. Rule out
9. Isolation unit
10. No significant findings
11. Past pertinent history
12. Within normal limits

1-G:

1. Within, into
2. Outside
3. Across; through
4. Above; upon; on
5. Below; under
6. Above; excessive

7. Before, forward
8. Back; again; backward
9. In; within
10. Behind
11. No; not; without
12. Out; away from

1-H:

1. Blood condition of increased sugar
2. Estimation of disease outcome
3. Process of cutting into
4. Study of cells
5. Malignant tumor arising from epithelial tissue
6. Increase in platelets or clotting cells
7. Study of the stomach and small intestine
8. Study of life
9. Pertaining to a short, wide head
10. Pertaining to caused by treatment
11. Pertaining to the eye
12. Inflammation of bone
13. Inflammation of the nose
14. Study of urine; study of the urinary tract

Chapter 2   Case Study and Exercises

stat:	Immediately	Lateral:	Pertaining to the side
pt.:	Patient	CBA:	Cat bite abscess
DLH:	Domestic long hair	MM:	Mucous membranes
Abdominal:	Pertaining to the abdomen	Anemia:	Decrease in red blood cells and/or hemoglobin
Evisceration:	Displacement of organ or tissue through the cavity that should contain it	Endotracheal:	Pertaining to within the windpipe
FVRCP:	Feline viral rhinotracheitis, Calicivirus, Panleukopenia	Dorsal recumbency:	Lying on its back
FeLV:	Feline leukemia virus	Viscera:	Internal organs
RV:	Rabies vaccine	Lavage:	Irrigation or washing out of an organ or cavity
P/E:	Physical examination	Peritonitis:	Inflammation of the peritoneum

2-A:

1. K
2. I
3. L
4. A
5. G
6. H
7. C
8. B
9. D
10. F
11. E
12. J

2-B:

1. Pathology
2. Neoplasm
3. Craniotomy
4. Visceral
5. Chondroma
6. Inguinal
7. Cytologist
8. Pharyngeal
9. Laryngitis
10. Intervertebral
11. Tracheotomy
12. Thoracotomy
13. Cranioplasty
14. Pelvic
15. Sacrocaudal
16. Lumbar
17. Chondralgia
18. Lavage
19. Benign
20. Physiology

2-C:

1. Diaphragm
2. Larynx
3. Diarrhea
4. Abscess
5. Cartilage
6. Malignant
7. Thoracic
8. Vertebrae
9. Cervical
10. Vomiting

2-D:

1. Surgical repair
2. Pertaining to; full of
3. Study of
4. Pain
5. Surgical puncture to remove fluid or gas
6. Specialist
7. Development; formation; growth
8. Process; condition
9. Abnormal condition
10. Pertaining to
11. Tumor; mass
12. Inflammation

2-E:

1. J
2. B
3. I, C
4. H
5. A
6. F or I
7. G
8. F
9. B
10. D

11. G
12. A
13. E

14. F
15. C

2-F:

1. Cat bite abscess
2. Feline infectious peritonitis
3. Vomiting/diarrhea
4. Immediately
5. Physical therapy
6. Negative
7. Feline immunodeficiency virus
8. Distemper, hepatitis, leptospirosis, parvo, parainfluenza, corona
9. Without
10. Positive
11. With
12. Mucous Membranes

2-G:

1. Deficient; below; under; less than normal
2. Between
3. Change
4. Down
5. Up
6. In; within
7. New
8. No; not; without

2-H:

1. The control center of the cell that contains chromosomes
2. Abnormal protrusion of an organ or tissue through a natural opening
3. Displacement of internal organs outside the cavity that should contain them
4. Process of building up complex proteins from simpler substances
5. Study of diseased tissue
6. Malignant tumor of cartilage arising from connective tissue
7. Cavity containing organs such as the stomach, intestines, spleen, and pancreas
8. Glands that secrete chemicals through tubes everywhere in the body
9. Glands that secrete hormones directly into the bloodstream
10. Tube that carries urine from the urinary bladder to the outside of the body
11. Thin, muscular partition separating the thoracic and abdominal cavities
12. Throat
13. Semi-permeable structure that surrounds and protects the cell
14. Process of breaking down complex food into simpler substances
15. Cartilage pad between vertebrae used for cushion and support

Chapter 3   Case Study and Exercises

Lameness:	Incapable of normal locomotion	ROM:	Range of motion
AAHA:	American Animal Hospital Association	Radiographs:	Instrument for recording X-rays
Gait:	Manner of walking	Osteitis:	Inflammation of bone
P/E:	Physical examination	Femoral:	Pertaining to the femur
bilat.:	Bilateral	Head:	Rounded articular process separated from the shaft of a bone by the neck
ACL:	Anterior cruciate ligament	Acetabulum:	Cup-like depression in the pelvis that helps form the hip joint
DVM:	Doctor of Veterinary Medicine	TPO:	Triple pelvic osteotomy
Anterior drawer:	Cranial movement of the proximal tibia in relation to distal femur to check for ACL injury	P.T.:	Physical therapy
TPLO:	Tibial plateau leveling osteotomy	CVT:	Certified veterinary technician
PROM:	Passive range of motion	Hydrotherapy:	Water treatment
®:	Right	NAVTA:	National Association of Veterinary Technicians of America
Coxofemoeral:	Hip		

3-A:

1. B
2. G
3. H
4. I
5. K
6. A

7. E
8. J
9. C
10. D
11. F
12. L

3-B:

1. Subcostal
2. Chondromalacia
3. Spondylitis
4. Fasciitis
5. Maxillary
6. Myopathy
7. Osteochondrosis
8. Tarsectomy
9. Osteosclerosis
10. Kinesiology

11. Abduction
12. Gait
13. Laxity
14. Flexion
15. Tetany
16. Condyle
17. Periosteum
18. Diaphysis
19. Dislocation or luxation
20. Olecranon

3-C:

1. Hypocalcemia: Blood condition of decreased calcium
2. Myasthenia: Muscle weakness
3. Rhabdomyoma: Tumor of skeletal muscle
4. Hypertrophy: Excessive development due to increased cell size
5. Fracture: Sudden breaking of bone
6. Dysplasia: Bad or abnormal development
7. Achondroplasia: Bones of the limbs fail to grow to normal size
8. Ankylosis: Abnormal condition of stiffening
9. Hemarthrosis: Abnormal condition of blood in the joint
10. Tenorrhaphy: Suture of a tendon

3-D:

1. Immature; embryonic
2. Surgical fixation
3. Softening
4. Measurement
5. Cell
6. Surgical fixation
7. Blood condition
8. Pertaining to
9. Formation
10. Movement
11. Instrument to cut
12. Growth

3-E:

1. All
2. Below, deficient, under, less than normal
3. Away from
4. Between
5. Around, surrounding
6. Bad, abnormal, painful, difficult
7. In, within
8. Above, upper

3-F:

1. American Veterinary Medical Association
2. Veterinary pharmaceuticals and biologicals
3. Registered veterinary technician
4. Total hip replacement
5. Orthopedic, orthopedic procedure
6. Electromyogram
7. Triple pelvic osteotomy
8. Tibial tuberosity advancement
9. Congenital articular rigidity
10. Cranial cruciate ligament
11. Physicians' Desk Reference
12. Tibial plateau leveling osteotomy

3-G:

1. Bursa
2. Subluxation
3. Skeletal
4. Myositis
5. Ligament
6. Kyphosis
7. Synovial
8. Amputation
9. Crepitation
10. Foramen

3-H:

1. Removal of a limb
2. Formation of bone
3. Abnormal condition of death
4. Pertaining to the fibula
5. Removal of part of the vertebral arch to relieve pressure from a ruptured IVD
6. Correction of a fracture
7. A joint; where two or more bones come together at a joint
8. Immature bone cell; bone cell that forms bone tissue
9. Pertaining to the patella
10. Pertaining to the phalanges; pertaining to the digits
11. Measurement of the pelvis
12. Malignant tumor of cartilage arising from connective tissue
13. Pertaining to below the ribs
14. Incision of a tendon; process of cutting into a tendon
15. Surgical fixation of a bone

3-I:

1.	Cardiac	Involuntary	Striated
2.	Skeletal	Voluntary	Striated
3.	Visceral	Involuntary	Smooth

Chapter 4   Case Study and Exercises

Melena
Hematemesis
Lethargy
Dehydration
Fecal
Ultrasound
Pancreatitis
Hepatomegaly
Intravenous catheter

Intravenous
Nothing by mouth
Antiemetic
Hyperglycemia
Alanine aminotransferase
Alkaline phosphatase
Drops
Injection

4-A:

1. fat
2. tooth
3. abnormal condition
4. mouth
5. gall; bile
6. tongue
7. lips
8. abdomen
9. blood
10. sugar

4-B:

1. Pharynx
2. Duodenum
3. Cecum
4. Descending colon
5. Anus
6. Liver

7. Esophagus
8. Gallbladder
9. Colon
10. Pancreas

11. Pancreas
12. Jejunum
13. Epiglottis
14. Trachea

4-C:

1. Anorexia: Lack of appetite
2. Steatorrhea: Fat in feces
3. Colostomy: New opening from the large intestine to the outside of the body
4. Gastrectomy: Removal of the stomach; excision of the stomach
5. Ascites: Abnormal accumulation of fluid in the abdomen
6. Dysphagia: Difficulty swallowing
7. Hepatitis: Inflammation of the liver
8. Fistula: Abnormal tube-like passageway that can occur all over the body
9. Peristalsis: Wave-like contractions of the tubes of the GI tract
10. Scours: Diarrhea of livestock

4-D:

1. Anastomosis
2. Cardiac sphincter
3. Pyloric stenosis
4. Peritonitis
5. Rugae
6. Diaphragm
7. Defecation; elimination
8. Emesis

9. Biopsy
10. Coprophagia
11. Jaundice
12. Megaesophagus
13. Shunt
14. Brachygnathia
15. Trichobezoar

4-E:

1. Visual examination of the abdomen
2. Anastomosis of the small and large intestine
3. Inflammation of the tongue
4. Blood condition of decreased sugar
5. Pertaining to below the lower jaw (mandible)
6. Inflammation of the gums
7. Removal of the gallbladder
8. Surgical repair of the palate
9. Blood condition of excessive bilirubin
10. Pertaining to the cheek

4-F:

1. cubic centimeter
2. grain
3. hemorrhagic gastroenteritis
4. gastric dilatation volvulus

5. milligram
6. gram
7. drop
8. intradermal

9. intramuscular
10. intravenous catheter
11. milliliter
12. left displaced abomasum

13. after meals
14. milliequivalents
15. by mouth

4-G:

1. parenteral
2. ulcer
3. regurgitation
4. bowel
5. intussusception

6. colic
7. gastropexy
8. gastrojejunostomy
9. deglutition
10. polydipsia

4-H:

1. $2\left[I\frac{3}{3}+C\frac{1}{1}+PM\frac{4}{4}+M\frac{2}{3}\right]=42$
2. 12
3. Liver
4. Rumen, reticulum, omasum, abomasum
5. Deciduous teeth

6. Ascending colon
7. F
8. Idiopathic
9. Icterus
10. F
11. F
12. Liver

4-I:

1. J
2. A
3. F
4. I
5. D

6. B
7. E
8. C
9. H
10. G

Chapter 5   Case Study and Exercises

1. C
2. C
3. B

4. C
5. B
6. C

5-A:

1. uterus
2. ovary
3. milk
4. vagina
5. egg

6. vulva
7. pregnancy
8. birth; labor
9. testes
10. penis

5-B:

1. Vulva
2. Spermatozoa; sperm
3. Uterine tube (Fallopian tube)
4. Seminiferous tubules
5. Scrotum
6. Semen
7. Glans penis
8. Endometrium
9. Cervix
10. Urethra
11. Os penis
12. Epididymis
13. Uterus
14. Amnion; amniotic sac

5-C:

1. Monorchid: One testicle has not descended
2. Coitus: Sexual intercourse
3. Vasectomy: Removal of vas deferens
4. Orchiectomy: Removal of testes
5. Ovarian: Pertaining to the ovary
6. Fetotomy: Surgical excision of the fetus
7. Fetus: Later stages of development
8. Castration: Removal of gonads
9. Meconium: First feces of newborn
10. Colostrum: First milk-like substance produced after delivery

5-D:

1. Cervix; neck
2. Semen; seed
3. Enlargement
4. First
5. Glans penis
6. None
7. Scanty
8. Hernia
9. Surgical fixation; to put in place
10. To bear; bring forth
11. Sharp; swift; rapid; acid; oxygen; quick
12. Pus

5-E:

1. Inflammation of the glans penis
2. Formation of sperm
3. Study of cells
4. Removal of mammary glands
5. After birth
6. Surgical fixation of testes
7. Removal of the prostate gland
8. Abnormal condition of the inner lining of the uterus
9. False pregnancy
10. Surgical puncture to remove fluid from the amnion

5-F:

1. Every night
2. Spay/ovariohysterectomy
3. Cesarean section
4. Spayed female
5. Castrated male
6. Once daily; every 24 hours

7. As needed
8. Abortion
9. Artificial insemination
10. Four times daily
11. Neutered male

12. Every day
13. Three times daily
14. Every other day
15. Pregnant

5-G:

1. viviparous
2. perineum
3. AB
4. ectopic
5. vaginal cytology

6. parturition
7. gamete
8. estrus
9. lactation
10. neonate

5-I:

1. H
2. J
3. G
4. D
5. B

6. A
7. C
8. F
9. I
10. E

Chapter 6   Case Study and Exercises

1. A
2. B
3. B
4. A
5. FALSE

6-A:

1. right atrium
2. left ventricle
3. pulmonary artery
4. lungs
5. pulmonary veins

6-B:

1. Atria
2. Angioplasty
3. Thrombolysis
4. Ischemia
5. Coronary arteries
6. Vena cava or vena cavae
7. Murmur
8. Pericardium

9. Auscultation
10. Vasoconstriction
11. Bicuspid valve or mitral valve
    or left AV valve
12. Shock
13. Embolus
14. Systole

6-C:

1. Arrhythmia: Abnormal heart rhythm
2. Stethoscope: Instrument used to listen to sounds within the body
3. Thrill: Vibrations felt on palpation of the chest
4. Hypertension: Increased blood pressure
5. Fibrillation: Rapid, random, and irregular contractions of the heart.
6. SA node: Pacemaker of the heart
7. Myocardium: Muscle layer of the heart
8. Cardiomegaly: Enlargement of the heart
9. Hypoxia: Lack of oxygen; lack of oxygen to tissues
10. Hypercapnia: Excessive CO_2

6-D:

1. O_2
2. Pressure
3. CO_2
4. Vein
5. Heart
6. Slow
7. Tightening; narrowing; stricture
8. Breakdown; destruction; separation
9. Clot
10. Plaque (fatty substance)
11. Vessel
12. Small; little

6-E:

1. Ventricular septal defect
2. Congestive heart failure
3. Ventricular fibrillation
4. Patent ductus arteriosus
5. Echocardiogram
6. Electrocardiogram
7. Premature ventricular contraction
8. Ventricular tachycardia
9. Aortic stenosis
10. Blood pressure
11. Beats per minute/breaths per minute
12. Carbon dioxide
13. Atrial fibrillation
14. Myocardial infarction
15. Premature atrial contraction

6-F:

1. pericardiocentesis
2. CRT
3. QRS
4. hypoxia (O_2 gives tissue its pink color)
5. ischemia
6. thrombolytic
7. stethoscope
8. thrill
9. venous congestion (heartworms infest the right side of the heart)
10. cardiac hypertrophy (athletes hearts are enlarged from usage)

6-G:

1. E
2. A
3. B
4. F
5. D
6. C

Chapter 7   Case Study and Exercises

1. A
2. B
3. C
4. B
5. B

7-A:

1. pleura
2. mediastinum
3. pharynx
4. nostrils
5. bronchi
6. alveoli
7. larynx
8. cilia
9. bronchioles
10. epiglottis
11. pleural cavity; pleural space
12. trachea

7-B:

1. Epistaxis: Nosebleed
2. Agonal: Respirations near death
3. Atelectasis: Incomplete dilation of the lungs
4. Inspiration: Breathing in; inhalation
5. Olfactory: Condition of smelling
6. Mucolytics: Substances to break down mucus
7. Percussion: Tapping a surface to determine the density of an underlying structure
8. Palliative: Relieving symptoms, but not curing
9. Bronchodilators: Substance to expand the bronchi
10. Diaphragm: Thin, muscular partition that separates the abdominal and thoracic cavities

7-C:

1. apnea
2. hypoxia
3. hemothorax
4. sinusitis
5. laryngoscopy
6. tracheostomy
7. pharyngeal
8. cyanosis
9. pneumonectomy
10. rhinoplasty
11. pyothorax
12. hypercapnia

7-D:

1. Arterial blood gas
2. Endotracheal tube
3. Cardiopulmonary cerebral resuscitation
4. Ovine progressive pneumonia
5. Bovine respiratory syncytial virus
6. Upper respiratory infection
7. Pulmonary embolism
8. Respiratory rate
9. Partial pressure of carbon dioxide
10. Pulse oximeter

7-E:

1. False. Aspiration inhales foreign material
2. False. Mucus
3. True
4. False. Air in chest cavity
5. True

6. False. Bronchodilators
7. True
8. True
9. False. Dyspnea is difficulty breathing; apnea is not breathing
10. True

7-F:

1. D
2. E
3. B

4. A
5. C

Chapter 8   Case Study and Exercises

1. C
2. False. It is the most common acquired bleeding disorder

8-A:

1. erythrocyte
2. eosinophils
3. lymphocytes
4. hemoglobin
5. erythropoietin
6. hemostasis

7. monoblast
8. coagulation
9. phlebotomy
10. leukemia
11. lipemia
12. hemorrhage

8-B:

1. Hemostasis: Stopping or controlling blood
2. Neutropenia: Deficiency or decrease in neutrophils
3. Eosinophilia: Increase in eosinophils
4. Morphology: Study of shape
5. Thrombosis: Abnormal condition of clots or clotting
6. Bilirubin: Metabolite of hemoglobin breakdown
7. Antigen: Foreign protein that stimulates the production of antibodies
8. Megakaryocyte: Precursor to a platelet formed in the bone marrow
9. Packed cell volume: Percentage of RBCs in a volume of blood
10. Dyscrasia: Any abnormal condition of blood.

8-C:

1. antigen
2. Von Willebrand's factor
3. no production
4. bacterial phagocyte

5. liver
6. liver, spleen, and bone marrow
7. plasma
8. leukemia is cancerous cells, leukocytosis has normal cells
9. polycythemia
10. PCV
11. False. Thrombosis is clots, thrombocytopenia is platelets or clotting cells
12. icteric

8-D:

1. Complete blood count
2. Disseminated intravascular coagulation
3. High power field
4. Quantity not sufficient
5. White blood cell differential

6. Hemoglobin
7. Autoimmune hemolytic anemia
8. Total protein
9. Immune mediated hemolytic anemia
10. Low power field

8-E:

1. Myeloid
2. Mononuclear
3. Hemolysis
4. Pancytopenia
5. Coagulopathy

6. Leukocytosis
7. Hypoalbuminemia
8. Anisocytosis
9. Homeostasis
10. Hemorrhagic

8-F:

1. C
2. D
3. E

4. A
5. B

Chapter 9   Case Study and Exercises

1. A
2. B
3. B

9-A:

1. zoonotic
2. histiocyte
3. lymph node
4. allergen
5. edema

6. B-lymphocytes
7. spleen
8. autoimmune disease
9. splenomegaly
10. toxin

9-B:

1. Lymphangioma: tumor of lymph vessels
2. Lymphadenitis: Inflammation of lymph nodes
3. Toxic: Pertaining to a poison
4. Resistant: Not easily affected
5. Tonsillitis: Inflammation of tonsils
6. Lymphocytosis: Increase in lymphocytes
7. Thymoma: Tumor on the thymus gland
8. Lymphoid: Resembling lymph
9. Immunosuppression: Impaired immune system
10. Interstitial fluid: Fluid in the spaces between cells

9-C:

1. FeLV or FIV
2. Groin
3. Suppressor T-cells
4. Passive immunity
5. Armpit

9-D:

1. Enzyme-linked immunosorbent assay
2. Immunofluorescent antibody test
3. Lymph node
4. Feline leukemia virus
5. Feline immunodeficiency virus
6. Prescription/medication
7. Metastasis
8. Biopsy
9. Treatment
10. Surgery

9-E:

1. C
2. A
3. D
4. E
5. B

Chapter 10   Case Study and Exercises

1. D
2. B
3. A

10-A:

1. Hypoadrenocorticism
2. Antidiuretic hormone
3. Hyperadrenocorticism
4. Epinephrine
5. Growth hormone
6. Pituitary gland
7. Corticosteroids
8. Noradrenaline
9. Tetraiodothyronine
10. Pituitary gland

10-B:

1. Adrenopathy: Disease condition of adrenal glands
2. Pancreatitis: Inflammation of the pancreas
3. Thymoma: Tumor of the thymus gland
4. Hyperglycemia: Blood condition of excessive sugar
5. Glucosuria: Sugar in the urine
6. Acromegaly: Enlargement of extremities
7. Hyponatremia: Blood condition of decreased sodium
8. Hyperkalemia: Blood condition of excessive potassium
9. Hormonal: Pertaining to hormones
10. Thyromegaly: Enlargement of the thyroid gland

10-C:

1.	GH	Anterior pituitary	Growth of bones and tissues
2.	Insulin	Pancreas	Decreases blood sugar
3.	PTH	Parathyroid glands	Regulates calcium and potassium
4.	ACTH	Anterior pituitary	Stimulates adrenal cortex to produce corticosteroids
5.	ADH	Posterior pituitary	Controls reabsorption of water by the kidney
6.	T4	Thyroid gland	Regulates metabolism
7.	LH	Anterior pituitary	Promotes ovulation
8.	Oxytocin	Posterior pituitary	Stimulates uterus contraction and milk secretion
9.	FSH	Anterior pituitary	Stimulates maturation of ovum
10.	Aldosterone	Adrenal cortex	Controls sodium reabsorption and potassium excretion by the kidney

10-D:

1. Polyuria/polydipsia
2. Thyroid-stimulating hormone
3. Parathormone
4. Diabetes mellitus
5. Diabetes insipidus
6. Diabetic ketoacidosis
7. Adrenocorticotropic hormone
8. Blood glucose
9. Prolactin
10. Low-dose dexamethasone suppression test

10-E:

1. C
2. E
3. B
4. D
5. A

Chapter 11   Case Study and Exercises

1. B
2. B
3. False

11-A:

1. Basal layer
2. Dermis
3. Sebaceous gland
4. Collagen
5. Melanin
6. Sebum
7. Pore
8. Subcutaneous layer
9. Hair follicle
10. Epidermis

11-B:

1. Percutaneous: Pertaining to through the skin.
2. Adipose: Pertaining to fat; full of fat
3. Pyoderma: Pus on the skin
4. Trichomycosis: Abnormal condition of fungus on the hair
5. Subungual: Pertaining to below the hoof
6. Lipoma: Tumor or mass of fat
7. Dermatoplasty: Surgical repair of the skin
8. Onychectomy: Removal of nails
9. Xeroderma: Dry skin
10. Pilosebaceous: Pertaining to the hair follicles and sebaceous glands

11-C:

1. Trichobezoar
2. Ulcer
3. Purulent
4. Petechiae
5. Ecchymosis
6. Hidrosis
7. Melanoma
8. Sebaceous cyst
9. Decubitus ulcers
10. Papilloma
11. Metastasis
12. Contusion
13. Pruritus
14. Alopecia
15. Atopy
16. Biopsy
17. Abscess
18. Albinism
19. Comedo
20. Fistula

11-D:

1. Cancer
2. Lupus erythematosus
3. Fine needle aspirate
4. Subcutaneous
5. Skin
6. Intradermal
7. Flea allergy dermatitis
8. Discoid lupus erythematosus
9. Subcutaneous
10. Systemic lupus erythematosus

11-E:

1. B
2. E
3. A

4. C
5. D

Chapter 12   Case Study and Exercises

M/N: Neutered male
Syncope: Fainting
Convulsions: Sudden, involuntary contractions of voluntary muscles
Tremors: Repetitive twitching of skeletal muscle
Phlebotomy: Venipuncture
EEG: Electroencephalogram; record of electricity in the heart
MRI: Magnetic resonance imaging, radiographic imaging technique showing a three-dimensional image of the brain
Extracranial: Pertaining to outside the skull
Intracranial: Pertaining to inside or within the skull
Epilepsy: Idiopathic brain disorder characterized by recurrent seizures
Seizure: Sudden, involuntary contractions of voluntary muscles
BAR: Bright, alert, responsive

1. D

12-A:

1. Gait
2. Lethargy
3. Cauda equina
4. Plexus
5. Neuron

6. Meninges
7. Cerebrum
8. Cerebellum
9. Dura mater
10. Aneurysm

12-B:

1. Encephalomalacia: Softening of the brain
2. Analgesia: Reducing pain
3. Bradykinesia: Slow movement
4. Hematoma: Mass or collection of blood
5. Neuropathy: Disease condition of nerves
6. Hemiplegia: Weakness of the right or left side of the body
7. Paraparesis: Paralysis of the rear limbs
8. Meningitis: Inflammation of the meninges
9. Comatose: Pertaining to a deep sleep
10. Poliomyelitis: Inflammation of the gray matter of the spinal cord

12-C:

1. Proprioception
2. Myelin sheath
3. Afferent

4. BBB
5. CNS
6. BSE

7. Spasticity
8. Narcolepsy
9. CT
10. Concussion
11. Sympathetic

12. Neurotransmitter
13. Innervation
14. Encephalocele
15. Brainstem

12-D:

1. Bovine spongiform encephalopathy
2. Lumbar puncture
3. Intracranial pressure
4. Blood brain barrier
5. Caprine arthritis encephalitis

6. Thromboembolic meningoencephalitis
7. Myasthenia gravis
8. Central nervous system
9. Cerebrospinal fluid
10. Seizure

12-E:

1. A
2. D
3. B
4. C
5. E

Chapter 13   Case Study and Exercises

1. A
2. B
3. A

13-A:

1. Iris
2. Tympanic membrane
3. Cerumen
4. Sclera
5. Optic disc
6. Pupil

7. Uvea
8. Canthus
9. Auricle
10. Ossicles
11. Nictitating membrane
12. Retina

13-B:

1. Tympanoplasty: Surgical repair of the eardrum
2. Blepharoptosis: Drooping of the eyelid
3. Conjunctivitis: Inflammation of the conjunctiva
4. Postauricular: Pertaining to behind the ear
5. Keratitis: Inflammation of the cornea
6. Lacrimation: Formation of the tears
7. Otorrhea: Discharge from the ears

8. Ophthalmology: Study of the eye
9. Otoscope: Instrument to visually examine the ear
10. Macrotia: Large ears

13-C:

1. Cataract
2. Proptosis
3. Nystagmus
4. Cochlea
5. Enucleation

6. Vitreous humor
7. Mydriasis
8. Tapetum lucidum
9. Esotropia
10. Photophobia

13-D:

1. Right eye
2. Both ears
3. Intraocular pressure
4. Both eyes

5. Right ear
6. Pupillary light reflex
7. Left eye
8. Left ear

13-E:

1. D
2. E
3. B

4. A
5. C

Chapter 14   Case Study and Exercises

1. B
2. B
3. C

14-A:

1. Nephron
2. Creatinine
3. Ureter
4. Renal cortex
5. Glomerulus

6. Urethra
7. Antidiuretic hormone
8. Bowman's capsule
9. Renal tubules
10. Micturition

14-B:

1. Lithotripsy: To crush stones
2. Nephrosclerosis: Hardening of the kidney
3. Pyelonephritis: Inflammation of the renal pelvis of the kidney
4. Cystocentesis: Surgical puncture to remove fluid from the urinary bladder
5. Erythropoiesis: Formation of red blood cells
6. Anuria: No urination
7. Polyuria: Excessive urination

8. Urethritis: Inflammation of the urethra
9. Ketosis: Abnormal condition of ketones
10. Glomerular: Pertaining to the glomerulus

14-C:

1. Renin
2. Oliguria
3. Albuminuria
4. Nephrolithotomy
5. Diuresis
6. Renal ischemia
7. Filtration
8. Sodium
9. BUN
10. Azotemia

14-D:

1. Antidiuretic hormone
2. Perineal urethrostomy
3. Sodium
4. Cystocentesis
5. Urinary tract infection
6. Urine specific gravity
7. Feline lower urinary tract disease
8. Feline urological syndrome
9. Blood urea nitrogen
10. Urinalysis

14-E:

1. E
2. B
3. C
4. D
5. A

Chapter 15   Exercises

15-A:

1. Coffin
2. P1 or proximal phalanx
3. Knee
4. Navicular
5. Fetlock
6. Distal interphalangeal
7. Cannon
8. Poll or occiput
9. Udder
10. Wolf teeth

15-B:

1. Ergot: Small mass of horny tissue in a small bunch of hair on the palmar and plantar aspects of the fetlock.
2. Chestnuts: Flattened, oval masses or horny tissue on the medial surface near the knee and hock
3. Lame: Unable to walk; deviation from the normal gait
4. Canter: Galloping at an easy pace.
5. Mare: Intact female horse 4 years or older
6. Gelding: Castrated male horse
7. Hindgut: The small intestine, cecum, and large intestine, collectively
8. Parrot mouth: Condition in which the maxilla in longer than the mandible

9. Laminitis: Inflammation of the lamina causing lameness
10. Cribbing: Habit in which the horse grasps an object with its incisors and applies pressure as it swallows air

15-C:

1. Frog
2. Halter
3. Dock
4. Draft
5. Croup
6. Blaze
7. Rasp
8. Lunging
9. Coronet
10. Withers

15-D:

1. Eastern equine encephalitis
2. Equine infectious anemia
3. Transmissible gastroenteritis
4. Vesicular stomatitis
5. Kicked by horse
6. Venezuelan equine encephalitis
7. Western equine encephalitis
8. Equine protozoal myeloencephalitis
9. Large animal
10. Equine influenza

15-E:

1. C
2. B
3. D
4. A
5. E

Chapter 16   Exercises

16-A:

1. Switch
2. Calving
3. Doe
4. Wether
5. Marbling
6. Heart girth
7. Flock
8. Carcass
9. Poll
10. Halter

16-B:

1. Offal: Non-edible products from slaughter.
2. Feedlot: Confined area where animals are fed and "fattened up" before going to slaughter.
3. Bolus: Mass of food or medication to be swallowed.
4. Heifer: Female bovine that has never given birth.
5. Lanolin: Commonly called wool fat or wool grease, this is the fatty substance produced by the sebaceous glands of sheep.
6. Mutton: Meat obtained from adult sheep.

7. Wattle: Appendages suspended by the mandibular area.
8. Hooks: Bony protrusions of the wing of the ilium dorsolaterally.
9. Pins: Bony protrusions of the ischium lateral to the tail base.
10. Kid: Young goat.

16-C:

1. Loin
2. Dewclaw
3. Gomer
4. Rendering
5. Docking
6. Balling gun
7. Chevon
8. Flank
9. Chine
10. Cull

16-D:

1. Bovine respiratory syncytial virus
2. Infectious bovine rhinotracheitis
3. Bovine viral diarrhea
4. Parainfluenzavirus

16-E:

1. C
2. A
3. E
4. B
5. D

Chapter 17   Exercises

17-A:

1. Sow
2. Ham
3. Gilt
4. Tusk
5. Boar
6. Snout
7. Farrowing
8. Needle teeth
9. Lard
10. Boar taint

17-B:

1. Rooting: Turning up of the ground using the snout to look for food.
2. Abbatoir: Building used for slaughter; also called a slaughterhouse.
3. Creep: Area that only young piglets can access.
4. Finish: Degree of fatness short of obesity.
5. Wallow: Area for pigs to rest and cool down; usually contains water or mud.
6. Farrowing crate: Pipework holding pen large enough to hold the sow, but narrow enough to prevent movement.
7. Brimming: Time of sexual receptivity when the female accepts the male.
8. Backfat: Thickness of fat along the back of a pig
9. Ear marking: Patterned pieces of cartilage punched out as a means of identification; ear notching.
10. Barrow: Castrated, young male pig

17-C:

1. Stillborn, mummification, embryonic death, infertility
2. Porcine respiratory and reproductive syndrome
3. Transmissible gastroenteritis
4. Porcine stress syndrome

17-D:

1. D
2. E
3. A

4. C
5. B

Chapter 18   Exercises

18-A:

1. Molt
2. Vent
3. Ventriculus
4. Crop
5. Tom

6. Columbiformes
7. Pin feather or blood feather
8. Albumen
9. Cere
10. Keel

18-B:

1. Clutch: Group of eggs.
2. Carapace: Dorsal aspect of the turtle's shell.
3. Ectotherm: Animal unable to regulate its own body temperature. Commonly called cold-blooded animals, they require the external environment to regulate their body temperature.
4. Urodeum: Portion of the cloaca in which the urogenital system opens.
5. Syrinx: Vocal organ in birds at the base of the trachea that produces sound
6. Primary feathers: Flight feathers connected to the metacarpus and phalanges of the wing
7. Cloaca: Common passage for fecal, urinary, and reproductive discharge in birds and lower vertebrates
8. Yolk: The yellow portion of the egg where nutrients and antibodies are stored for the developing embryo
9. Egg bound: Term used to describe the inability to pass an egg
10. 10. Ecdysis: Shedding of the external layer of skin

18-C:

1. Coverts
2. Remiges
3. Spectacle
4. Substrate
5. Preen

6. Fledgling
7. Furcula
8. Magnum
9. Psittacines
10. Parabronchi

18-D:

1. Protection
2. Insulate
3. Nesting

4. Mating
5. Flight

Chapter 19   Exercises

19-A:

1. Hob
2. Kit
3. Murine
4. Pup
5. Axenic

6. Propagate
7. Scurvy
8. Crepuscular
9. Progeny
10. Outbred

19-B:

1. Hybrid: Offspring from parents of different strains, varieties, or species.
2. Stock: Outbred animal lines and genetics.
3. Transgenic: An animal that has been genetically manipulated to contain DNA from another animal.
4. Gnotobiotic: Animals whose microflora and microfauna are known in complete detail.
5. Lapin: Neutered male rabbit.

19-C:

1. Institutional Animal Care and Use Committee
2. United States Department of Agriculture
3. National Institute of Health
4. American Association for Laboratory Animal Science
5. Animal and Plant Health Inspection Service
6. Animal Welfare Act
7. Food and Drug Administration
8. Public Health Safety
9. American College of Laboratory Animal Medicine
10. Association for Assessment and Accreditation of Laboratory Animal Care

19-D:

1. B
2. D
3. A
4. C

Index

Veterinary Medical Terminology Guide and Workbook, First Edition. Angela Taibo.
© 2014 John Wiley & Sons, Inc. Published 2014 by John Wiley & Sons, Inc.
Companion website: www.wiley.com/go/taibo/terminology